WORLD HEALTH ORGANIZ

INTERNATIONAL AGENCY FOR RESEARCH ON CANCER

STATISTICAL METHODS IN CANCER RESEARCH

VOLUME 1 - The analysis of case-control studies

BY

N.E. BRESLOW & N.E. DAY

TECHNICAL EDITOR FOR IARC

W. DAVIS

IARC Scientific Publications No. 32

INTERNATIONAL AGENCY FOR RESEARCH ON CANCER
LYON
1980

The International Agency for Research on Cancer (IARC) was established in 1965 by the World Health Assembly as an independently financed organization within the framework of the World Health Organization. The headquarters of the Agency are at Lyon, France.

The Agency conducts a programme of research concentrating particularly on the epidemiology of cancer and the study of potential carcinogens in the human environment. Its field studies are supplemented by biological and chemical research carried out in the Agency's laboratories in Lyon and, through collaborative research agreements, in national research institutions in many countries. The Agency also conducts a programme for the education and training of personnel for cancer research.

The publications of the Agency are intended to contribute to the dissemination of authoritative information on different aspects of cancer research.

First reimpression, 1982
Second reimpression, 1983
Third reimpression, 1989
Fourth reimpression, 1990
Fifth reimpression, 1992
Sixth reimpression, 1994
Seventh reimpression, 1998

ISBN 92 832 0132 9

International Agency for Research on Cancer 1980

REPRINTED IN THE UNITED KINGDOM

N.E. Breslow & N.E. Day (1980) *Statistical Methods in Cancer Research. Volume I – The Analysis of Case-Control Studies,* Lyon, International Agency for Research on Cancer (*IARC Scientific Publications* No. 32)

ERRATA

Page 47, line 8, should read "... in each age group in 1970,..."

Page 60, line 21, should read "... lines are larger than would be expected..."

Page 61, line 3, should read "... **x** = UK (Birmingham);..."

Page 75, line 33, should read "$(1 \times 0.2 + 6 \times 0.1)/(1 \times 0.2 + 3 \times 0.3 + 6 \times 0.1 + 18 \times 0.4) = 0.0899$"

Page 76, line 2, should read "$62.5 \times 0.0899 + 74.1 \times 0.9101 = 73.0\%$"
line 5, should read "73.0% of cancers by eliminating smoking, 60.6% by..."

Page 94, line 25, should read "... with both E and disease, then we should be..."

Page 141, line 4, delete the sentence beginning "Its only major drawback..."

Page 167, last line, should read "... = 0.98 corresponding to..."

Page 174, line 9, should read

$$= \frac{\left(|110-13| - \frac{5}{2} \right)^2}{302} = 29.57.$$

Page 180, last line, fourth box should read "$\frac{3}{M+1}$"

Page 200, line 22, should read "... variables $\mathbf{x} = (\mathbf{x}, ..., \mathbf{x_K})$"
last line, should read "$\mathbf{x}^*$ and $\mathbf{x}$ of risk variables is"

Page 201, line 1, should read "... with a standard $(\mathbf{x} = \mathbf{0})$"

Page 203, line 12, should read

$$= \frac{pr(z=1|y=1,\mathbf{x})pr(y=1|\mathbf{x})}{pr(z=1|y=0,\mathbf{x})pr(y=0|\mathbf{x}) + pr(z=1|y=1,\mathbf{x})pr(y=1|\mathbf{x})}$$

Page 204, line 21, should read "$\boldsymbol{\beta} = \Sigma^{-1} (\mu_1 \mu_0).$"
and throughout, β should read $\boldsymbol{\beta}$
line 17, should read "(Truett, Cornfield & Kannel, 1967)"
line 24, should read "... in place of μ_1, μ_0 and Σ,"
last line, should read "... likelihood..."

Page 205, line 1, should read "... and covariances for $\hat{\boldsymbol{\beta}}$ generated..."
line 18, should read "... $\boldsymbol{\beta}$ parameters of interest."

Page 206, line 28, should read "... The α and the $\boldsymbol{\beta}$'s are the..."
line 32, should read "... which are often denoted $\hat{\alpha}$ and $\hat{\boldsymbol{\beta}}$,"

Page 207, line 1, should read "... $\mathbf{S} = \mathbf{S}(\alpha,\boldsymbol{\beta})$, while..."
line 2, should read "... denoted $\mathbf{I} = \mathbf{I}(\alpha,\boldsymbol{\beta})$."
line 5, should read "Covariance matrix for $(\alpha,\boldsymbol{\beta}) = \mathbf{I}^{-1}(\alpha,\boldsymbol{\beta})$."
line 6, should read "... as the value $\alpha,\boldsymbol{\beta}$ for which..."

Page 212, last line, last column, should read "-0.125 ± 0.189"

Page 218, line 16, should read "... see Table 4.2),"

Page 225, line 8, should read "... of α parameters in (6.12)"

Page 229, line 7, should read "(G_3–G_6 = 0.4, p = 0.5; G_3–G_7 = 2.1, p = 0.15)"

Page 244, line 24, should read "*J. Am. stat. Assoc., 73,*"

Page 245, last two lines, should read "$\boldsymbol{\mu}_1$" and "$\boldsymbol{\mu}_0$"
insert before line beginning $\boldsymbol{\beta}_k$: "$\boldsymbol{\beta}$ vector of log relative risks associated with a vector $\mathbf{x}$ of risk factors"

Page 249, line 33, should read "... to all cells in the $2 \times 2 \times I$ dimensional..."

Pages 284–289, first column heading should read "YEAR OF BIRTH"

Page 314, line 15, should read "16   IF(CC(NDIAG).EQ.000)GOTO 11"

CONTENTS

Foreword 5

Preface 7

Acknowledgements 9

Lists of Symbols 12

1. Introduction 14

2. Fundamental Measures of Disease Occurrence and Association 42

3. General Considerations for the Analysis of Case-Control Studies 84

4. Classical Methods of Analysis of Grouped Data 122

5. Classical Methods of Analysis of Matched Data 162

6. Unconditional Logistic Regression for Large Strata 192

7. Conditional Logistic Regression for Matched Sets 248

Appendices 281

FOREWORD

Epidemiological and biostatistical studies on cancer and other chronic diseases have expanded markedly since the 1950s. Moreover, as recognition of the role of environmental factors in human cancer has increased, there has been a need to develop more sophisticated approaches to identify potential etiological factors in populations living in a wide variety of environments and under very different socioeconomic conditions.

Developments in many countries have required that appropriate governmental agencies establish regulations to control environmental cancer hazards. Such regulations may, however, have considerable social and economic impacts, which require that they be based on careful risk-benefit analyses. Epidemiological studies provide the only definitive information as to the degree of risk in man. Since malignant diseases are clearly of multifactorial origin, their investigation in man has become increasingly complex, and epidemiological and biostatistical studies on cancer require a correspondingly complex and rigorous methodology. Studies such as these are essential to the development of programmes of cancer control and prevention.

Dr N.E. Breslow and Dr N.E. Day and their colleagues are to be commended on this volume, which should prove of value not only to established workers but also to all who wish to become acquainted with the general principles of case-control studies, which are the basis of modern cancer epidemiology.

John Higginson, M.D.
Director,
International Agency for Research
on Cancer, Lyon, France

PREFACE

Twenty years have elapsed since Mantel and Haenszel published their seminal article on statistical aspects of the analysis of data from case-control studies. Their methodology has been used by thousands of epidemiologists and statisticians investigating the causes and cures of cancer and other diseases. Their article is one of the most frequently cited in the epidemiological literature, and there is no indication that its influence is on the wane; on the contrary, with the increasing recognition of the value of the case-control approach in etiological research, the related statistical concepts seem certain to gain even wider acceptance and use.

The last two decades have also witnessed important developments in biostatistical theory. Especially notable are the log-linear and logistic models created to analyse categorical data, and the related proportional hazards model for survival time studies. These developments complement the work done in the 1920s and 1930s which provided a unified approach to continuous data *via* the analysis of variance and multiple regression. Much of this progress in methodology has been stimulated by advances in computer technology and availability. Since it is now possible to perform multivariate analyses of large data files with relative ease, the investigator is encouraged to conduct a range of exploratory analyses which would have been unthinkable a few years ago.

The purpose of this monograph is to place these new tools in the hands of the practising statistician or epidemiologist, illustrating them by application to *bona fide* sets of epidemiological data. Although our examples are drawn almost exclusively from the field of cancer epidemiology, in fact the discussion applies to all types of case-control studies, as well as to other investigations involving matched, stratified or unstructured sets of data with binary responses. The theme is, above all, one of unity. While much of the recent literature has focused on the contrast between the cohort and case-control approaches to epidemiological research, we emphasize that they in fact share a common conceptual foundation, so that, in consequence, the statistical methodology appropriate to one can be carried over to the other with little or no change. To be sure, the case-control differs from the cohort study as regards size, duration and, most importantly, the problems of bias arising from case selection and from the ascertainment of exposure histories, whether by interview or other retrospective means. Nevertheless, the statistical models used to characterize incidence rates and their association with exposure to various environmental or genetic risk factors are identical for the two approaches, and this common feature largely extends to methods of analysis.

Another feature of our pursuit of unity is to bring together various methods for analysis of case-control data which have appeared in widely scattered locations in the epidemiological and statistical literature. Since publication of the Mantel-Haenszel procedures, numerous specializations and extensions have been worked out for particular types of data collected from various study designs, including: 1-1 matching with binary and polytomous risk factors; 1:M matching with binary risk factors; regression models for series of 2×2 tables; and multivariate analyses based on the logistic function. All these proposed methods of analysis, including the original approach based on stratification of the data, are described here in a common conceptual framework.

A second major theme of this monograph is flexibility. Many investigators, once they have collected their data according to some specified design, have felt trapped by the intransigences of the analytical methods apparently available to them. This has been a particular problem for matched studies. Previously published methods for analysis of 1:M matched data, for example, make little mention of what to do if fewer controls are found for some cases, or how to account for confounding variables not incorporated in the design. The tendency has therefore been to ignore the matching in some forms of analysis, which may result in considerable bias, or to restrict the analysis to a subset of the matched pairs or sets, thus throwing away valuable data. Such practices are no longer necessary nor defensible now that flexible analytical tools are available, in particular those based on the conditional logistic regression model for matched data.

These same investigators may have felt compelled to use a matched design in the first place in order simultaneously to control the effects of several potential confounding variables. We show here that such effects can often be handled adequately by incorporation of a few confounding variables in an appropriate regression analysis. Thus, there is now a greater range of possibilities for the control of confounding variables, either by design or analysis.

From our experiences of working with cancer epidemiologists in many different countries, on projects wholly or partly supported by the International Agency for Research on Cancer, we recognize that not all researchers will have access to the latest computer technology. Even if such equipment is available at his home institution, an investigator may well find himself out in the field wanting to conduct preliminary analyses of his data using just a pocket calculator; hence we have attempted to distinguish between analyses which require a computer and those which can be performed by hand. Indeed, discussion of the methods which require computer support is found mostly in the last two chapters.

One important aspect of the case-control study, which receives only minimal attention here, is its design. While we emphasize repeatedly the necessity of accounting for the particular design in the analysis, little formal discussion is provided on how to choose between various designs. There are at least two reasons for this restriction in scope. First, the statistical methodology for estimation of the relative risk now seems to have reached a fairly stable period in its development. Further significant advances in this field are likely to take place from a perspective which is quite different from that taken so far, for instance using cluster analysis techniques. Secondly, there are major issues in the design of such studies which have yet to be resolved completely; these include the choice of appropriate cases and controls, the extent to which individual matching should be used, and the selection of variables to be measured. While an understanding of the relevant statistical concepts is necessary for such design planning, it is not sufficient. Good knowledge of the particular subject matter is also required in order to answer such design questions as: What factors are liable to be confounders? How important are differences in recall likely to be between cases and controls? Will the exposure influence the probability of diagnosis of disease? Are other diseases liable to be related to the same exposure?

We are indebted to Professor Cole for providing an introductory chapter which reviews the role of the case-control study in cancer epidemiology and briefly discusses some of these issues.

N. E. Breslow and N. E. Day

ACKNOWLEDGEMENTS

Since the initial planning for this monograph in mid-1976, a number of individuals have made significant contributions to its development. Twenty epidemiologists and statisticians participated in an IARC-sponsored workshop on the statistical aspects of case-control studies which was held in Lyon from 12–15 December 1977 (see List of Participants). Funds for this were generously provided by the International Cancer Research Workshop (ICREW) programme, administered by the UICC. Several participants kindly provided datasets to be used for illustrative analysis and discussion during the meeting. Others sent written comments on a rough draft of the monograph which had been distributed beforehand. The discussion was very valuable in directing its subsequent development.

As various sections and chapters were drafted, they were sent for comment to individuals with expertise in the particular areas. Among those who generously gave of their time for this purpose are Professor D. R. Cox, Professor Sir Richard Doll, Dr M. Hills, Dr Kao Yu-Tong, Professor N. Mantel, Dr C. S. Muir, Professor R. Prentice, Professor D. Thompson and Dr N. Weiss. While we have incorporated many of the suggestions made by these reviewers, it has not been possible to accommodate them all; responsibility for the final product is, of course, ours alone.

An important feature of the monograph is that the statistical methods are illustrated by systematic application to data from recent case-control studies. We are indebted to Dr A. Tuyns, IARC, for contributing data from his study of oesophageal cancer in Ille-et-Vilaine, as well as for stimulating discussion. Similarly, we appreciate the generosity of Dr M. Pike and his colleagues at the University of Southern California for permission to use data from their study of endometrial cancer and for sharing with us the results of their analyses. Both these sets of data are given as appendices, as are data from the Oxford Childhood Cancer Survey which were previously published by Dr A. Stewart and Mr G. Kneale.

The data processing necessary to produce the illustrative analyses was ably performed by IARC staff, notably Mr C. Sabai and Miss B. Charnay. Mr P. Smith contributed substantial improvements to the programme for multivariate analyses of studies with 1:M matching (Appendix IV) and subsequently modified it to accommodate variable numbers of cases as well as of controls (Appendix V).

The response of the IARC secretarial staff to the requests for typing of innumerable drafts and redrafts has been extremely gratifying. We would like to thank especially Mrs G. Dahanne for her work on the initial draft and Miss J. Hawkins for shepherding the manuscript through its final stages. Valuable assistance with intermediate drafts was given by Miss M. McWilliams, Mrs A. Rivoire, Mrs C. Walker, Mrs A. Zitouni and (in Seattle) Mrs M. Shumard. The figures were carefully executed by Mr J. Déchaux. We are indebted to Mrs A. Wainwright for editorial assistance and to Dr W. Davis and his staff for final assembly of the manuscript.

During the last year of preparation of this monograph, both authors were on leave of absence from their respective institutions. NEB would like to thank his colleagues at the University of Washington, particularly Drs P. Feigl and V. Farewell for continuation of work in progress during his absence, and to the IARC for financial support during the year. NED would like to thank his colleagues at the IARC, in particular Dr J. Estève, for ensuring the uninterrupted work of the Biostatistics section of the IARC, and to the National Cancer Institute of the United States for financial support during the year.

LIST OF PARTICIPANTS AT IARC WORKSHOP
12–15 December 1977

Professor E. Bjelke
Division of Epidemiology
School of Public Health
University of Minnesota
Minneapolis, Minn., USA
(now at Institute of Hygiene and
    Social Medicine
University of Bergen
Bergen, Norway)

Professor N. E. Breslow
Department of Biostatistics
University of Washington
Seattle, Wash., USA

Professor P. Cole
Department of Epidemiology
Harvard School of Public Health
Boston, Mass., USA

Mr W. Haenszel
Illinois Cancer Council
Chicago, Ill., USA

Dr Catherine Hill
Institut Gustave-Roussy
Villejuif, France

Dr G. Howe
National Cancer Institute of Canada
Epidemiology Unit
University of Toronto
Toronto, Ont., Canada

Dr A. B. Miller
National Cancer Institute of Canada
Epidemiology Unit
University of Toronto
Toronto, Ont., Canada

Dr B. Modan
Department of Clinical Epidemiology
The Chaim Sheba Medical Center
Tel-Hashomer, Israel

Dr M. Modan
Department of Clinical Epidemiology
The Chaim Sheba Medical Center
Tel-Hashomer, Israel

Professor M. Pike
Professor of Community and Family
    Medicine, Department of Pathology
University of Southern California
Los Angeles, Calif., USA

Mr P. Smith
Imperial Cancer Research Fund
Cancer Epidemiology and
    Clinical Trials Unit
University of Oxford
Oxford, United Kingdom

Dr V. B. Smulevich
Department of Cancer Epidemiology
Cancer Research Center
Academy of Medical Sciences of
    the USSR
Moscow, USSR

Dr J. Staszewski
Institute of Oncology
Gliwice, Poland

IARC Participants:

Miss Bernadette Charnay
Dr N. E. Day
Dr J. Estève
Dr R. MacLennan
Dr C. S. Muir
Miss Annie Ressicaud
Mr C. Sabai
Dr R. Saracci
Dr J. Siemiatycki

LISTS OF SYMBOLS

To aid the less mathematically inclined reader we provide detailed descriptions of the various characters and symbols used in the text and in formulae. These are listed in order of appearance at the end of each chapter. You will notice that some letters or symbols have two different meanings, but these usually occur in different chapters; it will be clear from the context which meaning is intended.

The following mathematical symbols occur in several chapters:

$\times$ denotes multiplication: $3 \times 4 = 12$

Σ summation symbol: for a singly subscripted array of I numbers $\{x_i\}$,

$\sum_{i=1}^{I}$ or $\Sigma_i x_i = x_1 + \ldots + x_I$. For a doubly subscripted array $\{x_{ij}\}$, $\Sigma_i x_{ij}$ denotes summation over the i subscript $x_{1j} + \ldots + x_{Ij}$, while $\Sigma\Sigma$ denotes double summation over both indices.

Π product symbol. For a singly subscripted array of I numbers $\{x_i\}$, $\prod_{i=1}^{I} x_i$ or $\Pi_i x_i = x_1 \times x_2 \times \ldots \times x_I$.

log   the natural logarithm (to the base e) of the quantity which follows, which may or may not be enclosed in parentheses.

exp   the exponential transform (inverse of log) of the quantity which follows, which is usually enclosed in parentheses.

1. INTRODUCTION

1.1 The case-control study in cancer epidemiology

1.2 Objectives

1.3 Strengths

1.4 Limitations

1.5 Planning

1.6 Implementation

1.7 Interpretation

CHAPTER I

INTRODUCTION[1]

Only two decades ago the case-control study was an oddity; it was rarely performed, poorly understood and, perhaps for these reasons, not highly regarded. But this type of study design has increased steadily in use and in stature and today it is an important and perhaps the dominant form of analytical research in epidemiology, especially in cancer epidemiology. Nonetheless, as a form of research the case-control study continues to offer a paradox: compared with other analytical designs it is a rapid and efficient way to evaluate a hypothesis. On the other hand, despite its practicality, the case-control study is not simplistic and it cannot be done well without considerable planning. Indeed, a case-control study is perhaps the most challenging to design and conduct in such a way that bias is avoided. Our limited understanding of this difficult study design and its many subtleties should serve as a warning – these studies must be designed and analysed carefully with a thorough appreciation of their difficulties. This warning should also be heeded by the many critics of the case-control design. General criticisms of the design itself too often reflect a lack of appreciation of the same complexities which make these studies difficult to perform properly.

The two major areas where a case-control study presents difficulties are in the selection of a control group, and in dealing with confounding and interaction as part of the analysis. This monograph deals mainly with the analysis of case-control studies and with related quantitative issues. This introductory chapter has different objectives: (1) to give a perspective on the place of the case-control study in cancer epidemiology; (2) to describe the major strengths and limitations of the approach; (3) to describe some aspects of the planning and conduct of a case-control study; and (4) to discuss matching, a major issue in designating the control group.

1.1 The case-control study in cancer epidemiology

Definition

A case-control study (case-referent study, case-compeer study or retrospective study) is an investigation into the extent to which persons selected because they have

[1] Prepared by Philip Cole, M.D., Dr. P.H., Division of Epidemiology, Department of Public Health and the Comprehensive Cancer Center of the University of Alabama in Birmingham, USA. Supported by a contract (N01-CO-55195) from the International Cancer Research Data Bank, National Cancer Institute, USA, to the International Agency for Research on Cancer, Lyon, France.

a specific disease (the cases) and comparable persons who do not have the disease (the controls) have been exposed to the disease's possible risk factors in order to evaluate the hypothesis that one or more of these is a cause of the disease. This definition requires considerable expansion to provide a picture of all the major aspects of such studies and the common variations; some of the more important deserve mention.

First, while case-control studies usually include only one case group and one control group, there are three common departures from this situation. For efficiency an investigator may decide to study simultaneously, and in the same way, two or more diseases whose risk factors are thought to be similar. For example, we recently simultaneously studied cancer of the endometrium (Elwood et al., 1977) and benign breast disease (Cole, Elwood & Kaplan, 1978). In addition to the operational efficiencies of such "multi-disease" studies, the control groups may be able to be combined to give each case-control comparison increased power. (Of course, a multi-disease study could be considered as a series of case-control studies, each consisting of two groups.)

There are two more ways in which the use of more than one case series could be useful. In one, cases of a second cancer known to be caused by one of the factors under study could be included. If the factor is also found to be related to the second cancer, that case group would have served as a "positive control", revealing the sensitivity of the study. In another, several case series are included, but only one cancer is found to be related to the factor under study, and thus the other cancers would have a "negative control" function; this would provide some evidence that the association with the cancer of primary interest was not merely reflecting a built-in aspect of the study design.

The second way in which the number of groups is increased beyond two is rarely used in the study of cancer; but for some diseases, such as arteriosclerosis, hypertension and some mental illness, it may be useful to deal with a group of "para-cases" i.e., subjects who are intermediate between the clearly ill and the clearly healthy. The decision to designate such an intermediate group might, in fact, be made when the study is analysed.

The third, and most common, way in which case-control studies are expanded is by the use of more than one control group. Indeed, it has been suggested that a case-control study requires at least two control groups to minimize the possibility of accepting a false result (Ibrahim & Spitzer, 1979); the rationale is that if the same result is not achieved in the two case-control comparisons, both the apparent results are suspect. Inclusion of a second control group may, however, increase the cost and duration of a study by about 50% and this may not be worthwhile. Furthermore, it may be difficult to judge whether or not the results of the two comparisons are mutually supportive.

Usually, it seems judicious to use a single control group – the one which seems best suited to the needs of the particular study. But, there are two common circumstances in which a second control group may be indicated: (1) in the study of a cancer about which so little is known that no strong preference for one type of control group can be defended; (2) in the situation where one desirable control group has a specific deficiency which can be overcome by another desirable group. For example, in a case-control study to evaluate the hypothesis that tonsillectomy causes Hodgkin's disease, Gutensohn et al. (1975) wanted to control potential confounding by socioeconomic class in the study design. This presented a problem since it was not clear whether it was necessary to control for socioeconomic class in childhood or in adulthood or in both. They therefore used two control groups – the siblings and the spouses of the cases. It is useful to remember that if the two different case-control comparisons give different results the study is not necessarily uninterpretable. The explanation of the discrepancy, if one can be deduced, may be very informative. For example, in the study just mentioned, the relative risk of Hodgkin's disease among tonsillectomized persons was 1.4 using the sibling controls, but 3.1 using the spouses. This suggests that some factor(s), which is a correlate of the probability of having a tonsillectomy, which differs between spouses and which is over-controlled for by the use of sibling controls, is a cause of Hodgkin's disease. Thus, the hypothesis emerges, though not exclusively from this finding, that an aspect of lifestyle during childhood – perhaps the pattern of exposure to infectious agents – is a cause of Hodgkin's disease (Gutensohn & Cole, 1977).

The modes of analysis presented in this monograph relate exclusively to the comparison of a single group of cases and a single group of controls; simultaneous multi-group comparisons are not addressed. This, however, does not prevent use of the techniques presented for the analysis of a study with, say, two control groups. Each case group-control group comparison can be analysed using these techniques and the results "pooled" in a subjective way at the interpretation stage. Also, if the decision is made to pool the data from the control groups, one control group has, in effect, been created and the techniques are again appropriate.

A second aspect of case-control studies, which expands the definition offered, is that the exposures of interest are not limited to environmental factors; the genotype and endogenous factors may be investigated suitably with the case-control design. Similarly, a case-control study may relate to factors other than possible etiological agents, including possibly protective factors. Studies of the relationship of oral contraceptives to benign breast diseases exemplify this (Vessey, Doll & Sutton, 1971; Kelsey, Lindfors & White, 1974). Indeed, it may prove possible to extend the case-control design far afield from etiological investigations to such subjects as the evaluation of a health service. For example, Clarke and Anderson (1979) recently attempted to evaluate the efficacy of the Papanicolou smear by the case-control technique.

Finally, it is worth mentioning that although many techniques of survey research (e.g., questionnaire construction, subject selection) are used in case-control and other epidemiological studies, these studies are not examples of survey research. No etiological investigation, whether epidemiological or experimental, need describe a population; and, in a case-control study, neither the cases nor the controls need be representative of any population as conventionally designated. It is useful to consider, however, that even a case-control study which is not population-based does derive from a hypothetical population, being those individuals who, if they were to develop the cancer under study, would be included as cases but are otherwise potential controls. It is important that the vast majority, and preferably all, of the cases genuinely have the specified disease and that the controls are comparable to them; comparability implies the absence of bias, especially selection bias and recall bias.

While the case-control design can be modified in many ways, discussion is facilitated if it is limited to an etiological investigation employing only two groups of subjects, and this monograph is so restricted.

History

In 1926 Lane-Claypon reported a case-control study of the role of reproductive experience in the etiology of breast cancer (Lane-Claypon, 1926). This appears to be the first case-control study of cancer (and possibly of any disease) which meets the definition offered above; in fact the study is remarkably similar to a modern investigation. Lane-Claypon does not describe how or why she came to adopt this approach. Thereafter, until about 1950, there were no further case-control studies – at least of a cancer – similar in quality to that of Lane-Claypon. The design came to be used, however, for the investigation of outbreaks of acute diseases. For example, a comparison would be made between individuals with a foodborne disease and well persons with respect to specific foods eaten at a common meal.

In 1950 two case-control studies which linked cigarette smoking with lung cancer were published (Levin, Goldstein & Gerhardt, 1950; Wynder & Graham, 1950); and in ensuing years there were numerous similar studies of many cancers. Of these the smoking and lung cancer investigation by Doll and Hill warrants mention as the prototype case-control study (Doll & Hill, 1952). The 1950s also brought the first studies of case-control methodology. Especially important was Cornfield's demonstration that the exposure frequencies of cases and controls are readily convertible into a parameter of greater interest to most public health workers, namely the ratio of the frequency of disease among exposed individuals relative to that among the non-exposed (Cornfield, 1951). This parameter has several different names and somewhat different interpretations depending on the particular type of cases used in a case-control study; however, it is now widely referred to as the relative risk and is so described in this monograph. Another major paper of the 1950s was the synthesis of Mantel and Haenszel, which clarified the objectives of case-control studies, systematized the issues requiring attention in their performance and described two widely-used analytical techniques, a summary chi-square statistic and a pooled estimator of the relative risk (Mantel & Haenszel, 1959). It is encouraging that in 1977 an enumeration of the citation of papers published in the Journal of the National Cancer Institute showed the Mantel-Haenszel paper in sixth place and increasing in use (Bailar & Anthony, 1977).

Current perceptions of the epidemiological aspects of case-control studies are presented in a recent paper by Miettinen (1976), in the related correspondence (Halperin, 1977; Miettinen, 1977) and in the proceedings of a symposium on the topic (Ibrahim, 1979). This monograph represents a synthesis of recent progress regarding statistical aspects.

Present significance

From the mid-1950s to the mid-1970s the number of case-control studies (not necessarily cancer-related) published in two general and two epidemiology-related medical journals increased four- to sevenfold. In the mid-1970s, they comprised 7% of all papers published (Cole, 1979). More specifically pertinent to cancer, the 1979 edition of the *Directory of On-going Research in Cancer Epidemiology* (Muir & Wagner, 1979) includes 1 092 research projects compared with 622 in the 1976 edition (Muir & Wagner, 1976). Of the 1 092 current projects 320 (29%) were classified as case-control studies, while only 143 (13%) were classified as follow-up (cohort) studies. These figures make an impressive statement about the present and possible future role of the case-control study in cancer research. More persuasive, however, would be a favourable assessment of the results of case-control studies of cancer. While this has to be subjective and perhaps reflects only an individual point of view, it is contended that, with the exception of our knowledge of carcinogenic occupational exposures (attributable mainly to the perspicacity of clinicians and the results of non-concurrent follow-up studies), most of our epidemiological knowledge of cancer etiology was established or originated from case-control research. In the past few years alone, the case-control study has brought to light or improved our understanding of such associations as late first birth and breast cancer (MacMahon et al., 1970); diethylstilboestrol and vaginal cancer in young women (Herbst, Ulfelder & Poskanzer, 1971); exogenous oestrogens and cancer of the endometrium (Ziel & Finkle, 1975; Smith et al., 1975); alcohol and tobacco consumption and cancer of the oesophagus (Tuyns, Péquignot & Jensen, 1977); the hepatitis B virus carrier state and cancer of the liver (Prince et al., 1975; Trichopoulos et al., 1978); and the role of dietary factors in cancers of the stomach and large bowel (Haenszel et al., 1972, 1973, 1976; Modan et al., 1974, 1975).

Apart from their frequency and the importance of their results, there is a more direct justification for placing a high value on the role of the case-control study in cancer research: it will be indispensable for the foreseeable future. What could replace it? Experimental research can provide persuasive evidence of the carcinogenicity of some kinds of agents for animals, but a generalization is required before such evidence can be applied to man. For some agents, for example, 2-acetylaminofluorene, a potent bladder carcinogen for several animal species, the generalization is readily made by nearly everyone; for others, for example, saccharin, an animal carcinogen under special circumstances, the relevance to man is not clear. Furthermore, the experimental approach may prove to be nonpersuasive or even inapplicable to the study of the carcinogenicity of some aspects of human lifestyles. The concurrent follow-up (prospective cohort) study is too expensive and time-consuming to be done often or as an exploratory venture. The non-concurrent follow-up (retrospective cohort) study requires the good fortune of locating old information on exposure which is relevant to the question at hand. Furthermore, follow-up studies usually cannot address interaction and confounding because the necessary information does not exist or because too few subjects develop the cancer of interest.

It is not by chance that the case-control study developed rapidly in the 1950s and is so popular today. Rather, the case-control study is contemporaneous with, and results from, the emergence of the chronic diseases as major public health problems requiring etiological investigation. The case-control study is uniquely well-suited to the study of cancer and other diseases of long induction period, for it permits us to look back through time from effects to causes. This is the reverse of the observational sequence of experimental research and of follow-up studies whether concurrent or non-concurrent. Nonetheless, the case-control study needs no apology since it is not backward, unnatural or inherently flawed. Indeed, recent applications of case-control selection procedures and analytical methods to follow-up studies show that the same results are achieved as from the analysis of the whole cohort but that costs are reduced and efficiency improved (Liddell, McDonald & Thomas, 1977; Breslow & Patton, 1979). Furthermore, in everyday human affairs cause-effect relationships are often viewed in reverse temporal sequence, but there is no difficulty in recognizing them. Everyday affairs, however, usually have causal pathways that are short, simple and strong. When a causal pathway spans decades our ordinary perceptions may not suffice, and this is particularly true if the pathway is rather faint because the cause-effect relationship is weak, which it often is for cancers. Thus, we had to develop a more refined method of observation to look back through time; that refined and still evolving method is the case-control study.

None of the foregoing support of the case-control study deprecates other forms of research, experimental or non-experimental. Nor is it contended that the case-control study is flawless; poor case-control studies have been and will continue to be done, and even a well-designed and conducted case-control study may produce an erroneous result. Considering the frequency with which case-control studies are done, and the ease with which such studies can be launched for exploratory purposes, it is to be expected that some contradictory results will appear. In this respect, the case-control study is no different from other forms of research, including rigorous experimentation. Thus it seems inappropriate to use a smattering of conflicting results from case-control studies to justify the position that "Certain scientific problems of case-control studies are inherent in (their) architecture..." (Horwitz & Feinstein, 1979), especially when the "problems" are not described. On the other hand, most of us recognize that the case-control design is young and underdeveloped and that it presents many problems and challenges (Feinstein, 1979). Most would also agree with the participants in the Bermuda Case-Control Symposium that research into the case-control method *per se* should be encouraged and that a set of standards for such studies should be developed (Ibrahim, 1979 [Discussion]). These constructive suggestions reflect the realization that the case-control study is different from, and more complex than, most experimental research designs and that some criteria for a good experiment are not only irrelevant to it but would be counter-productive. Criticisms of the case-control design (Sommers, 1978) which appear to reflect a judgement based on criteria for experiments should not be accorded.

1.2 Objectives

The principal objective of an etiological case-control study is to provide a valid, and reasonably precise, estimate of the strength of at least one hypothesized cause-effect relationship. In practice, this objective is usually supplemented by several others. The more common of these are the evaluation of several hypotheses and the description of the circumstances under which the strength of a cause-effect relationship varies, that is, of biological interaction. These objectives are identical to those of follow-up studies and even of experimental investigations of etiology.

The identity of objectives of case-control studies and of, say, experiments emphasizes two important things. The first is that generalizability of results is not a principal objective, while validity is. This is an important distinction to bear in mind since the two objectives validity and generalizability can be in competition. To illustrate this, the validity objective suggests that a case-control study should be based on a rather narrowly-defined case series and on controls highly comparable with them. For example, rather than including all women with breast cancer a study could be restricted to premenopausal cases (and controls). Subject restriction of this type mimics the experimental situation in which homogenous animals are used in an effort to improve efficiency and to reduce the prospect that confounding could explain the results.

On the other hand, the wish to achieve the secondary objective of generalizability would result in an effort to identify all cases of a disease occurring in a designated population and to use a random (or stratified random) sample of that population as controls. Two considerations should be kept in mind before generalizability is sought. First, if the subjects are highly heterogeneous, the results for any subgroup are likely to be imprecise because of random variation. This imprecision leads to a lack of confidence in the validity of the results which, in turn, precludes generalization. Second, the willingness to generalize is ultimately subjective and dependent on knowledge of the subject matter, particularly of whether susceptibility to the cause is likely to differ between the group studied and the group to which one would like to generalize. Furthermore, few of us are willing to generalize the results of etiological research until there have been similar findings from at least two studies done in different demographic settings. These considerations suggest that validity should not be compromised in an effort to achieve generalizability; generalizability will follow from a valid result and especially from a series of valid results.

The second thing which follows from the similarity of objectives of case-control studies and experiments is the desirability of expressing results in terms which have a biological meaning and interpretation. In practice this means providing a measure of the difference, if any, in the frequency of disease between exposed and non-exposed persons, including, if possible, a description of the dose-response relationship. The measure to be provided is the relative risk and, if possible, the (absolute) difference in incidence rates or prevalences between exposed and non-exposed individuals. It is insufficient to provide only the exposure frequencies of the cases and controls with the related p-value or to provide only the coefficients and p-values derived from a multivariate model.

1.3 Strengths

The major strength of epidemiology compared with experimental research is that it applies directly to human beings. In an epidemiological study there is no species barrier to overcome in attempting to infer how applicable the results are to man. The major strength of the case-control design compared with other types of epidemiological research is its "informativeness". A case-control study can simultaneously evaluate many causal hypotheses whether they have been previously evaluated or are new. These studies also permit the evaluation of interaction – the extent and manner in which two (or more) causes of the disease modify the strength of one another. This design also permits the evaluation and control of confounding, that is, of an association resulting because the factor under study is associated with a known or suspected cause of the cancer. The reason for the informativeness is the large number of ill persons who are observed in a case-control study. In a follow-up study usually only a few subjects develop any one cancer. The others contribute relatively little information.

There is another way in which a case-control study is highly informative. If a population-based series of incident cases has been assembled, it is possible to describe the picture of the disease in that population. That is, one can describe incidence rates according to age, sex and various risk factors at a point in (in fact during a brief period of) time. This cannot be achieved in a follow-up study, even if a general population comprises the study group (which is uncommon), unless new sub-cohorts are periodically added to the persons under observation. The reason is that a follow-up study group gives a broad picture of a cancer only at the start of the study. Thereafter, the group evolves and certain subgroups, e.g., the young, "disappear"; another subgroup literally disappears from the study – those lost to follow-up. On the other hand, the population-based case-control study provides a "window" on the totality of a cancer. One example of such a study relates to cancer of the bladder (Cole, 1973).

A second advantage of the case-control design is its efficiency, which is particularly impressive in view of its high informativeness. Such studies may be done in a few weeks if pre-existing data are used, but more often they take a year or two especially if the subjects are interviewed. Furthermore, the cost of these studies has tended to be low because only pre-existing or anamnestic data were gathered on relatively few subjects; case-control studies usually include several hundred subjects compared with the many thousands in follow-up studies. However, this low cost is becoming less characteristic of case-control studies of cancer because the kind of data required is changing. Many studies now require that interviews be supplemented with complex biochemical or other types of analysis of biological specimens. Despite the increased cost, this change is welcome for it is due to improvement in our understanding of the causes of cancer. On the other hand, the use of biological specimens in case-control studies may sometimes contribute nothing, or even be inappropriate, because the changes found may reflect some pathophysiological effect of the cancer rather than a cause. The advantages, then, of speed and low cost, while a general attribute of case-control studies, are not characteristic of all of them. Moreover, speed and low cost are not unique to the case-control study, and indeed the non-concurrent follow-up study is usually superior in these aspects.

A third advantage of the case-control study is its applicability to rare as well as common diseases. In this context, all but the three most common cancers (those of the breast, lung and colon in the western world) are "rare". In addition, the more rare the cancer, the greater is the relative advantage of this design. A disease which is rare in general, however, may not be rare in a special exposure group. If this is suspected and if such a group can be identified from a period in the past, a non-concurrent follow-up study should be considered.

A fourth advantage is that case-control studies (as well as follow-up studies) permit evaluation of the causal significance of a rare exposure. This is often not appreciated, and it is a common misconception that a case-control study is inappropriate for study of a rare exposure. Insofar as the prevalence of an exposure makes it suitable or unsuitable for a case-control study, it is not the general prevalence (i.e., among potential controls) but that among the cases that is relevant. If a factor is rare, but nonetheless accounts for a high proportion of the cancer, that is, if the factor is related to a high population-attributable risk percent (Cole & MacMahon, 1971), it can be studied. Indeed this is a circumstance that maximizes the efficiency of the case-control design since it enables a small study to be quite powerful. One example is the case-control study of eight young women with clear-cell adnocarcinoma of the vagina and 32 controls (Herbst, Ulfelder & Poskanzer, 1971). Similarly, a large fraction of mesotheliomas of the pleura are related to exposure to asbestos (Greenberg & Lloyd Davies, 1974), and benign hepatomas in young women are related to use of the contraceptive pill (Edmondson, Henderson & Benton, 1976). On the other hand, a common exposure may prove unsuitable for a case-control investigation if it accounts for a small proportion of the cancer; in this situation a very large study will be required.

1.4 Limitations

One limitation suggested to characterize case-control studies is that they permit estimation only of relative disease frequency. This requires qualification. If a case-control study includes, as many have, an incidence or prevalence survey, it can provide risk factor-specific absolute measures of cancer frequency. For example, Salber, Trichopoulos and MacMahon (1969) provided incidence rates of breast cancer by marital status, and others have provided incidence rates of bladder cancer according to cigarette smoking status (Cole et al., 1971) and occupation (Cole, Hoover & Friedell, 1972). Even when a survey is not included it may be possible to estimate the absolute overall frequency of disease among the types of subjects studied and to infer risk factor-specific absolute frequencies. This is especially so with respect to cancer because of the information on incidence rates available from cancer registries. A method for doing this is described by MacMahon and Pugh (1970), and an example is the study of oral contraceptives and thromboembolic and gall-bladder disease from the Boston Collaborative Drug Surveillance Program (1973).

A second proposed limitation of case-control studies remains correct and is important. Namely, that these studies are highly susceptible to bias, especially selection bias which creates non-comparability between cases and controls. The problem of selection bias is the most serious potential problem in case-control studies and is discussed below. Other kinds of bias, especially that resulting from non-comparable information from cases and controls are also potentially serious; the most common of these is recall (anamnestic or rumination [Sackett, 1979]) bias which may result because cases tend to consider more carefully than do controls the questions they are asked or because the cases have been considering what might have caused their cancer. The weakness then of case-control studies is that, in the end, the investigator must appeal to subjective or only semi-quantitative arguments to the effect that the information that he has from cases and controls is equivalent in source and quality. Thus, to a great extent the problem of doing a persuasive case-control study is that of avoiding bias. In one sense this is a basis for optimism because the sources and nature of biases in epidemiological studies have only recently come under scrutiny (Sackett, 1979), and we can expect progress in developing methods for their identification and control. Yet, there will be biases peculiar to each cancer and to each exposure and even to each study. It may be possible, at least, to define the more important biases that commonly affect certain kinds of case-control studies; Jick and Vessey (1978) have attempted this for case-control studies of drug exposures.

1.5 Planning

The case series

When a problem has been defined and a case-control study decided upon, attention is usually given first to designating the cases. The goal should be to designate a group of individuals who have a malignancy which is, as far as possible, a homogeneous etiological entity. It will be easier to unravel a single causal web rather than several at one time. For example, only a very limited level of knowledge can be reached in the study of the epidemiology of "cancer of the uterus"; but, if adenocarcinoma of the uterine corpus is distinguished from squamous-cell carcinoma of the cervix and if research is directed at one or the other, considerable progress can be made. We can go further in making these distinctions by not defining diseases solely in terms of mani-festational characteristics, no matter how refined we consider them to be. Definitions of disease based on their clinical or histological appearance suffice when there is a one-cause/one-manifestational-entity relationship. But they do not suffice for cancer. To study the complex cause-effect relationships of cancer we should attempt to use all existing knowledge, manifestational and epidemiological, to designate a restricted case series which is as homogeneous as possible with respect to etiology. The inadequacy of using only organ site and histological appearance or cell type to specify an etiological entity is made clear from one of the ideas about multiple-causation. In this, it is suggested that one type of cancer may have more than one independent set of causes. In order to identify cases likely to have the same set of causes the case series could be restricted according to age, sex, race or some other appropriate factor.

The restriction of case characteristics may bring benefits besides providing a series homogeneous with respect to cause. For one, the narrower range of possible causative factors is more likely to exclude false causes from consideration – "causes" which turn out to have no association with the cancer, or an association due only to confounding.

Another and especially important benefit is that the problem of selection bias may be reduced. When there is no association between the factor and the cancer of interest, there are nonetheless many ways in which an association may appear in the data of a case-control study. (The reverse situation, of no apparent association when in fact there is one, may also occur for similar reasons, but is not illustrated here.) One of the most important ways in which a false association can be created is by a selection bias. The question of selection bias must be considered simultaneously for both the case and the control series, since it is a question of their comparability; however, the problem of selection bias can most easily be appreciated with reference to case selection. Some mechanisms of selection bias may best be minimized by appropriate methods of case selection, thus the topic is presented here. By selection bias, I mean the bias which results when cases (or controls) are included in (or excluded from) a study because of some characteristic they exhibit which is related to exposure to the risk factor under evaluation. Often, for cases, the characteristic will be a sign or symptom of the cancer under study which is not always due to the cancer. This definition makes it clear that selection bias is not a single or simple phenomenon. It may, for example, represent a selection force towards inclusion in the study which operates on cases or on controls, or on both but unequally. Nor is this selection a conscious one; indeed, the parties applying the force will usually not even be aware (because it is usually not known) that the selection characteristic is associated with the factor under study. An example of a proposed selection bias follows. In 1975 two groups reported a rather strong association between the use of exogenous oestrogens and cancer of the endometrium (Ziel & Finkle, 1975; Smith et al., 1975). Later, Horwitz and Feinstein (1978) proposed that the association was due to a selection bias. They pointed out that women who use exogenous oestrogens are more likely than those who do not to experience vaginal bleeding, a moderately frequent but not serious side effect of the medication. However, vaginal bleeding in a postmenopausal woman is a matter of concern since it is a common sign of cancer of the endometrium. Thus, a postmenopausal woman who exhibits vaginal bleeding is likely to be examined closely for endometrial cancer whether or not she takes oestrogens. Usually, this includes a histological examination of tissues taken from her endometrium. The basis for this proposed bias is complete if one accepts the suggestion that in a high proportion of apparently normal postmenopausal women there is a condition which, morphologically, mimics cancer of the endometrium or which "is" cancer of the endometrium of an indolent type. Thus, Horwitz and Feinstein (1978) proposed that the use of oestrogens was merely attracting attention to a large number of these indolent conditions by causing vaginal bleeding and diagnostic evaluations. (If correct, this would serve as an excellent example of selection bias. However, Hutchison (1979) reviewed the Horwitz-Feinstein proposal and concluded on several bases that, while the proposed selection bias is credible and may even occur, it is unlikely to be sufficiently strong to account for any but a small part of the approximately sevenfold excess risk of endometrial cancer among oestrogen users. The fact that the association persists when the base series is restricted to women with frankly invasive cancer (Gordon et al., 1977) supports this view).

This type of selection bias is not likely to be a problem in case-control studies of cancer. For one reason, virtually by definition, cancer tends to be a progressive condition which ultimately comes to diagnosis. The bias is much more likely to operate in studies of non life-threatening conditions which produce no, or tolerable, symptoms. The bias is also more likely to operate in studies of drug exposure than in those of etiological agents in general, for drugs produce many adverse effects some of which cause a patient to be subjected to a battery of diagnostic tests.

The status of cases to be included in a case-control study must also be decided. There are three types that are often used – incident, prevalent and, occasionally, decedent. The use of decedent cases will not be discussed except to point out that their study brings the same problems as the study of prevalent cases plus additional ones. Decedent cases probably should not be used except in a preliminary study of a disease based on medical record review or in the study of a disease which becomes manifest by causing sudden death.

Incident or newly-diagnosed cases are to be preferred and are the type usually used in case-control studies of cancer. They have several advantages over prevalent (previously diagnosed) cases. For one, the time of disease onset is closer to the time of etiological exposure than is any later time. Thus, an incident case should recall better than a prevalent case the experience or exposures under evaluation. Similarly, recent medical, employment or other records are likely to be available and more informative than older records. In addition, a series of incident cases has not been acted upon by the determinants of survival whereas a series of prevalent cases has. That is, the cases prevalent at any point in time are the survivors of a larger series of incident cases diagnosed in a preceding period. If incident and prevalent cases differ with respect to risk factors, the use of prevalent cases would give an erroneous result. For example, using prevalent cases there appeared to be an association between the HLA antigen A2 and acute leukaemia (Rogentine et al., 1972). A second study, however, showed that this association was due to improved survival among cases with HL-A2, rather than to an increased risk of developing the disease among persons with HL-A2 (Rogentine et al., 1973). A third advantage of incident cases is that the effects of the disease are less likely to appear as causes. If a case has been prevalent for several years he may have changed his environment or lifestyle in a number of ways. Then, unless care is taken to restrict inquiry to the pre-morbid circumstances, a false characterization will occur. A final advantage of incident cases is that they relate more directly to the usual objective of an etiological investigation; i.e., with incident cases one evaluates the way in which exposure relates to the incidence rate of a cancer not to its prevalence.

There is only one advantage to the use of prevalent cases over the use of incident cases: they are already available. This might be considered a major advantage, since most cancers are sufficiently uncommon that it could take several years of ascertainment at several medical centres to assemble an adequate number of incident cases. However, the case-fatality of cancer remains sufficiently high that, usually, a large series of prevalent cases cannot be assembled unless cases diagnosed long ago are included. This may provide abundant opportunity for determinants of survival to act. For these reasons there is usually no appreciable advantage to the exclusive use of prevalent cases.

When the case series has been defined in terms of characteristics and type, a source must be located. In most case-control studies cases are identified by monitoring of pathology department log books, hospital operating-room schedules, or discharge lists. Less frequently, the office records of a number of physicians are used. In cancer research, an additional source of cases is the hospital or regional cancer registry. However, unless a special effort is made, regional cancer registries usually cannot identify cases until three months or more after diagnosis.

The control series

The designation of the type, number and size of the control group or groups and the problem of selecting the specific control subjects are perhaps the most important and most difficult tasks in planning a case-control study. The issue of the number of control groups was addressed above. Here the issues of the type and size of the group are discussed. The method of selecting the individual control subjects will not be discussed as it is almost entirely dependent on study-specific circumstances. One general question, however, relates to whether, when using a hospital-based control series, subjects with conditions known to be associated with the exposure under study should be eligible as controls. Most epidemiologists consider it reasonable to exclude them if the exposure-related illness is the reason for their current hospitalization.

There is no one type of control group suitable for all studies and, it must be acknowledged, there are no firm criteria for what is an acceptable group. The major factors which contribute to choice of a control group are the characteristics and source of the cases and knowledge of the risk factors of the cancer to be studied and of how these might confound or interact with the exposure to be investigated.

The characteristics and source of the case series must heavily influence the type of control selected if comparability of the two series is to be achieved, that is, if selection bias is to be avoided. In general, if a population-based series of cases has been assembled, a random or (age and sex) stratified random sample of the population will prove to be a suitable control series. If cases have come from a restricted source it is usually appropriate to select controls from the same source. In an extension of the latter notion, Horwitz and Feinstein (1978) suggested that reduction of selection bias would be achieved if controls were selected from among persons who had undergone the same diagnostic test as the cases and found not to have cancer. This is intended to overcome bias due to selecting cases from among those who are excessive users of medical services. Such people may be highly likely to have had diagnostic tests performed, even on marginal indications, and may also have an unusual exposure experience. However, if controls are also drawn from those who have had the diagnostic test, then they should be more closely comparable with cases in terms of medical service use and exposure experience. An example of this approach to the control of selection bias is the study by Horwitz and Feinstein (1978) of cancer of the endometrium; controls were drawn from among women who had been evaluated by uterine dilatation and curettage, just as the cases had been. This type of control group would appear inappropriate because agents which cause one disease in an organ often cause other diseases of that organ, or signs or symptoms referable to it. If such a procedure is followed in a study of, say, lung cancer, individuals with chronic pulmonary diseases would comprise a high proportion of the control series. An association of lung cancer with cigarette smoking would still be perceived, because it is a strong association, but it would be muted because smoking causes many diseases of the lung. Despite this difficulty, the use of a diagnostic register as a source of controls may be a useful way to reduce the possible "medical consumerism" bias described above. However, to be appropriate, such rosters of potential controls should relate to procedures for the diagnosis of conditions of organs other than that organ which is the site of the cancer afflicting the cases.

It has been suggested, for yet another reason, that the control series should have undergone or be subjected to the same diagnostic procedures as the cases. The reason proposed is that it would permit exclusion of early cases or "cases-to-be" from the control series and thus permit a more appropriate comparison. This exclusion is contrary to principle since even cases-to-be are a portion of the at-risk population (whether a real or hypothetical population), and their exclusion would distort the estimated frequency of exposure among the group as a whole (Miettinen, 1976). The exclusion is also difficult to accept in practice since it would be expensive, would pose practical problems, and for some procedures would be ethically unacceptable. Furthermore, since the remaining lifetime risk of developing any specific cancer is 10% or less (for most cancers much less) very few potential controls would be excluded in this way.

Another consideration in designating the control series is related to the persistent opinion that the controls must be like the cases in every respect apart from having the disease of interest. The historical basis of this misconception is clear; it comes from the axiom of experimental research that control subjects must be treated in every respect like exposed subjects. But in a case-control study this axiom is inapplicable. The consequences of selecting controls to be like cases with respect to some correlate of the exposure under study but to a correlate which is not a risk factor, that is, of "overmatching", are now recognized and are discussed in the section on matching.

A second aspect of control selection is the size of the series. When the number of available cases and controls is large and the cost of gathering information from a case and a control is about equal, then the selection ratio of controls to cases would be unity. The standard issues would then be invoked to estimate the acceptable minimum study size. The question becomes more complex when the size of either group is severely limited or the cost of obtaining information is greater for either cases or controls. For example, it occurs frequently that only a small number of cases is available for study. In this circumstance, the selection ratio should be increased to two, three or even four controls per case. This is not commonly done, and it is regrettable to see otherwise good case-control studies which are non-persuasive because of the unnecessarily small size of the control series. The selection ratio should be permitted to vary according to the circumstances of the study. But, one must be wary; it is wise to stay within the bounds of 4 : 1, except when the data are available at little cost or when they were collected for another purpose, and especially if they are in the form of a machine-readable file. The reasons for this have been presented by Gail et al. (1976) and by Walter (1977) and relate mainly to the small increase in statistical power as the ratio increases beyond four.

A third aspect of the designation of controls and a major factor in case-control studies is the source of the control group. Most studies use either hospital patients or the general population; restricted population groups, e.g., neighbours of cases or special groups such as associates or relatives of cases are much less often used.

The general population has a major strength as the source of the control series. Such controls will be especially comparable with the cases when a population-based series of cases has been assembled. This often makes for the most persuasive type of case-control study because of the high comparability of the two series and because a high level of generalizability of results is achieved. Even when a hospital-based series of cases is assembled, the population controls have the attribute of being, in general, well, and so causes of disease are not inordinately prevalent among them. Thus, one usually need exclude nobody from a population control series. (There are some exceptions to this. For one, it is reasonable to exclude people who do not have the organ in which the cancer develops. This is of some significance in studies of cancer of the uterus, at least in the United States where 30% or more of women aged about 50 years do not have a uterus. For another, it seems reasonable to exclude a control who has been previously diagnosed with the cancer under study.) There are, however, three disadvantages associated with use of the general population as a control group. Firstly, it can be extremely expensive and time-consuming to select and to obtain information from such a group. Secondly, the individuals selected are often not cooperative and response tends to be worse than that from other types of controls. This second disadvantage is especially important because it detracts from the presumed major strength of a general population control group. A third disadvantage of a population-based control series may arise if it is used in the study of a disease with mild symptoms for which medical attention need not be sought. In this instance the factors which lead to seeking medical care, such as, perhaps, affluence, will appear to be correlated with the disease. This problem is a small one in studies of cancer in countries where medical care is generally available.

Other kinds of general population control groups besides a random sample are sometimes used. Probably the most common of these is a neighbourhood control series. If these controls are obtained by having the interviewer actually move physically through each neighbourhood, the cost of the study may be extremely high. Furthermore, it may be difficult or impossible to characterize or even to enumerate the non-respondents (not at home) or the non-cooperators (those who decline to participate). It appears that non-cooperation is high when this approach is used. A recent example of a study using a neighbourhood control group is that of Clarke and Anderson (1979). For each control finally obtained, an average of 12 household contact efforts were required, one of which led to a non-cooperator. Thus, the effective proportion of cooperators in this study was about 50% and even that was obtained from among a self-selected group of respondents. On the other hand, if neighbourhood controls can be selected by use of some type of directory or listing and the initial contact made by telephone or letter, response should be acceptable. Even so, it is usually difficult to accept the rationale offered to justify the use of close neighbourhood controls. Generally, this is stated to be the wish to match the controls to the cases with respect to socioeconomic class. But, people who live in the same neighbourhood are likely to be similar in more respects than socioeconomic class and so the potential for overmatching is great. A random sample of the general population is usually less costly to obtain and may be superior as well. If a factor such as socioeconomic class is to be controlled, this can be done in the analysis of a study using controls from the general population, provided the relevant information is obtained.

The use of hospital patients as a control group has several advantages. Such people are readily available, have time to spare and are cooperative. Moreover, since they are hospitalized (or have been recently) they may have a "mental set" similar to that of the cases. This should reduce anamnestic bias, one of the most serious potential problems in a case-control study. The use of hospital patients as controls may also make the cases and controls similar with respect to determinants of hospitalization. This is probably useful if the cases have a disease for which hospitalization is elective. Probably it is not very important in the study of cancer, unless the case series is assembled from one, or a few, highly specialized institutions which have a wide referral area. The use of hospital patients as controls has one possibly serious limitation. The controls may be in hospital for a condition which has etiological features in common with the disease under study. To minimize this problem, controls should be selected from patients with conditions in many diagnostic categories. Another limitation of hospital controls has arisen only over the past few years, particularly in the United States. Before approaching hospital patients it is usually necessary to have the approval of a responsible physician or surgeon; this is becoming difficult to obtain, presumably because of growing concern about the confidentiality of medical information.

Matching

In planning a case-control study it must be decided whether the controls are to be matched to the cases and, if so, with respect to what factors and how closely. This warrants careful consideration because the decision will have implications for virtually every subsequent aspect of the study. Furthermore, an inappropriate decision will prove costly in time and money and may lead to an unsatisfactory study result. The issues underlying the question of matching received little attention until about ten years ago; but recently there have been several efforts at clarification, for example, those of Billewicz (1965), Miettinen (1976), McKinlay (1977), and Rubin (1979). These efforts have provided an appreciation of the complexity of what at first appears to be a straightforward approach to improving a study. This is an overview of some basic considerations relating to matching. In addition to being restricted to the case-control setting, this presentation is limited in that it deals primarily with factors which are dichotomous and only with matched pairs. These limitations do not distort the essential issues and permit them to be expressed more simply. In Chapters 5 and 6 ordinal scale exposures and multiple- and variable-ratio matching are considered.

In a case-control study the main purpose of matching is to permit use of efficient analytical methods to control confounding by the factors matched for. By confounding I mean the factor of interest is associated with the cancer under study, but this association is at least to some extent, and possibly entirely, non-causal. The association occurs because the factor of interest (the confounded factor) is associated with a true cause (the confounding factor) of the disease. Confounding can be illustrated by the concern expressed about the relationship between exogenous oestrogens and endometrial cancer. Steckel (1976) suggested that among women who will develop cancer of the endometrium at a later age, a fairly high proportion might have a rather difficult menopause. This is reasonable since cancer of the endometrium is probably caused by some hormonal difficulty, as are the signs and symptoms of the menopause. It is also reasonable to suggest that women who have a difficult menopause would be more likely than others to seek medical attention and to receive treatment with oestrogen, which is often prescribed for menopausal problems. If this were true, then oestrogens would (validly) appear to be associated with endometrial cancer in a case-control study (or in a follow-up study, for that matter). The association, however, would be non-causal, being confounded by a true cause of endometrial cancer, the hormonal aberration, which also "causes" women to receive oestrogens. (This particular proposed "constitutional confounding" was chosen as an example because it is quite illustrative, but it is almost certainly not correct since: (1) there is a dose-response relationship between oestrogen use and the relative risk of endometrial cancer; (2) the incidence rate of endometrial cancer has risen concurrently with the increase in oestrogen use; (3) the strength of the association between oestrogen use and endometrial cancer is similar in populations which are very dissimilar in their frequency of oestrogen use; and (4) cessation of oestrogen use is followed by a reduction in endometrial cancer incidence.)

A simpler, and correct, example of confounding is the association of cancer of the mouth with the occupation "bartender". Mouth cancer is caused by excessive alcohol and tobacco consumption, both of which are relatively common among bartenders. As can be seen from these two examples, for a factor to be confounding, it must be associated *both* with the cancer under study (as a cause of the cancer must be) and with the exposure of interest.

Confounding can be controlled in the analysis of a study or it may be eliminated by design in one of several ways. Of these ways, matching is by far the most often used, probably because it appears to be a direct and intuitive approach. In addition, when there are only dichotomous (exposed, non-exposed) factors under evaluation, the match- ed-pairs (one control per case) design permits a straightforward estimation of the rel- ative risk and its statistical significance. These features probably explain why pair match- ing was the first technique widely used to control confounding and remains popular today. But since there are now effective ways to control confounding in the analysis of the data the desirability of matching warrants reassessment.

Matching in a case-control study is an attempt to mimic blocking in an experiment, that is, randomizing animals within categories of a factor known (or suspected) to in- fluence the outcome under evaluation. However, any analogy between blocking and matching is false in one crucial respect. In experimental work, no matter how extensive the blocking, the investigator manipulates exposure to the factor under study (usually by randomization). This guarantees that the blocking factors will not be correlated with the exposure of interest. However, exposure is not manipulated in a case-control study, and so a matching factor, unlike a blocking factor, will be associated with any exposure which differs between cases and controls. This must include the exposure under study if the matching is justified. For, if the matching is justified it will be with respect to a confounding factor, necessarily a correlate of the exposure under study. This means that any mode of analysis which fails to accommodate the fact that the matching process has forced the controls to be more like the cases than they otherwise would be, with respect to the exposure of interest, will lead to an estimate of the relative risk which is too close to unity. And, if the matching has been carried sufficiently far by matching on several variables, the cases and controls will be virtually identical with respect to the exposure to be studied. Effectively, time and money will have been spent in a counter- productive effort; the study will provide no information or, worse, an erroneous result. Thus it is necessary to avoid overmatching, that is, matching for a variable which is relat- ed to the exposure under study but which is not an independent risk factor and so can- not be a confounding factor.

It is useful to distinguish between two types of overmatching. One type occurs when the investigator matches for a factor which is part of the mechanism whereby the factor under study produces cancer. As an example, consider the prospect of matching con- trols to cases for the presence or absence of endometrial hyperplasia in a study of exog- enous oestrogens and endometrial cancer. Hyperplasia is a condition which is caused by exogenous oestrogen and which may progress to cancer. The controls will thus be made very like the cases in exposure history, and the data, even when appropriately analysed, will lead to a relative risk biased towards unity. The second type of overmatching relates to matching for a variable which is a correlate of the factor under study, not an inde- pendent risk factor and not a part of the causal mechanism. In this instance an appropri- ate analysis will provide an inferentially valid estimate of the relative risk. However, the study will be inefficient, that is, imprecise, and there may be little confidence in the estimate obtained. The way this inefficiency comes about is described below.

Even matching which is indicated can be expensive and may prolong the data-gather- ing phase of a study. The number of matching "strata" is one of the determinants of cost and this increases sharply as the number of variables increases. For example, if a study involves matching for sex (two categories) and age (say, five categories) there will be ten strata. If matching for religion (say, three categories) is added there will be 30 strata, and formation of matched pairs will become difficult. The addition of one more matching variable, bringing the total number of strata to a minimum of 60, will make the search for a matched control tedious even for the more common types of subject. And for the less frequent types it may prove impossible to form matched pairs, with the consequent exclusion of some cases from the study. In addition to the number of strata, the specific variables chosen for matching will also influence the cost and time necessary to do the matching. Efforts have been made to match even for variables for which information must be obtained by interviewing the potential controls; if a control does not match the case for which be was being considered, the cost of contacting and interviewing him will usually be wasted. Generally, rather than expending resources in following an elaborate matching scheme, it will prove more efficient to gather data from a reasonably large number of potential controls and to evaluate and control confounding when the data are analysed. This approach can be especially efficient if the range of the subjects is restricted (perhaps one sex and a narrow age range) and if advance information is available as to whether individuals meet the restricted characteristics.

Matching can be envisioned as an effort to increase the contribution (or informativeness) of each subject to the study. Thus, while there may be relatively few subjects in a matched study, any matched pair which is discordant for exposure (one member exposed, the other not) makes a moderately large contribution to the evaluation of the relative risk and its statistical significance. However, each matched pair which is exposure-concordant makes no contribution at all. This illustrates the need to avoid matching for factors which are correlates of exposure but which do not confound the association of interest. The effect of such matching is to create an excessive number of uninformative exposure-concordant pairs.

A final cost of matching may have to be paid when the data are analysed. The matching process requires that the data first be analysed with the matching taken into account. If a stratified analysis is used (see Chapter 5), control for the confounding effect of factors other than those matched for will lead to the elimination of much of the data. However, if it is necessary to control such factors it may be possible to demonstrate that, as is often so, only age and sex are pertinent as matching factors and that the matching can be ignored as long as age and sex are carefully controlled in the analysis or the results are derived for specific age-sex groups. The analysis may then proceed and the effect of an unmatched confounding factor controlled for. If regression methods are used in the analysis (see Chapter 7) unmatched and matched factors can be controlled directly.

Some of the problems associated with matching are illustrated by an unusual case-control study done to evaluate the hypothesis that tonsillectomy is associated with increased risk of Hodgkin's disease (Johnson & Johnson, 1972). The study included 85 persons with Hodgkin's disease and, as their controls, 85 siblings, each sibling being matched to the respective case for sex and for age as well as, inherently, for sibship. The study was interpreted as showing no association between tonsillectomy and Hodgkin's disease. It seemed likely to others, however, that although the study consisted of a control series closely matched to the cases for likely strong correlates of tonsillectomy, especially sibship, the matching had been ignored in the analysis (the analysis had not been described). The data were then reanalysed (Cole et al., 1973) and a relative risk of 2.1 with p = 0.07 was found – a positive result consistent with an earlier report. This illustrates the need to accommodate the matching with an appropriate form of analysis. In fact the 85 matched pairs were a subset of a larger series of 174 cases and their 472 siblings. The reduction to the 85 matched pairs, presumably to control potential confounding by sex and age, had caused 74% of the available data to be discarded. When all the data were analysed, thus ignoring age and sex, the relative risk was 2.0 (p = 10^{-4}). The near identity of the two relative risks is evidence that, in this series of subjects, there was no confounding by age and sex and that matching for those factors was irrelevant and wasteful.

The following should be considered when matching is contemplated for a case-control study. First, matching is only justified for factors which are known or suspected to confound the association of interest; that a factor may be related to the exposure of interest is not sufficient justification for matching. Second, matching may also be justified for factors which could interact with the exposure of interest in producing disease, since it provides more efficient estimates of relative risk within subgroups homogeneous with respect to suspected interacting factors. Third, it is usually possible to justify the costs in time and money of matching for age, sex and nominal scale variables with a large number of realizations (sibship, neighbourhood). However, such nominal scale variables should be matched for only if they meet one of the first two criteria, and this is uncommon. Fourth, when it is decided to match for a factor the matching should be as close as possible, with expense being the constraint to making an ever tighter match. For example, age is usually matched for arbitrarily in (plus or minus) five- or ten-year units. Frequently, it would cost very little more to match on year of birth or perhaps two-year age units. With respect to matching for age in particular it would be appropriate to modify the closeness of the match to the age of the subjects studied. For children and young adults a very close match is indicated because experiences change rapidly at these ages and because a discrepancy of a given magnitude, say one year, is a relatively greater proportion of the lifespan than it is in middle or old age. Since the principal objective of matching is to eliminate a potential confounder as such, the tighter match is to be desired since it minimizes the prospect that there would be "residual confounding" within the matching strata.

1.6 Implementation

Information gathering

The methods and problems of gathering information for a case-control study, as for other studies, greatly depend on the locale in which the study is done and the information sources used (interview, postal questionnaire, medical or other type of record review). Only a few general suggestions are offered. A case-control study usually begins with the investigator seeking cooperation from several hospitals or medical practitioners. This usually amounts to a request to identify cases, and perhaps controls, from available records. At least in the United States, this cooperation is becoming more difficult to obtain for several reasons, the major one being concern about litigation by a patient who believes that confidentiality has been breached. It is remarkable how deep and widespread this concern is, considering the rarity of the problem. For example, in the Department of Epidemiology at the Harvard School of Public Health during a period in which at least 15 000 subjects identified from hospital records were requested to provide information, there was no such litigation nor serious threat of it. Despite this experience, which seems typical of epidemiological research, it is often not possible to persuade hospital administrators to cooperate. When non-cooperation is anticipated it is useful to make initial contact with a hospital through a staff physician who supports the research.

The next stage is to abstract the medical records of the cases, and of potential controls, at locations where cooperation was received. If possible the items on the record abstract form should follow the sequence of the medical record, but this may not be possible if several different hospitals are involved. If the medical record abstract involves information pertinent to the exposures under evaluation, as occurs when the role of drugs is in question, it is important to blind the abstractor to the case-control status of the record. It is also important to delete from the record or to mask any information relating to exposures sustained after the case's cancer was diagnosed, and during the equivalent time for the controls. These things will usually prove difficult and will involve at least two people in the record abstracting process. Nonetheless, both are usually justifiable.

It is best to conduct interviews concurrently for cases and controls. This should minimize the likelihood that learning by those gathering the data will influence the results. It would also minimize any effects of short-term changes, such as those of the seasons, or of some unexpected publicity about the cancer or the factors under study.

It is often recommended that, when they are involved, there should be as few interviewers as possible, preferably one. The rationale of this is that it will introduce uniformity into data collection. But, if the quality of the work is poor or if the interviewer is biased, a study would be ruined by having only one interviewer. It seems wiser, when practical, to have several well-trained interviewers. When more than one interviewer is used, it may be informative to analyse the principal study factors on an interviewer-specific basis. A positive result based on information from only a small proportion of the interviewers would be a cause for concern.

There are several suggestions concerning interviewers which are sound but difficult to meet. One of these is to keep the interviewers, and all study staff, unaware of the principal hypothesis(es) under evaluation. But even if the investigator attempts this, the interviewers usually become aware of what is important from the interview form itself or from sources external to the study. Another suggestion is that the interviewers be unaware of the status (case or control) of each subject they interview. One way of doing this is to have one person arrange the interview and another conduct it. This may prove effective for interviews conducted in hospital but is rarely even possible for those done at home. The reason is that the subjects, both cases and controls, usually want more information than was given them about the objectives of the study and the reason for their inclusion. In order to answer such questions in an honest, even if ambiguous, way the interviewer usually has to know the subject's status. The need for ambiguity often arises because many physicians still do not want their patient told of the diagnosis of cancer. Another reason is that the interviewer does not know, or should not inform the subjects, about the specific purpose of the study. A third suggestion concerning interviewers can and should be met: each of them should deal with the same ratio of controls to cases as exists in the study as a whole.

When a postal questionnaire is used to gather data an effort should be made to make the form as simple as possible in both appearance and use. This can be implemented by aligning the various insets so that there are as few different margins as possible. It is also useful to make the format of the response as uniform as possible, e.g., all boxes to be checked or alternatives to be circled, but not both. The instructions to the subject should be as brief and clear as possible. There is no disadvantage, however, in terms of response frequency, in making the questionnaire itself as long as required, within reason, nor does there seem to be any disadvantage (in terms of response frequency) in using franked as opposed to stamped mail, nor in using second or third class as opposed to first class service. In general, it appears that age and socioeconomic status of the subjects are determinants of response (younger and better-off subjects respond better), while features of the postage and questionnaire are relatively unimportant (Kaplan & Cole, 1970).

In both an interview form and a postal questionnaire, each item should deal with one question – compound questions should be avoided. It is usually advisable, especially in an interview, to permit unstructured responses; in such cases the space for the response should be followed by an indication of the units in which the response is to be expressed. Prescribed ranges to classify a response (e.g., <2, 2–4, 4–6, 7+ years) should be avoided; it is rarely justified to degrade information in this way at the time of collection. Note also that the responses in this example are ambiguous: the second and third are not mutually exclusive. All forms should be tested repeatedly to remove ambiguities and queries which elicit vague or ambiguous responses. Completed interviews should be reviewed by an experienced supervisor and the interviewers informed of the assessment of their work; part of this process should be undertaken by the investigator.

Information management

Information management commences well when good information-gathering forms and high-quality gathering and editing procedures are used. One aspect which relates particularly to information management is the use of "self-coding" forms. This term used to refer to several different formats, including one requiring the subject or interviewer to select a response and enter a corresponding code into a designated space. Generally, mixing information gathering with information management in this way is ill-advised; it is conducive to error and may reduce rapport in the interview setting. It is better to have all the coding done by two (or more) people (including, if convenient, the interviewers themselves) in a setting free of the stress of information gathering.

The information gathered must be translated into a series of numeric (or, rarely, alphabetic) codes. Generally, one item in the code will correspond with one item on the form. Each code item should consist of a series of mutually exclusive, collectively exhaustive categories. Virtually every item will require the categories "other" and "unknown", and rarely is it justified to combine these. No code item should be a "derived variable", i.e., a variable whose value is determined from two or more other variables. Computing the value of a derived variable is done more accurately, objectively, and at lower cost, by a computer. Just as there is no reason to degrade information at the gathering stage there is no need to degrade it at the coding stage. In fact, modern analytical techniques argue for the use of highly refined data throughout the study, degradation to conventional ranges being reserved for the presentation of the results.

The early responses should be encoded by a highly experienced person and, if necessary, the code modified to permit designation of unanticipated responses or for other improvements. The need for this will be minimal if the forms have been well-designed and tested. The early work of the coders should be checked carefully to reveal any systematic problem resulting from a misunderstanding of how certain responses are to be encoded.

It is still common to have information encoded by one person and checked by another. The information is then key-punched and key-verified and a file created on a tape (usually for storage or transportation) or on a disc (for analysis). This procedure may serve for studies which gather an enormous amount of information and which can tolerate a modest amount of error, as is usually true of a follow-up study. However, most case-control studies gather a relatively small amount of information at relatively high cost. For these it is better to have each form coded by two people working independently. The code sheets prepared by one are then key-punched and a file created; no key-verification is done. The file is then printed out as a listing which is as easy to read as possible: triple spacing between lines, blank spaces between items. This printout is then checked against the code sheet of the second coder and errors are resolved. In this way all errors are caught by a single checking procedure, including coding errors which are often missed by the conventional procedure. Finally, a few of each of the computer-generated, derived variables are checked against the values generated by one person. While these procedures seem tedious they are not much more so than the usual ones, and they virtually guarantee that analysis can proceed in the knowledge that, as far as is humanly possible, the disc file is an accurate image of the information gathered.

1.7 Interpretation

The interpretation of a study involves evaluating the likelihood that the result reflects: one or more biases in design or conduct, the role of confounding, the role of chance or the role of causality. An approach to interpretation is presented here which is similar to that presented in Chapter 3 but is less concerned with quantification.

The most common basis for suggesting that a case-control study has produced an erroneous (biased) result (a suggestion which, of course, usually comes from a reviewer, not from the investigators) is that subject selection was inappropriate. This usually implies a selection bias but may refer to inclusion of non-cases in the case series (rarely a problem in the study of cancer) or "cases-to-be" in the control series. A second common basis for proposing a biased result is that there has been a systematic error in data collection such as that due to recall bias or to the interviewers knowing the case-control status of the subjects. A third basis for suggesting error is that there may have been an inordinate amount of random error in the data gathering. This suggestion is commonly offered for studies in which no apparent association emerges in relation to a factor acknowledged to be difficult to describe or quantify, such as diet. A fourth basis for suggesting error is that an inappropriate analysis has been done. Often the critic will suggest that the results are in error and imply that it is because of one or more of these reasons. Though it is not commonly done, it would be far more constructive if, in addition to invoking one problem or another, the critic would go further and, in discussion with the investigators, attempt to determine in which direction and to what extent the study result might be altered by correction of the proposed flaw. It is not rare for the critic of a positive study to imply that the correct result is the absence of association and to defend his proposal on the basis of a perceived bias which, if it truly existed and could be corrected, would probably cause the study result to be even more strongly positive.

A second interpretation to be considered is that the study result reflects confounding by some known (or suspected) cause of the cancer. This interpretation, it should be remembered, does not imply that the results are false. Rather, it implies that a valid but non-causal association exists between the cancer and the factor under study. Until recently, efforts were made to exclude confounding as an explanation of study results by showing that the proposed confounding factor was not associated to a statistically significant extent with the cancer under study. While it is understandable how this approach came to be used it is now unacceptable. The question of confounding is not dealt with in this way. Instead it is necessary to show to what extent the relative risk changes, or does not change, when the effect of the proposed confounding factor(s) is controlled. This change (if any) in the relative risk is an index of the degree of confounding. The relative risk estimate which persists after control of the confounding factor is the one which describes the specific association at issue.

When an unconfounded estimate of relative risk is available, interpretation turns to the possible role of chance. The issue, of course, is the possible role that chance effects in subject selection may have played in producing the unconfounded, not the crude, estimate of relative risk. This is addressed by estimating the significance level, or p-value, associated with the difference observed between cases and controls in their exposure histories. If this value is small, say, less than 0.05, it is usually concluded that the role of chance is unlikely to explain the observed departure of the relative risk from unity. There is nothing wrong with this, but it is a rather limited way to describe the role of chance. The confidence limits of the relative risk are more informative, especially in a study which shows no association. Use of the p-value and use of confidence limits are not mutually exclusive, but there are objections to the use of the p-value alone (Cole, 1979).

Finally, interpretation moves to the prospect that a valid causal association would explain the results. Occasionally, the causal inference is made as a "diagnosis of exclusion". That is, if the result is not perceived as biased and not due to chance or confounding, then it must be causal. But causality has at least three positive criteria and these should be reviewed, in addition to excluding alternative explanations. The *strength* of the association relates to causality. Relative risks of less than 2.0 may readily reflect some unperceived bias or confounding factor, those over 5.0 are unlikely to do so. The *consistency* of the association is germane to causality. Is the association seen in all subgroups where expected, and is there a dose-response relationship? Both these considerations relate to internal consistency. The extent to which the study is externally consistent, i.e., consistent with previous reports, can also be evaluated to support or refute a causal inference. That is, when a similar finding appears in different, especially very different, settings the notion of causality is favoured even if only because alternative explanations are less credible. A third criterion of causality is *biological credibil-*

ity; is it understood in biological terms how the exposure under study could produce the cancer of interest? However, while pertinent, the response to this question is not especially convincing one way or another; it has proven all too easy to propose credible biological mechanisms relating most exposures to most cancers; and, on the other hand, the failure to perceive such a mechanism may reflect only our ignorance of the state of nature.

For the sake of completeness another criterion of causality is mentioned: this relates to how the *frequency* of disease changes when the proposed cause is removed from (or added to) the environment. No doubt the response to manipulation of the exposure is the most cogent type of causal argument, but it does not concern the investigator dealing with the results of a particular case-control study.

Finally, there are two further considerations to bear in mind when interpreting a result. First, as an alternative to the four interpretations discussed, it could be decided that a study is "unevaluable". This decision is usually arrived at by exclusion, that is, there may be no basis for placing confidence in any of the other interpretations. The most frequent situation occurs when a study has no detectable flaw but its results are consistent with a chance effect. While the judgement of "unevaluable" may be tenable, it does not mean that the study is in error or has no value. Unless the study is so small as to be hopelessly imprecise, it can still make a contribution, in the context of other studies, to evaluating the hypothesis in question. Secondly, it is useful to keep in mind that the interpretation decided upon is not immutable. An investigator and the scientific community may favour one interpretation today and a different one later, in the light of knowledge acquired in the interim.

REFERENCES

Bailar, J.C. & Anthony, G.B. (1977) Most cited papers of the Journal of the National Cancer Institute 1962–75. *J. natl Cancer Inst., 59,* 709–714

Billewicz, W.Z. (1965) The efficiency of matched samples: an empirical investigation. *Biometrics, 21,*623–643

Boston Collaborative Drug Surveillance Program (1973) Oral contraceptives and venous thromboembolic disease, surgically confirmed gall-bladder disease, and breast tumours. *Lancet, i,* 1399–1404

Breslow, N.E. & Patton, J. (1979) *Case-control analysis of cohort studies.* In: Breslow, N. & Whittemore, A., eds, *Energy and Health,* Philadelphia, Society for Industrial and Applied Mathematics, pp. 226–242

Clarke, E.A. & Anderson, T.W. (1979) Does screening by "Pap" smears help prevent cervical cancer? A case-control study. *Lancet, ii,* 1–4

Cole, P. (1973) *A population-based study of bladder cancer.* In: Doll, R. & Vodopija, I., eds, *Host Environment Interactions in the Etiology of Cancer in Man,* Lyon, International Agency for Research on Cancer *(IARC Scientific Publications No. 7),* pp. 83–87

Cole, P. (1979) The evolving case-control study. *J. chron. Dis., 32,* 15–27

Cole, P. & MacMahon, B. (1971) Attributable risk percent in case-control studies. *Br. J. prev. soc. Med., 25,* 242–244

Cole, P., Elwood, J.M. & Kaplan, S.D. (1978) Incidence rates and risk factors of benign breast neoplasms. *Am. J. Epidemiol., 108,* 112–120

Cole, P., Hoover, R. & Friedell, G.H. (1972) Occupation and cancer of the lower urinary tract. *Cancer, 29,* 1250–1260

Cole, P., Mack, T., Rothman, K., Henderson, B. & Newell, G. (1973) Tonsillectomy and Hodgkin's disease (Letter to the Editor). *New Engl. J. Med., 288,* 634

Cole, P., Monson, R.R., Haning, H. & Friedell, G.H. (1971) Smoking and cancer of the lower urinary tract. *New Engl. J. Med., 284,* 129–134

Cornfield, J. (1951) A method of estimating comparative rates from clinical data. Application to cancer of the lung, breast and cervix. *J. natl Cancer Inst., 11,* 1269–1275

Doll, R. & Hill, A.B. (1952) A study of the aetiology of carcinoma of the lung. *Br. med. J., ii,* 1271–1286

Edmondson, H.A., Henderson, B. & Benton, B. (1976) Liver-cell adenomas associated with use of oral contraceptives. *New Engl. J. Med., 294,* 470–472

Elwood, J.M., Cole, P., Rothman, K.J. & Kaplan, S.D. (1977) Epidemiology of endometrial cancer. *J. natl Cancer Inst., 59,* 1055–1060

Feinstein, A.R. (1979) Methodologic problems and standards in case-control research. *J. chron. Dis., 32,* 35–41

Gail, M., Williams, R., Byar, D.P. & Brown, C. (1976) How many controls? *J. chron. Dis., 29,* 723–731

Gordon, J., Reagan, J.W., Finkle, W.D. & Ziel, H.K. (1977) Estrogen and endometrial carcinoma. An independent pathology review supporting original risk estimate. *New Engl. J. Med., 297,* 570–571

Greenberg, M. & Lloyd Davies, T.A. (1974) Mesothelioma Register 1967–68. *Br. J. ind. Med., 31,* 91–104

Gutensohn, N. & Cole, P. (1977) The epidemiology of Hodgkin's disease among the young. *Int. J. Cancer, 19,* 595–604

Gutensohn, N., Li, F., Johnson, R. & Cole, P. (1975) Hodgkin's disease, tonsillectomy and family size. *New Engl. J. Med., 292,* 22–25

Haenszel, W., Kurihara, M., Segi, M. & Lee, R.K.C. (1972) Stomach cancer among Japanese in Hawaii. *J. natl Cancer Inst., 37,* 969–988

Haenszel, W., Berg, J.W., Segi, M., Kurihara, M. & Locke, F.B. (1973) Large-bowel cancer in Hawaiian Japanese. *J. natl Cancer Inst., 51,* 1765–1779

Haenszel, W., Correa, P., Cuello, C., Guzman, N., Burbano, L.C., Lores, H. & Muñoz, J. (1976) Gastric cancer in Colombia. II. Case-control epidemiologic study of precursor lesions. *J. natl Cancer Inst., 57,* 1021–1026

Halperin, M. (1977) Estimability and estimation in case-referent studies (Letter to the Editor). *Am. J. Epidemiol., 105,* 496–498

Herbst, A.I., Ulfelder, H. & Poskanzer, D.C. (1971) Adenocarcinoma of the vagina. Association of maternal stilbestrol therapy with tumor appearance in young women. *New Engl. J. Med., 284,* 878–881

Horwitz, R.I. & Feinstein, A.R. (1978) Alternative analytic methods for case-control studies of estrogens and endometrial cancer. *New Engl. J. Med., 299,* 1089–1094

Horwitz, R.I. & Feinstein, A.R. (1979) Methodologic standards and contradictory results in case-control research. *Am. J. Med., 66,* 556–564

Hutchison, G.B. (1979) Re: "Estrogens and endometrial carcinoma" (Letter to the Editor). *New Engl. J. Med., 300,* 497

Ibrahim, M.A., ed. (1979) The case-control study: consensus and controversy. *J. chron. Dis., 32,* 1–144

Ibrahim, M.A. & Spitzer, W. (1979) The case-control study: the problem and the prospect. *J. chron. Dis., 32,* 130–144

Jick, H. & Vessey, M.P. (1978) Case-control studies in the evaluation of drug-induced illness. *Am. J. Epidemiol., 107,* 1–7

Johnson, S.K. & Johnson, R.E. (1972) Tonsillectomy history in Hodgkin's disease. *New Engl. J. Med., 287,* 1122–1125

Kaplan, S. & Cole, P. (1970) Factors affecting response to postal questionnaires. *Br. J. prev. soc. Med., 24,* 245–247

Kelsey, J.L., Lindfors, K.K. & White, C. (1974) A case-control study of epidemiology of benign breast diseases with reference to oral contraceptive use. *Int. J. Epidemiol. 3,* 333

Lane-Claypon, J.E. (1926) *A Further Report on Cancer of the Breast. Reports on Public Health and Medical Subjects 32,* London, Her Majesty's Stationery Office

Levin, M.L., Goldstein, H. & Gerhardt, P.R. (1950) Cancer and tobacco smoking. A preliminary report. *J. Am. med. Assoc., 143,* 336–338

Liddell, F.D.K., McDonald, J.C. & Thomas, D.C. (1977) Methods of cohort analysis: appraisal by application to asbestos mining. *J. R. stat. Soc. Ser. A, 140,* 469–491

McKinlay, S.M. (1977) Pair matching – a reappraisal of a popular technique. *Biometrics, 33,* 725–735

MacMahon, B. & Pugh, B. (1970) *Epidemiologic Methods,* Boston, Little Brown

MacMahon, B., Cole, P., Lin, T.M., Lowe, C.R., Mirra, A.P., Ravnihar, B., Salber, E.J., Valaoras, V.G. & Yuasa, S. (1970) Age at first birth and breast cancer risk. *Bull. World Health Org., 43,* 209–221

Mantel, N. & Haenszel, W. (1959) Statistical aspects of the analysis of data from retrospective studies of disease. *J. natl Cancer Inst., 22,* 719–748

Miettinen, O.S. (1976) Estimability and estimation in case-referrant studies. *Am. J. Epidemiol., 103,* 226–235

Miettinen, O.S. (1977) Estimability and estimation (Letter to the Editor). *Am. J. Epidemiol., 105,* 498–502

Modan, B., Lubin, F., Barell, V., Greenberg, R.A., Modan, M. & Graham, S. (1974) The role of starches in the etiology of gastric cancer. *Cancer, 34,* 2087–2092

Modan, B., Barell, V., Lubin, F., Modan, M., Greenberg, R.A. & Graham, S. (1975) Low-fiber intake as an etiologic factor in cancer of the colon. *J. natl Cancer Inst., 55,* 15–18

Muir, C.S. & Wagner, G., eds (1976) *Directory of On-going Research in Cancer Epidemiology 1976,* Lyon, International Agency for Research on Cancer

Muir, C.S. & Wagner, G., eds (1979) *Directory of On-going Research in Cancer Epidemiology 1979,* Lyon, International Agency for Research on Cancer *(IARC Scientific Publications No. 27)*

Prince, A.M., Szmuness, W., Michon, J., Demaille, J., Diebolt, G., Linhard, J., Quenum, C. & Sankale, M. (1975) A case-control study of the association between primary liver cancer and hepatitis B infection in Senegal. *Int. J. Cancer, 16,* 376–383

Rogentine, G.N., Yankee, R.A., Gart, J.J., Nam, J. & Trapani, R.J. (1972) HLA antigens and disease: acute lymphocytic leukemia, *J. clin. Invest., 51,* 2420–2428

Rogentine, G.N., Trapani, R.J., Yankee, R.A. & Henderson, E.S. (1973) HLA antigens and acute lymphocytic leukemia: the nature of the association. *Tissue Antigens, 3,* 470–476

Rubin, D.R. (1979) Using multivariate matched sampling and regression analysis to control bias in observational studies. *J. Am. stat. Assoc., 74,* 318–328

Sackett, D.L. (1979) Bias in analytic research. *J. chron. Dis., 32,* 51–63

Salber, E.J., Trichopoulos, D. & MacMahon, B. (1969) Lactation and reproductive histories of breast cancer patients in Boston. *J. natl Cancer Inst., 43,* 1013–1024

Smith, D.C., Prentice, R., Thompson, D.J. & Herrmann, W.L. (1975) Association of exogenous estrogens and endometrial cancer. *New Engl. J. Med., 293,* 1164–1167

Sommers, S.C. (1978) *Postmenopausal estrogens and endometrial cancer: a pathologist's overview.* In: Silverberg, S.G. & Major, F.J., eds, *Estrogens and Cancer,* New York, Wiley, pp. 45–53

Steckel, R.J. (1976) Re: "Estrogens and endometrial carcinoma" (Letter to the Editor). *New Engl. J. Med., 294,* 848

Trichopoulos, D., Tabor, E., Gerety, R.J., Xirouchaki, E., Sparros, L., Muñoz, N. & Linsell, C.A. (1978) Hepatitis B and primary hepatocellular carcinoma in a European population. *Lancet, ii,* 1217–1219

Tuyns, A.J., Péquignot, G. & Jensen, O.M. (1977) Le cancer de l'oesophage en Ille-et Vilaine en fonction des niveaux de consommation d'alcool et de tabac. Des risques qui se multiplient. *Bull. Cancer, 64,* 45–60

Vessey, M.P., Doll, R. & Sutton, P.M. (1971) Investigation of the possible relationship between oral contraceptives and benign and malignant breast disease. *Cancer (Philad.), 28,* 1395

Walter, S.D. (1977) Determination of significant relative risks and optimal sampling procedures in prospective and retrospective comparative studies of various sizes. *Am. J. Epidemiol., 105,* 387–397

Wynder, E.L. & Graham, E.A. (1950) Tobacco smoking as a possible etiologic factor in bronchogenic carcinoma. A study of six hundred and eighty-four proved cases. *J. Am. med. Assoc., 143,* 329–336

Ziel, H.K. & Finkle, W.D. (1975) Increased risk of endometrial cancer among users of conjugated estrogens. *New Engl. J. Med., 293,* 1167–1170

2. FUNDAMENTAL MEASURES OF DISEASE OCCURRENCE AND ASSOCIATION

2.1 Measures of disease occurrence

2.2 Age- and time-specific incidence rates

2.3 Cumulative incidence rates

2.4 Models of disease association

2.5 Empirical behaviour of the relative risk

2.6 Effects of combined exposures

2.7 Logical properties of the relative risk

2.8 Estimation of the relative risk from case-control studies - basic concepts

2.9 Attributable risk and related measures

CHAPTER II

FUNDAMENTAL MEASURES OF DISEASE OCCURRENCE AND ASSOCIATION

The occurrence of particular cancers varies remarkably according to a wide range of factors, including age, sex, calendar time, geography and ethnicity. Etiological studies attempt to explain such variation by relating disease occurrence to genetic markers, or to exposure to particular environmental agents, which may have a similar variation in time and space. The cancer epidemiologist studies how the disease depends on the constellation of risk factors acting on the population and uses this information to determine the best measures for prevention and control. This process requires a quantitative measure of exposure, as well as one of disease occurrence, and some method of associating the two.

In this chapter we introduce the fundamental concepts of disease incidence rates, cumulative incidence, and risk. These will allow us to make a precise comparison of disease occurrence in different populations. Relative risk is defined and shown to have both empirical and logical advantages as a measure of disease/risk factor association, especially in connection with case-control studies. The close connection between cohort and case-control studies is emphasised throughout.

2.1 Measures of disease occurrence

Two measures of disease frequency, incidence and prevalence, are commonly introduced in textbooks on epidemiology. *Point prevalence* is the proportion of a defined population affected by the disease in question at a specified point in time. The numerator of the proportion comprises all those who have the disease at that instant, regardless of whether it was contracted recently or long ago. Thus, diseases of long duration tend to have a higher prevalence than short-term illnesses, even if the total numbers of affected individuals are about equal.

Incidence refers to new cases of disease occurring among previously unaffected individuals. This is a more appropriate measure for etiological studies of cancer and other chronic illnesses, wherein one attempts to relate disease occurrence to genetic and environmental factors in a framework of causation. The duration of survival of patients with a given disease, and hence its prevalence, may be influenced by treatment and other factors which come into play after onset. Early reports of an association between the antigen HL-A2 and risk for acute leukaemia (Rogentine et al., 1972), for example, were later corrected when it was shown that the effect was on survival rather than on incidence (Rogentine et al., 1973). Since causal factors necessarily operate prior to diagnosis, a more sensitive indication of their effects is obtained by using incidence as the fundamental measure of disease.

Rates, as opposed to frequencies, imply an element of time. The rate of occurrence of an event in a population is the *number of events which occur during a specified time interval, divided by the total amount of observation time accumulated during that interval.* For an incidence rate, the events are new cases of disease occurring among disease-free individuals. The denominator of the rate can be calculated by summing up the length of time during the specified interval that each member of the population was alive and under observation, without having developed the disease. It is usually expressed as the number of person-years of observation. Mortality rates, of course, refer to deaths occurring among those who remain alive.

The annual incidence rate for a particular calendar year is the number of new cases diagnosed during the year, divided by an approximation of the person-years of observation, such as the midyear population. If the disease is a common one, the denominator should refer more specifically to the subjects who are disease-free at midyear and hence at risk of disease development. This correction is rarely needed for cancer occurring at specific sites because the number of people alive with disease will be relatively small. One exception to this which illustrates the general principle is that of uterine cancer. In societies where a substantial fraction of older women have undergone a hysterectomy, the denominators used to calculate rates of cervical or endometrial cancer should include only women with an intact uterus, as the remainder are no longer at risk for the particular disease. This adjustment is particularly important when comparing cancer incidence among populations with different hysterectomy rates.

In calculating incidence rates *time* is usually taken to be *calendar time.* An annual rate is thus based on all cases which occur between January 1 and December 31 of a given year. However, there are other ways of choosing the origin of the time-scale besides reference to a particular date on the calendar.

Chronological age, for example, is simply elapsed time from birth. The fact that cancer incidence rates are routinely reported using age as the fundamental "time" variable reflects the marked variation of incidence with age which is found for most cancer sites. A typical practice is to use $J = 18$ age intervals, each having a constant length of five years (0–4, 5–9, ... 80–84, 85–89), ignoring cases occurring at age 90 or over. Sometimes the first interval is chosen to be of length $l_1 = 1$ (first year of life), the second of length $l_2 = 4$ (ages 1–4) and the remainder to have a constant length of 5 years. Cases of disease are allocated to each interval according to the age at diagnosis. Since individual ages will change during the period of observation, the same person may contribute to the person-years denominators for several age intervals.

Yet another possibility for the time variable is *time on study.* In prospective epidemiological investigations of industrial populations, for example, workers may enter the study after two or five years of continuous employment. Time is then measured as years elapsed since entry into the study. *Survival rates* for cancer and other diseases are presented in terms of elapsed months or years since diagnosis or definitive treatment. Here of course the endpoint is death for patients with disease. When using time on study as the fundamental time variable it is usually quite important to account also for the effects of age, whether one is calculating survival rates among cancer patients or cancer incidence rates among a cohort of exposed workers.

Fig. 2.1 Schematic illustration of age-specific incidence rates. (D = diagnosis of cancer; W = withdrawn, disease free.)

	Period 1	Period 2	Period 3
Number of events	2	4	3
Total observation time	59.7	93.5	43.6
rate	0.034	0.043	0.069

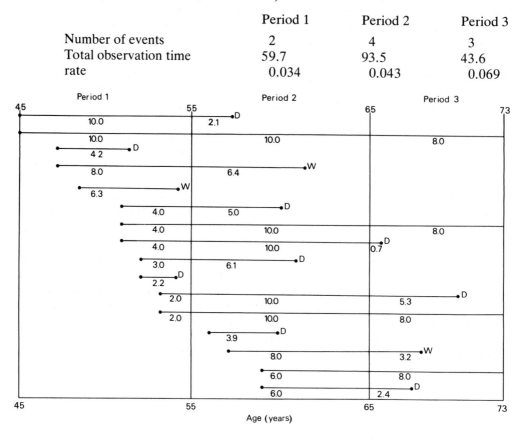

Figure 2.1 illustrates schematically the method of calculation of incidence rates for a study in which the time axis is divided into intervals: 45–54, 55–64 and 65–72 years inclusive. In this case time in fact means age. Subjects are arranged according to their age at entry to the study, which for simplicity has been taken to correspond to a birthday. The first subject, who entered the study on his 45th birthday and developed the disease (D) early in his 57th year, contributes 10 years of observation and no events to the 45–54 age period and 2.1 years and one event to the 55–64 age period. The third subject, who entered the study at age 47, was withdrawn (W) from observation during his 61st year (perhaps due to death from another disease) and hence contributes only to the denominator of the rate.

The least ambiguous definition of a rate results from making the time intervals short. This is because populations themselves change over time, through births, deaths or migrations, so that the shorter the time interval, the more stable the denominator used in the rate calculations. Also, the rate itself may be changing during the interval. If the change is rapid it makes sense to consider short intervals so that information about the magnitude of the change is not lost; but if the intervals are too short only a few events will be observed in each one. The instability of the denominator must be balanced against statistical fluctuations in the numerator when deciding upon an appropriate time interval for calculation of a reasonably stable rate.

If an infinite population were available, so that statistical stability was not in question, one could consider making the time intervals used for the rate calculation infinitesimal. As the length of each interval approaches zero, one obtains in the limit an *instantaneous rate* $\lambda(t)$ defined for each instant t of time. This concept has proved very useful in actuarial science, where, with the event in question being death, $\lambda(t)$ represents the *force of mortality*. In the literature of reliability analysis, where the event is failure of some system component, $\lambda(t)$ is referred to as the *hazard* rate. When the endpoint is diagnosis of disease in a previously disease-free individual, we can refer to the instantaneous incidence rate as the *force of morbidity*.

The method of calculation of the estimated rate will depend upon the type of data available for analysis. It is perhaps simplest in the case of a longitudinal follow-up study of a fixed population of individuals, for example: mice treated with some carcinogen who are followed from birth for appearance of tumours; cancer patients followed from time of initial treatment until relapse or death; or employees of a given industry or plant who are followed from date of employment until diagnosis of disease. A common method of estimating incidence or mortality rates with such data is to divide the time axis into J intervals having lengths l_j and midpoints t_j. Denote by n_j the number of subjects out of the original population of n_0 who are still under observation and at risk at t_j. Let d_j be the number of events (diagnoses or deaths) observed during the jth interval. Then the incidence at time t_j may be estimated by

$$\lambda(t_j) = \frac{d_j}{l_j \times n_j} \tag{2.1}$$

that is, by the number of events observed *per subject, per unit time* in the population at risk during the interval. Of course the denominator in equation (2.1) is only an approximation to the total observation time accumulated during the interval, which should be used if available.

Example: An example of the calculation of incidence rates from follow-up studies is given in Table 2.1 which lists the days until appearance of skin tumours for a group of 50 albino mice treated with benzo[a]-pyrene (Bogovski & Day, 1977). For the purpose of illustration, the duration of the study has been divided into four periods of unequal length: 0–179 days, 180–299 days, 300–419 days and 420–549 days. These are rather wider than is generally desirable because of limited data. Nineteen of the animals survived the entire 550 days without developing skin tumours, and are listed together at the bottom of the table. The contribution of each animal to the number of tumours and total observation time for each period are shown. Thus, the mouse developing tumour at 377 days contributes 0 tumours and 180 days observation to Period 1, 0 tumours and 120 days observation to Period 2, and 1 tumour and 78 days observation to Period 3.

Tumour incidence rates shown at the bottom of Table 2.1 were calculated in two ways. The first used the actual total observation time in each period, while the second used the approximation to this based on the number of animals alive at the midpoint (equation 2.1). Thus the incidence rate for Period 1 is 0 as no tumours were observed. For Period 2, 7 tumours were seen during 5 415 mouse-days of observation for a rate of $(7/5\,415) \times 1\,000 = 1.293$ per 1 000 mouse-days. The approximate rate is $[7/(47 \times 120)] \times 1\,000 = 1.241$ tumours per 1 000 mouse-days. The rate increases during the third period and then falls off.

Except in rare instances, cancer incidence rates are not obtained by continuous observation of all members of a specified population. Since the production of stable rates for cancers at most individual sites requires a population of at least one million subjects, the logistic and financial problems of attempting to maintain a constant sur-

Table 2.1 Calculation of incidence rate of skin tumours in mice treated with benzo[a]pyrene[a]

No. of animals if greater than one	Day of tumour appearance or day of death without tumour (*)	No. of animals at risk at start of each day	Contribution to rate calculation by period							
			Period 1 (0–179 days)		Period 2 (180–299 days)		Period 3 (300–419 days)		Period 4 (420–549 days)	
			No.[b]	Days[c]	No.	Days	No.	Days	No.	Days
	178*	50		179						
	187	49		180	1	8				
	194	48		180	1	15				
(3)	243	47		540	3	192				
	257	44		180	1	78				
	265*	43		180		86				
	297	42		180	1	118				
	297*	41		180		118				
(2)	327	40		360		240	2	56		
(2)	336	38		360		240	2	74		
	377	36		180		120	1	78		
	379	35		180		120	1	80		
	390*	34		180		120		91		
(2)	399	33		360		240	2	200		
	413	31		180		120	1	114		
	431*	30		180		120		120		12
	432*	29		180		120		120		13
(2)	444*	28		360		240		240		50
	482*	26		180		120		120		63
	495*	25		180		120		120		76
	515*	24		180		120		120		96
	522*	23		180		120		120		103
(2)	544*	22		360		240		240		250
	549	20		180		120		120	1	130
(19)	550*	19		3 420		2 280		2 280		2 470
Totals			0	8 999	7	5 415	9	4 293	1	3 263
No. animals at risk at midpoint				50		47		36		25
Length of interval (days)				180		120		120		130
Rate[d] (per 1 000 mouse-days)				0		1.293		2.096		0.306
Rate[e] (per 1 000 mouse-days)				0		1.241		2.083		0.308

[a] From Bogovski and Day (1977)
[b] No. of tumours observed during period
[c] Contribution to observation time during period
[d] Rate calculated using total observation time in denominator
[e] Rate calculated from equation (2.1)

veillance system are usually prohibitive. The information typically available to a cancer registry for calculation of rates includes the cancer cases, classified by sex, age and year of diagnosis, together with *estimates* of the population denominators obtained from the census department. How good the estimated denominators are depends on the frequency and accuracy of the census in each locality.

Example: Table 2.2 illustrates the calculation of the incidence of acute lymphatic leukaemia occurring among males aged 0–14 years in Birmingham, UK, during 1968–72 (Waterhouse et al., 1976). The numbers of cases (d_j), classified by age, and the number of persons (n_j) in each age group in 1971, the midyear of the observation period, are shown. In order to approximate the total person-years of observation, n_j is multiplied by the length of the observation period, namely five years. While this is adequate if the population size and age distribution remain fairly stable, this procedure would not suffice for times of rapid change in population structure. A better approximation to the denominator for the 1–4 year age group, for example, would be to sum up the numbers of 1–4 year-olds in the population at mid–1968 plus those at mid–1969 and so on to 1972. As is standard for cancer incidence reporting, the rates are expressed as numbers of cases per 100 000 person-years of observation. Table 2.3 presents the calculated rates for three additional sites and a larger number of age groups.

Table 2.2   Average annual incidence rates of acute lymphatic leukaemia for males aged 0–14 Birmingham region (1968–72)[a]

Age (years)	Interval length (l)	No. of cases (d)	Population (1971) (n)	No. of years of observation (1968–72)	Rate[b] (per 100 000 person-years)
0	1	2	45 300	5	0.88
1–4	4	47	182 400	5	5.15
5–9	5	30	228 300	5	2.63
10–14	5	13	202 500	5	1.28

[a] From Waterhouse et al. (1976)

[b] Rate $= \dfrac{d}{n \times 5} \times 100\ 000$

2.2 Age- and time-specific incidence rates

If the population has been under observation for several decades, cases of disease and person-years at risk may be classified usefully by both calendar year and age at diagnosis. The situation is illustrated in Figure 2.2. As each study subject is followed forward in time, he traces out a 45° trajectory in the age × time plane. Person-years of observation are allocated to the various age × time cells traversed by this path, and diagnoses of cancer or other events are assigned to the cell in which they occur. Thus, the upper left-hand cell in Figure 2.2, corresponding to ages 50–54 years and the 1940–44 time period, contains 1 death and 6 person-years of observation for a rate of $1/6 \times 100 = 16.7$ events per 100 person-years. An analysis of age-specific rates averaged over a certain calendar period would ignore the time axis in this diagram (as in Figure 2.1), while an analysis of time-specific rates would ignore the age classification. Typical practice is to consider five-year intervals of age and time, so as to be

Fig. 2.2 Schematic diagram of a follow-up study with joint classification by age and
year. (D = diagnosis of cancer; W = withdrawn, disease free.)

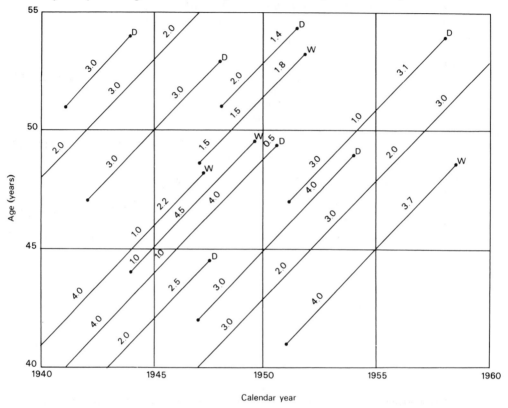

able to study the reasonably fine details of the variation in rates; but this will depend
on the amount of data available.

A *cross-sectional* analysis results from fixing the calendar periods and examining the
age-specific incidences. Alternatively, in a *birth-cohort* analysis, the same cancer
cases and person-years are classified according to year of birth and age. This is possible since any two of the three variables (1) year of birth, (2) age and (3) calendar
year determine the third. In Figure 2.2, for example, the 1890–99 birth cohort would
be represented by the diagonal column of 45° lines intersecting the vertical axis between 40 and 50 years of age in 1940.

Example: Figure 2.3 shows the age-specific incidence of breast cancer in Iceland during the three
calendar periods 1910–29, 1930–49 and 1950–72 (Bjarnasson et al., 1974). While the three curves show
a general increase in incidence with calendar time, they also have rather different shapes. There was a
decline in incidence with age after 40 years during the 1911–29 period, a fairly constant incidence during
1930–49 and an increase in incidence with age during the latest calendar period.

If the data are rearranged into birth cohorts, a more coherent picture emerges. Figure 2.4 shows
the age incidence curves for three cohorts of Icelandic women born in 1840–79, 1880–1909 and 1910–49,

Fig. 2.3 Age-specific incidence of breast cancer in Iceland for the three time periods 1911–29, 1930–49, 1950–72. From Bjarnasson et al. (1974).

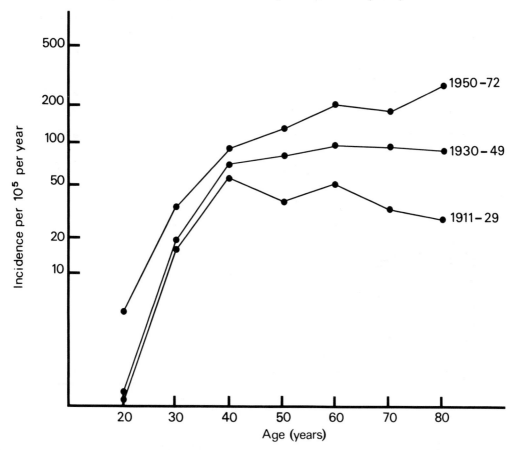

respectively. Because the period of case ascertainment was limited to the years 1910–72, the age ranges covered by these three curves are different. However, their shapes are much more similar than for the cross-sectional analysis of Figure 2.3; there is a fairly constant distance between the three curves on the semi-logarithmic plot. Since the ratios of the age-specific rates for different cohorts are therefore nearly constant across the age span, one may conveniently summarize the inter-cohort differences in terms of ratios of rates.

2.3 Cumulative incidence rates

While the importance of calculating age- or time-specific rates using reasonably short intervals cannot be overemphasized, it is nevertheless often convenient to have a single synoptic figure to summarize the experience of a population over a longer time span or age interval. For example, in comparing cancer incidence rates between different countries, it is advisable to make one comparison for children aged 0–14, another for

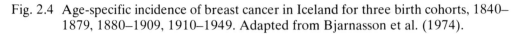

Fig. 2.4   Age-specific incidence of breast cancer in Iceland for three birth cohorts, 1840–
1879, 1880–1909, 1910–1949. Adapted from Bjarnasson et al. (1974).

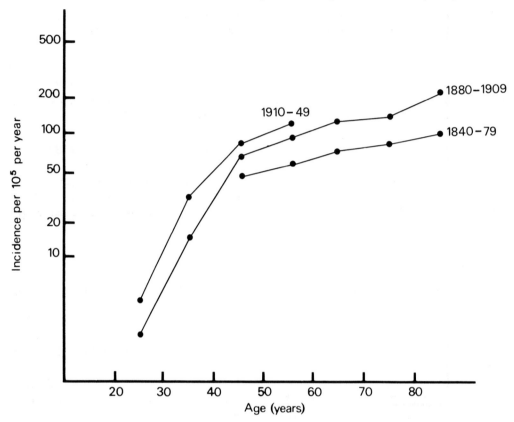

young adults aged 15–34, and a third for mature adults aged 35–69. Comparison of
rates among the elderly may be inadvisable due to problems of differential diagnosis
among many concurrent diseases.

The usual method of combining such age-specific rates for comparison across different
populations is that of direct standardization (Fleiss, 1973). The *directly standardized*
(adjusted) rate consists of a weighted average of the age-specific rates for each study
group, where the weights are chosen to be proportional to the age distribution of some
external standard population. Hypothetical standard populations have been constructed
for this purpose, which reflect approximately the age structure of World, European or
African populations (Waterhouse et al., 1976); however, the choice between them
often seems rather arbitrary.

An alternative and even simpler summary measure is the *cumulative incidence rate*,
obtained by summing up the annual age-specific incidences for each year in the
defined age interval (Day, 1976). Thus the cumulative incidence rate between 0 and t
years of age, inclusive, is

$$\Lambda(t) = \sum_{n=0}^{t} \lambda(n)$$

where the $\lambda(n)$ give the annual age-specific rates. In precise mathematical terms, the cumulative incidence rate between time 0 and t is expressed by an integral

$$\Lambda(t) = \int_{0}^{t} \lambda(u)du \tag{2.2}$$

where $\lambda(u)$ represents the instantaneous rate. The cumulative incidence between 15 and 34 years, inclusive, would be obtained from yearly rates as

$$\Lambda(34) - \Lambda(14) = \sum_{n=15}^{34} \lambda(n).$$

In practice, age-specific rates may not be available for each individual year of life but rather, as in the previous example, for periods of varying length such as 5 or 10 years. Then the age-specific rate $\lambda(t_i)$ for the ith period is multiplied by its length l_i before summing:

$$\hat{\Lambda}(t_j) = \sum_{i=1}^{j} l_i \lambda(t_i).$$

When calculating the cumulative rate from longitudinal data, we have, using (2.1),

$$\hat{\Lambda}(t_j) = \frac{d_1}{n_1} + \dots + \frac{d_j}{n_j}, \tag{2.3}$$

where the d_i are the deaths and the n_i are the numbers at risk at the midpoint of each time interval.

One reason for interest in the cumulative incidence rate is that it has a useful probabilistic interpretation. Let P(t) denote the net *risk*, or *probability*, that an individual will develop the disease of interest between time 0 and t. We assume for this definition that he remains at risk for the entire period, and is not subject to the *competing risks* of loss or death from other causes. The instantaneous incidence rate at time t then has a precise mathematical definition as the rate of increase in P(t), expressed relative to the proportion of the population still at risk (Elandt-Johnson, 1975). In symbols

$$\lambda(t) = \frac{1}{1 - P(t)} \times \frac{dP(t)}{dt}.$$

From this it follows that

$$1 - P(t) = \exp\{-\Lambda(t)\}, \tag{2.4}$$

or, using logarithms[1] rather than exponentials,

$$\Lambda(t) = -\log\{1 - P(t)\}.$$

---

[1] log denotes the natural logarithm, i.e., to the base e, which is used exclusively throughout the text.

These equations tell us that when the disease is rare or the time period short, so that the cumulative incidence or mortality is small, then the probability of disease occurrence is well approximated by the cumulative incidence

$$P(t) \approx \Lambda(t). \qquad (2.5)$$

Example: To illustrate the calculation of a cumulative rate, consider the age-specific rates of urinary tract tumours (excluding bladder) for Birmingham boys between 0 and 14 years of age (Table 2.3). These are almost entirely childhood tumours of the kidney, i.e., Wilms' tumours or nephroblastomas. The period cumulative rate is calculated as $(1 \times 2.2) + (4 \times 1.0) + (5 \times 0.4) + (5 \times 0.0) = 8.20$ per 100 000 population. Note that the first two age intervals have lengths of 1 and 4 years, respectively, while subsequent intervals are five years each. Table 2.4 shows the cumulative rates for all four tumours in Table 2.3 using three age periods: 0–14, 15–34 and 35–69. Also shown are the cumulative risks, i.e., probabilities, calculated from the rates according to equation (2.4). With the exception of lung cancer, which has a cumulative rate approaching 0.1 for the 35–69 age group, the rates and risks agree extremely well.

Table 2.3   Average annual incidence per 100 000 population by age group for Birmingham region, 1968–72 (males)[a]

Age (years)	Tumour site			
	Urinary tract (excl. bladder)	Stomach	Lung	Lymphatic leukaemia
0	2.2	0.0	0.0	0.9
1–4	1.0	0.0	0.0	5.2
5–9	0.4	0.0	0.0	2.6
10–14	0.0	0.0	0.0	1.3
15–19	0.1	0.0	0.1	1.0
20–24	0.2	0.1	0.7	0.4
25–29	0.1	0.7	0.8	0.3
30–34	0.5	0.7	3.3	0.6
35–39	1.2	4.3	9.1	0.6
40–44	4.0	7.6	25.6	0.9
45–49	4.6	18.1	71.4	1.5
50–54	7.1	31.3	137.4	1.6
55–59	11.8	64.1	257.5	4.3
60–64	16.7	100.6	404.9	7.0
65–69	21.7	150.2	520.3	11.2

[a] From Waterhouse et al. (1976)

Estimates of the cumulative rate are much more stable numerically than are estimates of the component age- or time-specific rates, since they are based on all the events which occur in the relevant time interval. This stability makes the cumulative rate the method of choice for reporting results of small studies. An estimate of $\Lambda(t)$ for such studies may be obtained by applying equation (2.3), with the chosen intervals so fine that each event occupies its own separate interval. In other words, we simply sum up, for each event occurring before or at time t, the reciprocal of the number of subjects remaining at risk just prior to its occurrence.

Table 2.4 Cumulative rates and risks, in percent, of developing cancer between the indicated ages: calculated from Table 2.3

Age period (years)		Tumour site			
		Urinary tract (excl. bladder)	Stomach	Lung	Acute lymphatic leukaemia
0–14	Rate	0.0082	0.0	0.0	0.0412
	Risk	0.0082	0.0	0.0	0.0412
15–34	Rate	0.0045	0.0075	0.0245	0.0115
	Risk	0.0045	0.0075	0.0245	0.0115
35–69	Rate	0.3355	1.8810	7.1310	0.1355
	Risk	0.3349	1.8634	6.8827	0.1355

Example: Consider the data on murine skin tumours shown in Table 2.1. Since 49 animals remain at risk at the time of appearance of the first tumour, t = 187 days, the cumulative rate is estimated as $\hat{\Lambda}(187) = 1/49 = 0.020$. The estimate at t = 243 days is given by

$$\hat{\Lambda}(243) = \frac{1}{49} + \frac{1}{48} + \frac{1}{47} + \frac{1}{46} + \frac{1}{45} = 0.106.$$

Note that the contribution from the three tumours occurring at 243 days, when 47 animals remain at risk, is given by $(1/47) + (1/46) + (1/45)$ rather than $(3/47)$. This is consistent with the idea that the three tumours in fact occur at slightly different times, which are nevertheless too close together to be distinguished by the recording system.

Only 20 animals remain at risk at the time of the last observed tumour, 549 days, the others having already died or developed tumours. Hence this event contributes $1/20 = 0.05$ to the cumulative rate, bringing the total to

$$\frac{1}{49} + \frac{1}{48} + \frac{1}{47} + \frac{1}{46} + \frac{1}{45} + \dots + \frac{1}{20} = 0.457.$$

The risk of developing a skin tumour in the first 550 days is thus estimated to be $1 - \exp(-0.457) = 0.367$ for mice in this experiment who survive the entire study period. Figure 2.5 shows the cumulative incidence rate plotted as a function of days to tumour appearance.

In summary, three closely related measures are available for expressing the occurrence of disease in a population: the instantaneous incidence rate defined at each point in time; the cumulative incidence rate defined over an interval of time; and the probability or risk of disease, also defined over an interval of time. Our next task is to consider how exposure of the population to various risk factors may affect these same rates and risks of disease occurrence.

2.4 Models of disease association

The simplest types of risk factors are the *binary* or "all or none" variety, as exemplified by the presence or absence of a particular genetic marker. Environmental variables are usually more difficult to quantify since individual histories vary widely with respect to the onset, duration and intensity of exposure, and whether it was continuous or intermittent. Nevertheless it is often possible to make crude classifications into an

Fig. 2.5 Cumulative incidence of skin tumours in mice after treatment with benzo[α]-
pyrene. From Bogovski and Day (1977).

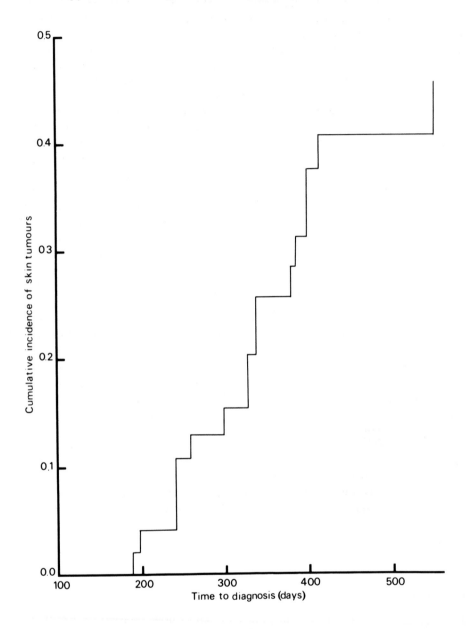

exposed *versus* a non-exposed group, for example by comparing confirmed cigarette smokers with non-smokers, or lifelong urban with lifelong rural residents. In order to introduce the concept of risk factor/disease association, we suppose here that the population has been divided into two such subgroups, one exposed to the risk factor in question and the other not exposed.

As shown in the earlier examples, incidence rates may vary widely within the population according to such factors as age, sex and calendar year of observation. Thus whatever measure is used to compare incidence rates in the exposed *versus* non-exposed subgroups, this too is likely to vary by age, sex and time. What is clearly desired in this situation is a measure of association which is as stable as possible over the various subdivisions of the population; the more nearly constant it is, the greater is the justification for expressing the effect of exposure in a single summary number; the more it varies, the greater is the necessity to describe how the *effect* of exposure is *modified* by demographic or other relevant factors on which information is available.

Suppose that the population has been divided into I strata on the basis of age, sex, calendar period of observation, or combinations of these and other features. Denote by λ_{1i} the incidence rate of disease in the ith stratum for the exposed subgroup and by λ_{0i} the rate for the non-exposed subgroup in that stratum. The first measure of association we consider is the *excess risk* of disease, defined as the *difference* between the stratum-specific incidences

$$b_i = \lambda_{1i} - \lambda_{0i}. \tag{2.6}$$

Since the measure is defined in terms of incidence rates, rather than risks, it would perhaps be more accurate to refer to it as the excess rate of disease. We follow convention by allowing the distinction between risks and rates to be blurred somewhat in discussing measures of association, except when it is critical to the point in question.

The intuitive idea underlying this approach is that cases contributing to the "natural" or background disease incidence rate in the ith stratum are due to the presence of general factors which operate on exposed and non-exposed individuals alike. Cases caused by exposure to the particular agent under investigation are represented in the excess risk b_i (Rothman, 1976). If these two causes of disease, the general and the specific, were in some sense operating independently of each other, one might expect the number of excess cases of disease occurring per person-year of observation to reflect only the level of exposure and to be unrelated to the underlying natural risk. Thus the excess risk would be relatively constant from stratum to stratum, apart from random statistical fluctuations.

The idea of a constant excess risk due to the particular exposure may be formally expressed by hypothesizing an *additive model* for the two dimensional sets of rates. With b representing the *additive effect* of exposure, the model states

$$\lambda_{1i} = \lambda_{0i} + b. \tag{2.7}$$

Unfortunately the concept of independence leading to this model is rather simplistic and breaks down when one considers plausible mechanisms for the disease process (Koopman, 1977). Suppose, for example, that a disease was caused in infancy or early childhood but took many years to develop. If the age distribution of the cases produced by the specific exposure were the same as that of the spontaneous cases, the differences in age-specific rates would be greater for the ages in which the spontaneous incidence was higher, even if the general and specific exposures had operated independently of each other early on. Nonetheless (2.7) may be postulated *ad hoc,* and if it appears to correspond reasonably well to the data, the estimate of b derived from the fitted model may be used as an overall measure of the effect of exposure.

In technical statistical terms, this model states that there are no *interactions* between the additive effects of exposure and strata on incidence rates; exposure to the risk factor has the same effect on disease incidence rates in each of the population strata. More generally, the absence of interactions between two factors, A and B, means that the effects of Factor B on outcome do not depend on the levels of Factor A. It is important to recognize, however, that what we mean by the effect of a factor depends very much on the scale of measurement. Since the rates are expressed on a simple arithmetic scale in (2.7), we speak of additive effects. As the following example shows, whether or not there are statistical interactions in the data may depend on the scale on which the outcome or response variable is measured.

Fig. 2.6 Schematic illustration of concept of statistical interaction.

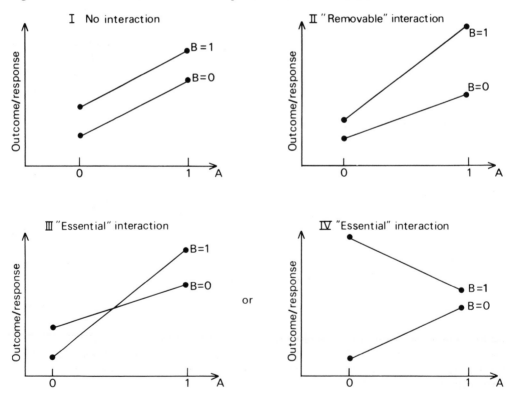

Example: Figure 2.6 illustrates the concept of interaction schematically. Conditions for no interaction hold when the two response curves are parallel (Panel I). Note that the definition of interaction is completely symmetric; the diagram shows also that the effect of Factor A is independent of the level of Factor B.

The non-parallel response curves shown in Panel II of the figure indicate that Factor B has a greater effect on outcome at level 1 of Factor A than it does at level 0. It is apparent, however, that if the outcome variable were expressed on a different scale, for example a logarithmic or square root scale which tended to bring together the more extreme outcomes, the interaction could be made to disappear. In this sense we may speak of interactions which are "removable" by an appropriate choice of scale.

The situation in Panels III and IV, characterized by the response curves either crossing over or having slopes of different signs, allows for no such remedy. In Panel III the effect of Factor B is to increase the response at one level of Factor A, and to decrease it at another, while in Panel IV it is the sign of the A effect which changes with B. In the present context this would mean that exposure to the risk factor increased the rate of disease for one part of the population and decreased it for another. No change of the outcome scale could alter this essential difference.

While the excess risk is a useful measure in certain contexts, the bulk of this monograph deals with another measure of association, for reasons which will be clarified below. This is the *relative risk* of disease, defined as the *ratio* of the stratum-specific incidences:

$$r_i = \frac{\lambda_{1i}}{\lambda_{0i}} \, .$$

The assumed effect of exposure is to *multiply* the background rate λ_{0i} by the quantity r_i. Absence of interactions here leads to a *multiplicative model* for the rates such that, within the limits of statistical error, these may be expressed as the product of two terms, one representing the underlying natural disease incidence in the stratum and the other representing the relative risk r. More precisely, the model states

$$\lambda_{1i} = \exp(\beta)\lambda_{0i} \qquad (2.8)$$

where $\beta = \log(r)$. Alternatively, if the incidence rates are expressed on a logarithmic scale, it takes the form

$$\log \lambda_{1i} = \log \lambda_{0i} + \beta.$$

Comparing this with equation (2.7) it is evident that they have precisely the same structure, except for the choice of scale for the outcome measure (incidence rate). In other words, the multiplicative model (2.8) is identical to an additive model in log rates. Such models are called *log-linear*.

While excess and relative risk are defined here in terms of differences and ratios of stratum-specific incidence rates, analogous measures for the comparison of cumulative rates and risks may be deduced directly from equations (2.2) and (2.4). Suppose, for example, that the two sets of incidence rates have a (constant) difference of 10 cases per 100 000 person-years observation for each year of a particular 15-year time period. Then the difference between the cumulative rates over this same period will be $10 \times 15 = 150$ cases per 100 000 population. On the other hand, if the two sets of rates have a (constant) ratio of 5 for each year, the ratio of the cumulative rates will also equal 5.

Because there is an exponential term in equation (2.4), the derived relationships between the probabilities, or risks, for this same time period are not so simple. Let $P_0(t)$ denote the net probability that a non-exposed person develops the disease during the time period from 0 to t years, and let $P_1(t)$ denote the analogous quantity for the exposed population. If the corresponding incidence rates satisfy the multiplicative equation $\lambda_1(u) = r\lambda_0(u)$ for all u between 0 and t, then

$$P_1(t) = 1 - \{1 - P_0(t)\}^r.$$

This relationship is well approximated by that for the cumulative rates

$$P_1(t) \approx rP_0(t),$$

providing the disease is sufficiently rare, or the time interval sufficiently short, so that both risks and rates remain small. In general, the ratio of disease risks is slightly less extreme, i.e., closer to unity, than is the ratio of the corresponding rates.

We have now introduced the two principal routes by which one may approach the statistical analysis of cancer incidence data: the additive model, where the fundamental measure of association is the excess risk, and the multiplicative model, where the effect of exposure is expressed in relative terms. In order to arrive at a choice between these two, or indeed to decide upon any particular statistical model, several considerations are relevant. From a purely empirical viewpoint, the most important properties of a model are simplicity and goodness of fit to the observed data. The aim is to be able to describe the main features of the data as succinctly as possible. Clarity is enhanced by avoiding models with a large number of parameters which must be estimated from the data. If, in one type of model many interaction terms (see § 6.1) are required to fit the data adequately, whereas with another only a few are required, the latter would generally be preferred.

The empirical properties of a model are not the only criteria. We also need to consider how the results of an analysis are to be interpreted and the meaning that will be attached to the estimated parameters. Excess and relative risks inform us about two quite different aspects of the association between risk factor and disease. Since relative risks for lung cancer among smokers *versus* non-smokers are generally at least five times those for coronary heart disease, one might be inclined to say that the lung cancer-smoking association is stronger, but this ignores the fact that the differences in rates are generally greater for heart disease. From a public health viewpoint the impact of smoking on mortality from heart disease may be more severe than its effect on lung cancer death rates. This fact has led some authors to advocate exclusive use of the additive measure (Berkson, 1958). Rothman (1976), as noted earlier, has argued that it is the most natural one for measuring interaction.

In spite of these considerations, the relative risk has become the most frequently used measure for associating exposure with disease occurrence in cancer epidemiology, both because of its empirical behaviour and because of several logical properties it possesses. Empirically it provides a summary measure which often requires little qualification in terms of the population to which it refers. Logically it facilitates the evaluation of the extent to which an observed association is causal. The next two sections explore these important properties of the relative risk in some detail. We merely point out here that, once having obtained an estimate of the relative risk, it is certainly possible to interpret that estimate in terms of excess risk provided one knows the disease incidence rates for unexposed individuals in the population to which it refers. For example, if the baseline disease incidence is 20 cases per year per 100 000 population and the relative risk is 9, this implies that the difference in rates between the exposed and unexposed is $(9-1) \times 20 = 160$ cases per 100 000. In our opinion, the advantages of using the relative measure in the analysis far outweigh the disadvantage of having to perform this final step to acquire a measure of additive effect, if in fact that is what is wanted. No measure of association should be viewed blindly, but instead each should be interpreted using whatever information exists about the actual magnitude of the rates.

2.5 Empirical behaviour of the relative risk

Several examples from the literature of cancer epidemiology will illustrate that the relative risk provides a stable measure of association in a wide variety of human populations. When there are differences in the (multiplicative) effect of exposure for different populations, it is often true that the levels of exposure are not the same, or that there are definite biological reasons for the discrepancies in the response to the same exposure.

Temporal variation in age-specific incidence

Table 2.5 shows the age-specific incidence rates for breast cancer in Iceland for two of the birth cohorts represented in Figure 2.4. The ratios of these rates for the two cohorts are remarkably stable in the range 1.66–1.81, whereas the differences between them triple over the 50-year age span. Thus, while one can describe the relationship between birth cohort and incidence by saying that the age-specific rates for the later cohort are roughly 1.7 times those for the earlier one, no such simple summary is possible using the excess risk as a measure of association. Note that the ratio of the cumulative rates summarizes that for the age-specific ones, and that the cumulative risk ratio is only slightly less than the rate ratio despite the 50-year age span.

Table 2.5 Average annual incidence rates for breast cancer in Iceland, 1910–72, per 100 000 population[a]

Year of birth	Age (years) 40–49	50–59	60–69	70–79	80–89	Cumulative (ages 40–89) Rate (%)	Risk (%)
1880–1909	65.90	95.10	129.50	140.10	227.90	6.59	6.38
1840–1879	38.70	53.80	71.70	81.10	136.90	3.82	3.75
Difference	27.20	41.30	57.80	59.00	91.00	2.77	2.63
Ratio	1.70	1.78	1.81	1.73	1.66	1.73	1.70

[a] From Bjarnasson et al. (1974)

Geographical variation in age-specific incidence

Figure 2.7 gives a plot of incidence rates against age for stomach cancer occurring in males in three countries (Waterhouse et al., 1976). In calculating these rates, six 5-year age intervals were used: 35–39, 40–44, 45–49, 50–54, 55–59, 60–64. Since a logarithmic scale is used for both axes, the plotted points appear to lie roughly on three parallel straight lines, each with a slope of about 5 or 6. This quantitative relationship, which is common for many epithelial tumours, may be expressed symbolically as follows. Denote by $\lambda_i(t)$ the average annual incidence rate for the ith area at age t, where t is taken to be the midpoint of the respective age interval: t = 37.5, 42.5, etc. The fact that the log-log plots are parallel and linear means that approximately

$$\log \lambda_i(t) = \alpha + \beta_i + \gamma \log(t), \tag{2.9}$$

where we arbitrarily set $\beta_1 = 0$, thus using country 1 as a baseline for comparison. Raising each side of this equation to the power e, the relationship may also be expressed as

$$\lambda_i(t) = e^\alpha r_i t^\gamma, \tag{2.10}$$

where $r_i = \exp(\beta_i)$.

The values of the parameters in (2.9) which give the best "fit" to the observed data points, using a statistical technique known as 'weighted least squares regression' (Mosteller & Tukey, 1977, p. 346), are $\alpha = -18.79$, $\beta_1 = 0$, $\beta_2 = 0.67$, $\beta_3 = 1.99$ and $\gamma = 5.49$. Although the deviations of the plotted points about the fitted regression lines are slightly larger than would be expected from purely random fluctuations, the equations well describe the important features of the data.

The parameters r $(= \exp \beta)$ describe the relative positions of the age-incidence curves for the three countries. By considering ratios of incidence rates, the relative risk of stomach cancer in males in Japan *versus* those in Connecticut is

$$\frac{\lambda_3(t)}{\lambda_1(t)} = \frac{r_3 t^\gamma}{r_1 t^\gamma} = \exp(\beta_3 - \beta_1) = 7.3$$

while the relative risk in Birmingham *versus* that in Connecticut is

$$\exp(\beta_2 - \beta_1) = 1.9.$$

The most important feature of the above relationships is that, to the extent that equations (2.9) or (2.10) hold, the relative risks between different areas *do not vary with age*. The chance that a Birmingham male of a given age contract stomach cancer during the next year is roughly twice that of his New England counterpart, and the same applies whether he is 45, 55 or 65 years old. On the other hand, the absolute differences in the age-specific rates, i.e., $\lambda_2(t) - \lambda_1(t)$, vary markedly with age. The percentage increase in incidence associated with each 10% increase in age is related to the parameter γ through the equation

$$\left(\frac{\lambda_i(1.1t)}{\lambda_i(t)} - 1\right) \times 100\% = \left((1.1)^\gamma - 1\right) \times 100\% = \left((1.1)^{5.49} - 1\right) \times 100\% = 69\%,$$

and varies neither with age nor with area.

Fig. 2.7 Age-specific incidence of stomach cancer in three populations. From Water-house et al. (1976). Number of cases shown by each point. (▲ = Japan (Miyagi); × = UK (Birmingham); ● = US (Connecticut).)

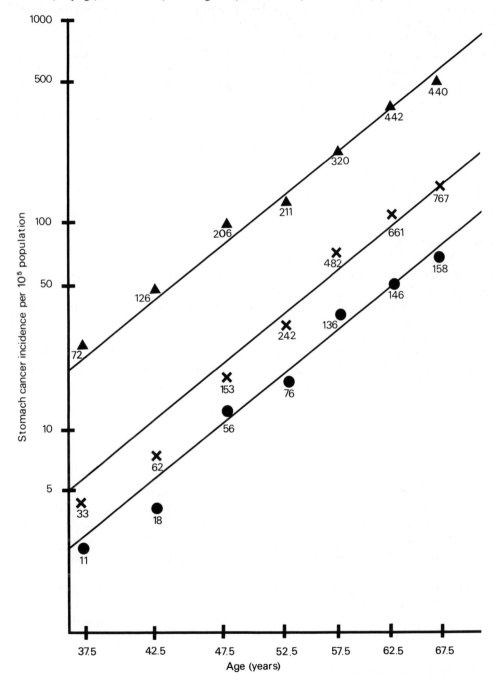

As shown by Cook, Doll & Fellingham (1969), most epithelial tumours have age-incidence curves of a similar shape to that of gastric cancer, differing between populations only by a proportionality constant, i.e., relative risk. This is a good technical reason for choosing the ratio as a measure of association, since it permits the relationship between each pair of age-incidence curves to be quite accurately summarized in a single number.

The two epithelial tumours which deviate most markedly from this pattern are those of the lung and the breast. For breast cancer we have already shown how irregularities in the cross-sectional age curves reflect a changing incidence by year of birth, and that a basic regular behaviour is seen when the data are considered on a cohort basis (Figures 2.3 and 2.4; Bjarnasson et al., 1974). A similar phenomenon has been noted for lung cancer, where a large part of the inter-cohort differences are presumably due to increasing exposure to tobacco and other exogenous agents (Doll, 1971).

Risk of cancer following irradiation

Radiation induces tumours at a wide range of sites, and its carcinogenic effects have been studied in a variety of population groups, including the atomic bomb survivors in Japan and people treated by irradiation for various conditions. As discussed in the previous example, the "natural" incidence of most cancers varies widely with age at diagnosis. Here we examine how the carcinogenic effect of radiation varies according to *age at exposure,* i.e., the age of the individual when irradiated.

In the mid 1950s, Court Brown and Doll (1965) identified over 14 000 individuals who had been treated by irradiation for ankylosing spondylitis between 1935 and 1954 in the United Kingdom. The latest report analyses the mortality of this group up to 1 June 1970 (Smith, 1979). In Figure 2.8 we show the change with age at exposure of the relative risk and of the absolute risks for leukaemia and for other heavily irradiated sites. For both types of malignancy, the relative risk varies little with age at exposure, whereas the absolute risk increases rapidly as age at treatment increases. The effect of the radiation is thus to multiply the incidence which would be expected among people in the general population of the same age by a factor of roughly 4.8 for leukaemia and 1.5 for other heavily irradiated sites. As a function of *time since exposure,* the relative risk for leukaemia appears to reach a peak after 3–5 years and then decline to zero, whereas the effect on heavily irradiated sites may persist for 20 or more years after exposure.

An analysis of the mortality among atomic bomb survivors for the period 1950–74 (Beebe, Kato & Land, 1977) demonstrates a similar uniformity of relative risk with age at exposure, and the corresponding sharp increase in absolute risk. There is, however, one major exception to the uniformity of the relative risk. For those aged less than ten years at exposure the relative risks are considerably higher than in subsequent age groups, which presumably indicates greater susceptibility among young children.

Studies of breast cancer induced by radiation include those of atomic bomb survivors (MacGregor et al., 1977) and of women treated by irradiation for tuberculosis (Boice & Monson, 1977) or a range of benign breast conditions (Shore et al., 1977). The relative risk appears higher among women exposed at younger ages and is particularly high among those exposed in the two years preceding menarche or during their first

Fig. 2.8 Ratio of observed to expected numbers of deaths and excess death rates from leukaemia and cancers of heavily irradiated sites according to age at first treatment with X-rays for ankylosing spondylitis. From Smith (1979).

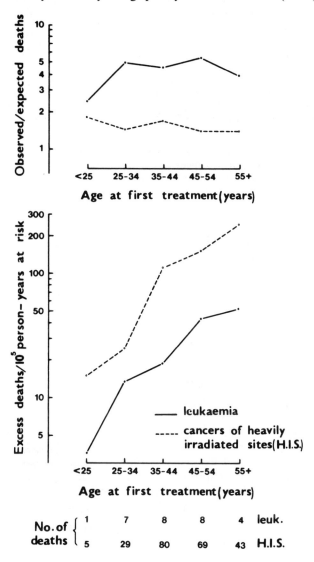

pregnancy (Boice & Stone, 1979). The proliferation of breast tissue during menarche or first pregnancy would suggest an increased susceptibility to carcinogenic hazards.

The relative risk thus seems to provide a fairly uniform measure of the carcinogenic effect of radiation as a function of age at exposure, except where a difference in the relative risk probably reflects differences in tissue susceptibility.

Lung cancer and cigarette smoking

Smoking and irradiation are perhaps the most extensively studied of all carcinogenic exposures. Cigarette smoking is related to tumours at a number of sites including the respiratory tract, the oral cavity and oesophagus, and the bladder and pancreas. The relationship with cancer of the lung has been the most extensively studied, and the results of several large prospective studies have quantified the association in some detail.

Table 2.6 presents the change in incidence with age among continuing smokers and among non-smokers, as given by Doll (1971), the data for consecutive five-year age groups being averaged. The excess risk increases sharply with age, whereas the relative risk, although increasing, changes only slowly.

Table 2.6 Incidence of bronchial carcinoma among non-smokers and continuing smokers, per 100 000 person-years[a]

Age at risk (years)	Non-smokers	Smokers	Relative risk	Excess risk
35–44	2.8	5.2	1.9	2.4
45–54	5.8	67.0	11.6	61.2
55–64	13.9	221.8	16.0	207.9
65–74	25.6	482.2	18.8	456.6
75–84	49.4	860.5[b]	17.4	811.1

[a] From Doll (1971)
[b] Likely to be unreliable due to under-reporting

A more appropriate way of looking at the risk of lung cancer associated with cigarette smoking, however, is in terms of duration of smoking rather than simply age. Figure 2.9 presents the incidence of lung cancer for non-smokers as a function of age, and for smokers as a function of both age and duration of smoking. The increase in relative risk with age is clear, but more striking is the parallellism of the lines for non-smokers and for smokers when incidence is related to duration of smoking. Since for non-smokers we might regard exposure as lifelong, one could consider that the two time scales both refer to duration of exposure. The figure thus displays a constant relative difference in incidence when the more relevant time scales are used.

Breast cancer and age at first birth

The large international study by MacMahon and associates (MacMahon et al., 1970) showed that age at first birth is the major feature of a woman's reproductive life which influences risk for breast cancer. Table 2.7, taken from their work, shows the uniformity of the relationship between risk and age at first birth over all centres in a collaborative study. Furthermore (not shown in the table), these relative risks change little with age at diagnosis. The populations included in the study showed a wide range of incidence levels, and had age-incidence curves of quite different shapes. The ability of the

Fig. 2.9 Age-specific mortality rates from lung cancer for smokers and non-smokers. From Doll (1971). (● —— ● = cigarette smokers by duration of smoking; ○——○ = cigarette smokers by age; ×——× = non-smokers by age.)

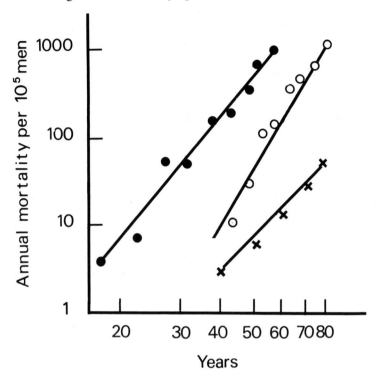

Table 2.7 Estimates of relative risk of breast cancer, by age at first birth[a, b]

Centre	Nulliparous	Parous, age at first birth (years):				
		<20	20–24	25–29	30–34	35+
Boston	100	32	55	76	90	117
Glamorgan	100	38	49	67	73	124
Athens	100	51	71	79	106	127
Slovenia	100	81	74	94	112	118
Sao Paulo	100	49	65	94	84	175
Taipei	100	54	45	37	89	106
Tokyo	100	26	49	78	100	138
All centres	100	50	60	78	94	122

[a] From MacMahon et al. (1970)
[b] Estimated risk relative to a risk of 100 for the nulliparous; adjusted for age at diagnosis

relative risk to summarize the relationships among so wide an array of incidence patterns indicates that, at least in this situation, it reflects a fundamental feature of the disease. The absolute differences in age-specific incidence rates by age at first birth vary widely between the populations.

The failure of previous work on the influence of reproductive factors on risk of breast cancer to identify the basic importance of age at first birth was probably due to inappropriate measures of disease association. As MacMahon et al. concluded, "Previous workers seem not to have considered the differences of sufficient importance to warrant detailed exploration. An apparent lack of interest in the relationship may have resulted from failure to realize the magnitude of the differences in relative risk that underlie it. This lack of recognition of the strength of the relationship can be attributed primarily to analyses using summary statistics such as means ...".

2.6 Effects of combined exposures

The previous examples have illustrated the extent to which the relative risk remains constant over different age strata, or among different population groups. We shall now examine the extent to which the relative risk associated with one risk factor varies with changing exposure to a second risk factor, and we shall see that in this situation one also frequently observes relative uniformity. Consider the simplest situation, with two dichotomous variables A and B. There are four incidence rates, denoted λ_{AB}, λ_A, λ_B and λ_0 according to whether an individual is exposed to both, one or neither of the factors. The three relative risks, expressed using λ_0 as the baseline incidence, are $r_{AB} = \lambda_{AB}/\lambda_0$, $r_A = \lambda_A/\lambda_0$ and $r_B = \lambda_B/\lambda_0$, respectively.

Among those exposed to B, the relative increase in risk incurred by also being exposed to A is given by $\lambda_{AB}/\lambda_B = r_{AB}/r_B$. If the relative risk associated with exposure to A is the same, whether or not there is exposure to B, we say that the effects of the two factors are independent or do not interact (Figure 2.6). In this case $r_{AB}/r_B = r_A$, from which $r_{AB} = r_A r_B$. Thus, the independence of relative risks for two or more exposures implies a multiplicative combination for the joint effect. But, if the two risk factors each have additive rather than multiplicative effects on incidence, then similar calculations show that the relative risk for the joint exposure under the no interaction assumption is $r_{AB} = r_A + r_B - 1$.

The uniformity of relative risk for the exposures considered in the earlier examples can also be interpreted as a multiplicative combination of effects. Since the spontaneous incidence of leukaemia increases with age and radiation affects the spontaneous incidence proportionately, the joint effect is simply the product of the spontaneous rate and the radiation risk. Women in the United States have an incidence of breast cancer about six times higher than that of Japanese women. The joint action of the factor responsible for the elevated risk among United States women, whatever it may be, and age at first birth is clearly multiplicative.

Example: As an example of the joint effects of two risk factors, Table 2.8 summarizes results from a case-control study of oral cancer as related to alcohol and tobacco consumption (Rothman & Keller, 1972). The 483 cases and 492 controls were cross-classified according to four levels of consumption of each risk factor and also two age categories, under and over 60 years of age. Using methods which will be introduced in Chapter 4, age-adjusted relative risks of oral cancer were calculated for each of the 16

Table 2.8 Joint effect of alcohol and tobacco consumption on risk for oral cancer[a,b]

Alcohol (oz/day)	Tobacco (cigarette equiv./day)				Alcohol risk (adjusted for tobacco)
	0	1–19	20–39	40+	
0	1.0	1.6	1.6	3.4	1.0
0.1–0.3	1.7	1.9	3.3	3.4	1.8
0.4–1.5	1.9	4.9	4.9	8.2	2.9
1.6+	2.3	4.8	10.0	15.6	4.2
Tobacco risk (adjusted for alcohol)	1.0	1.4	2.4	4.2	

[a] From Rothman and Keller (1972)
[b] Relative risks adjusted for age at diagnosis

alcohol/tobacco categories shown. These may be denoted r_{ij}, where i refers to tobacco level and j to alcohol level. Since the category of lowest exposure to both factors is used as a baseline for comparison with other groups, $r_{11} = 1.0$.

The multiplicative hypothesis in this framework takes the form

$$r_{ij} = r_{i1}r_{1j}, \qquad (2.11)$$

whereby the relative risk for a given category of tobacco/alcohol consumption is obtained as the product of a relative risk for the tobacco level times that for the alcohol level. Again, this expresses the idea that relative risks for different tobacco levels do not vary according to alcohol consumption, and vice versa. Of course the r_{ij} presented in Table 2.8 do not satisfy this requirement exactly. Procedures are presented in Chapter 6 for finding estimates of r_{i1} and r_{1j} which yield the *best fit* to the observed data under the model. These estimates, shown in the margins of Table 2.8, were used to calculate the expected number of cases in Table 2.9. Comparison of the observed numbers of cases with those expected under the model shows that agreement between the model and the data is about as good as can be expected, given the errors inherent in random sampling.

Table 2.9 Observed number of cases and controls by smoking and drinking category, and the number expected under the multiplicative model[a]

Alcohol (oz/day)	Tobacco. (cigarette equiv./day)											
	0			1–19			20–39			40+		
	Cases	Controls	Expected cases	Cases	Controls	Expected cases	Cases	Controls	Expected cases	Cases	Controls	Expected cases
0	10	38	7.67	11	26	9.91	13	36	17.54	9	8	7.87
0.1–0.3	7	27	7.36	16	35	16.34	50	60	47.08	16	19	18.21
0.4–1.5	4	12	5.14	18	16	15.64	60	49	61.37	27	14	26.86
1.6+	5	8	5.82	21	20	24.11	125	52	122.00	91	27	90.06

[a] From Rothman and Keller (1972)

The multiplicative effects of alcohol and tobacco have been demonstrated by Wynder and Bross (1961) for cancer of the oesophagus, and for cancer of the mouth in an earlier publication (Wynder, Bross & Feldman, 1957).

Example: A second example concerns the joint effect of asbestos exposure and cigarette smoking on risk for bronchogenic carcinoma. Selikoff and Hammond (1978) followed 17 800 asbestos insulation workers prospectively from 1 January 1967 to 1 January 1977. Smoking histories were obtained for the majority of the cohort. Risk estimates for smoking obtained from the American Cancer Society prospective study (Hammond, 1966) were applied to generate expected numbers of deaths from lung cancer among the insulation workers. Table 2.10 gives the observed and expected numbers of lung cancer deaths among continuing smokers and among non-smokers.

Since the asbestos-related risks in the two groups are about equal, it follows that the risk for cigarette smoking asbestos insulation workers, compared with non-smokers not exposed to asbestos, is the product of their smoking risk, from which the expected numbers were derived, and their asbestos risk. Similar results have been reported by Berry, Newhouse and Turok (1972) and reviewed by Saracci (1977).

Table 2.10 The joint effect of cigarette smoking and asbestos exposure on risk for lung cancer. Lung cancer mortality among 17 800 asbestos insulation workers, 1967–77[a]

Lung cancer deaths			
	Observed	Expected[b]	Relative risk
Non-smokers	8	1.82	4.40
Smokers	228	39.7	5.74

[a] From Hammond, Selikoff and Seidman (1979)
[b] Based on age-specific general population rates for men smoking equivalent numbers of cigarettes

The epidemiology of cancer thus provides empirical reasons for choosing relative risk as the natural measure of association of cancer and exposure. On many occasions similar exposures lead to similar relative risks, almost independent of the population group exposed. When appreciable differences in relative risk are observed, these often can be expected to reflect real differences in susceptibility or exposure which may not be immediately apparent. As an interesting contrast, Table 2.11 gives data for ischaemic heart disease (Doll & Peto, 1976), where the biological processes are presumably different. The relative risks change markedly with age, and a different measure of association might be more appropriate.

Table 2.11 Smoking and risk for ischaemic heart disease, by age[a]

Age (years)	Annual death rate per 100 000 men[b] (no. of deaths in parentheses)											
	Non-smokers			Current smokers, smoking cigarettes only (no./day)								
			RR	1–14		RR	15–24		RR	25+		RR
< 45	7	(3)	1.0	46	(12)	6.6	16	(22)	2.3	104	(18)	14.9
45–54	118	(32)	1.0	220	(38)	1.9	368	(90)	3.1	383	(69)	3.3
55–64	531	(79)	1.0	742	(91)	1.4	819	(123)	1.5	1 025	(125)	1.9
< 65	166	(114)	1.0	278	(141)	1.7	358	(235)	2.2	427	(212)	2.6
65–74	1 190	(83)	1.0	1 866	(134)	1.6	1 511	(101)	1.3	1 731	(81)	1.5
75+	2 432	(92)	1.0	2 719	(113)	1.1	2 466	(50)	1.0	3 247	(27)	1.3

[a] From Doll and Peto (1976)
[b] Indirectly standardized for age to make the four entries in any one line comparable

2.7 Logical properties of the relative risk

In addition to an empirical justification for its use, the relative risk has some properties of a logical nature which are useful for appraising the extent to which the observed association may be explained by the presence of another agent, or may be specific to a particular disease entity. Cornfield et al. (1959) gave a precise statement and formal proof of these properties (see also § 2.9).

> "If an agent, A, with no causal effect upon the risk of disease, nevertheless, because of a positive correlation with some other causal agent, B, shows an apparent risk, r, for those exposed to A, relative to those not so exposed, then the prevalence of B, among those exposed to A, relative to the prevalence among those not so exposed, must be greater than r."

Thus, in order that the smoking-lung cancer association be explained by a tendency for people with a cancer-causing genotype to smoke, the putative genetic trait must carry a risk of at least ninefold in addition to being at least nine times more prevalent among smokers. Spurious associations due to confounding are always weaker than the underlying genuine associations when strength of association is measured by relative risk.

Cornfield et al. also note that the relative measure is a sensitive indicator of the *specificity* of the association with a particular disease entity:

> "If a causal agent A increases the risk for disease I and has no effect on the risk for disease II, then the relative risk of developing disease I, alone, is greater than the relative risk of developing disease I and II combined, while the absolute measure is unaffected."

Thus, if the agent in question increases the risk of a certain histological type of cancer at a given site (e.g., "epidermoid" as opposed to other types of lung cancer) but has little or no effect on other types, a greater relative risk is obtained when the calculation is restricted to the particular histological type than when all cancers at that site are considered. But, it makes no difference to the excess risk if the other histological types are included or not.

Finally, from the point of view of case-control studies, there is one compelling reason for adopting the relative risk as the primary measure of association even in the absence of other considerations. This is simply that, as shown in the next section, the *relative risk is in principle directly estimable from data collected in a case-control study*. Additional information, namely knowledge of actual incidence rates for at least one of the exposed or non-exposed populations, is required to estimate the excess risk.

2.8 Estimation of the relative risk from case-control studies – basic concepts

A full understanding of how the data from a case-control study permit estimation of the relative risk requires careful description of how cases and controls are sampled from the population. The studies whose analysis is considered in this monograph involve the ascertainment of new (incident) cases which occur in a defined study period. Ideally these cases are identified through a cancer registry or some other system which covers a well-defined population; with hospital-based studies the referent population, consisting of all those "served" by the given hospital, may be more imaginary than real. Most commonly the sample will contain all new cases arising during the study period, or at least all those successfully interviewed. Otherwise they are assumed to be a random sample of the actual cases.

The controls in a case-control study are assumed to represent a random sample of the subjects who are disease-free, though otherwise at risk. The control sample may be stratified, for example on the basis of age and sex, so that it has roughly the same age and sex distribution as the cases. Or, the controls may be individually matched to cases on the basis of family membership, residence or other characteristics. Under such circumstances the controls are assumed to constitute a random sample from within each of the subpopulations formed by the stratification or matching factors.

If infinite resources were available, one would ideally conduct a prospective investigation of the entire population. Subjects would be classified at the beginning of the study period on the basis of exposure to the risk factor, and at the end of the period according to whether or not they had developed the disease. Suppose that a proportion p of the individuals at risk in a particular stratum were exposed at the beginning of the study. Denote by $P_1 = P_1(t)$ the probability that an exposed person in this stratum develops the disease during a study period of length t, and by $P_0 = P_0(t)$ the analogous quantity for the unexposed. Let $Q = 1-P$ and $q = 1-p$. Then the *expected* proportions of individuals who fall into each of the resulting four categories or cells may be represented thus:

	Exposed	Unexposed	Total
Diseased	pP_1	qP_0	$pP_1 + qP_0$
Disease-free	pQ_1	qQ_0	$pQ_1 + qQ_0$
Total	p	q	1

$$(2.12)$$

If the study period is reasonably short, which means of the order of a year or two for most cancers and other chronic disease, the probabilities P_1 and P_0 will be quite small. According to § 2.4, their ratio will thus be a good approximation to the ratio r of stratum-specific incidence rates averaged over the study period. In other words, we have as an approximation $r = \lambda_1/\lambda_0 \approx P_1/P_0$. Since $Q_1 \approx Q_0 \approx 1$ under these same circumstances, it follows that $P_1/Q_1 \approx P_1$ and $P_0/Q_0 \approx P_0$, and thus that the relative risk is also well approximated by the *odds ratio* ψ of the disease probabilities:

$$\psi = \frac{P_1 Q_0}{P_0 Q_1} \approx \frac{P_1}{P_0} \approx r. \qquad (2.13)$$

The term "odds ratio" derives from the fact that ψ may also be written in the form $(P_1/Q_1) \div (P_0/Q_0)$, i.e., as the ratio of the "odds" of disease occurrence in the exposed and non-exposed sub-groups.

Example: Suppose the average annual incidence rates for the exposed and non-exposed substrata are $\lambda_1 = 0.02$ and $\lambda_0 = 0.01$ and that the study lasts three years. Then the cumulative rates are $\Lambda_1 = 0.06$ and $\Lambda_0 = 0.03$, while the corresponding risks (2.4) are $P_1 = 1 - \exp(-0.06) = 0.05824$ and $P_0 = 1 - \exp(-0.03) = 0.02956$. It follows that the odds ratio is

$$\psi = \frac{0.05824 \times 0.97044}{0.02956 \times 0.94176} = 2.03,$$

as compared with a relative risk $r = \lambda_1/\lambda_0$ of exactly 2.

As Cornfield (1951) observed, the approximation (2.13) provides the critical link between prospective and retrospective (case-control) studies *vis-à-vis* estimation of the relative risk. If the entire population were kept under observation for the duration of the study, separate estimates would be available for each of the quantities p, P_1 and P_0, so that one could determine all the probabilities shown in (2.12). If we were to take samples of exposed and unexposed individuals at the beginning of the study and follow them up, this would permit estimation of P_1 and P_0 and thus of both excess and relative risks, but not of p; of course such samples would have to be rather large in order to permit sufficient cases to be observed to obtain good estimates. With the case-control approach, on the other hand, sampling is done according to disease rather than exposure status. This ensures that a reasonably large number of diseased persons will be included in the study. From such samples of cases and controls one may estimate the exposure probabilities given disease status, namely:

$$p_1 = \text{pr(exposed}\,|\,\text{case)} = \frac{pP_1}{pP_1 + qP_0} \quad \text{and}$$

$$p_0 = \text{pr(exposed}\,|\,\text{control)} = \frac{pQ_1}{pQ_1 + qQ_0}.$$

It immediately follows that the odds ratio calculated from the exposure probabilities is identical to the odds ratio of the disease probabilities, or in symbols:

$$\psi = \frac{p_1 q_0}{p_0 q_1} = \frac{P_1 Q_0}{P_0 Q_1}. \tag{2.14}$$

Consequently the ratio of disease incidences, as approximated by the odds ratio of the corresponding risks, can be directly estimated from a case-control study even though the latter provides no information about the absolute magnitude of the incidence rates in the exposed and non-exposed subgroups.

Example: As an illustration of this phenomenon, suppose the incidence rates from the previous example applied to a population of 10 000 persons, of whom 30% were exposed to the risk factor. If the entire population were kept under observation for the study period one would expect to find $P_1 \times 3\,000 = 175$ exposed cases and $P_0 \times 7\,000 = 207$ non-exposed cases. The data could thus be summarized:

	Exposed	Unexposed	Total
Diseased	175	207	382
Disease-free	2 825	6 793	9 618
Total	3 000	7 000	10 000

If, instead of making a complete enumeration of the population, one carried out a case-control study in which all 382 cases of disease were ascertained along with a 10% sample of controls, the expected distribution of the study data would be:

	Exposed	Unexposed	Total
Diseased	175	207	382
Disease-free	282	679	961

From this we calculate the exposure odds ratio for the case-control sample:

$$\frac{p_1 q_0}{p_0 q_1} = \frac{(175/382) \times (679/961)}{(282/961) \times (207/382)}$$

$$= \frac{175 \times 679}{282 \times 207}$$

$$= 2.04,$$

which differs from the previous figure of $\psi' = 2.03$ only because the expected values in the table have been rounded to whole numbers.

One fundamental sampling requirement to which attention is drawn is that the *sampling fractions for cases and controls must be the same regardless of exposure category.* If exposed subjects are more or less likely to be included in the sample than are the unexposed, serious bias can result. In the previous example, if only 5% of the unexposed control population had been sampled rather than 10% as for the exposed, the computed odds ratio would be 1.02, indicating no apparent effect. This source of bias is especially serious when using "hospital-based" controls, since exposure may be related to other diagnoses besides those under investigation.

In studies for which the period of case acquisition is longer than a year or two, several potential problems arise. First, the odds ratio approximation to the relative risk does not hold when the cumulative rates and risks on which it is based are large. Second, the classification of cases and controls according to variables which change over time becomes confused; it is not immediately clear, for example, whether a subject's age should be recorded at the beginning of the study, at the end, or at the time of diagnosis and interview. And finally, whereas the preceding development implicitly assumed that the controls remained disease-free for the duration of the study, in practice controls are usually sampled continuously throughout the study period, along with the cases. This raises the possibility that someone interviewed as a control during the first year of the study will turn up as a case later on; thus, we must decide whether such a person is to be treated in the analysis as a case, a control, both or neither.

In fact the resolution of these queries and potential difficulties is surprisingly easy. *We simply divide up the time period of the study into a number of shorter intervals and use time interval as one of the bases for stratification of the population.* Yearly intervals are probably more than satisfactory in most instances. Suppose, for example, that the population at risk was initially divided into six 5-year age groups from 35–39 through to 60–64 years. With a 5-year study there would thus be $30 = 5 \times 6$ age-time strata. Most individuals would move from one age group to the next at some point during the study, unless its start happened to correspond exactly with their 35th, 40th or similar birthday. A separate estimate of the relative risk would be obtained for each stratum by computing the odds ratio of the exposure probability of cases and controls in the usual fashion. If the 30 estimates appeared reasonably stable with respect to age and time, they would be combined into a single summary of relative risk for the entire population. Otherwise variations in the relative risk could be *modelled* as a function of age and/or time in the statistical analysis.

Partition of the study period into several time intervals resolves each of the problems mentioned above. First, by making the intervals sufficiently short, the cumulative incidence rates over each one are guaranteed to be so small as to be virtually indistinguishable from the cumulative risks; this means that the odds ratio approximation to each relative risk will involve negligible error. Second, the fact that ages are changing throughout the study period is explicitly accounted for in that each case and control is assigned to the appropriate age category in which he finds himself at the time of ascertainment; in practice this means that ages are recorded at the time of interview, as is commonly done anyway. Finally, while such an event would usually be rare, a person could be included as both a case and a control; having been sampled as a disease-free control at one time, he might develop the disease later on and thus be re-interviewed as a case. Exclusion of either of his interview records from the statistical analysis would, technically speaking, bias the result.

It is of interest to consider the limiting form of such a partition of the study period in which the time intervals become arbitrarily small. The effect is that each case is matched with one or more controls who are disease-free at the precise moment that the case is diagnosed. Such controls are usually chosen to be of the same age and sex and may have other features in common as well. This approach, which in fact accords reasonably well with the actual conduct of many studies, avoids completely the odds ratio approximation to the relative risk since the relevant time periods are infinitesimally small. It implies, however, that the resultant data are analysed so as to preserve intact the matched sets of case and control(s). Prentice and Breslow (1978) present a more mathematical account of this idea, while in Chapters 5 and 7 we discuss methods of analysis appropriate for matched data collected in this fashion [see also Liddell et al. (1977)].

In the sequel we will use repeatedly and without further comment the odds ratio approximation to the relative risk, assuming that the conditions for its validity as outlined here have been met for the data being analysed.

2.9 Attributable risk and related measures

Case-control studies provide direct estimates of the relative increase in incidence associated with an exposure. They may also yield unbiased estimates of the distribution of exposure levels in the population, provided of course that the control samples have been drawn from the population at risk according to a well-defined sampling scheme, rather than on the basis of matching to individual cases. By combining the information about the distribution of exposures with the estimates of relative risk, one can determine the degree to which cases of disease occurring in the population are explained by the exposure. Likewise, knowledge of the differences in the distribution of exposure among two or more populations permits calculation of the extent to which differences in risk between them are due to confounding by the exposure. In this section we explore briefly a few such auxiliary measures derived from the relative risk. While these are useful in interpreting the results of a study, questions on the statistical significance of the results should be directed primarily towards the relative risk.

In order to simplify the discussion, let us ignore the possible age/sex/time variation in incidence rates. Suppose that λ_0 and λ_1 denote the overall incidence rates for the non-exposed and exposed subgroups and let $r=\lambda_1/\lambda_0$ represent the relative risk. Then the proportion of the cases of disease occurring among exposed persons which is in excess in comparison with the non-exposed is

$$\frac{\lambda_1-\lambda_0}{\lambda_1} = \frac{r-1}{r},$$

a quantity which has been labelled by Cole & MacMahon (1971) as the *attributable risk for exposed persons*. If p denotes the proportion of persons in the population exposed to the risk factor, then the total disease incidence is

$$\lambda = p\lambda_1 + (1-p)\lambda_0.$$

The excess among the exposed is given by $p(\lambda_1-\lambda_0)$, from which one arrives at the expression

$$AR = \frac{p(\lambda_1-\lambda_0)}{p\lambda_1 + (1-p)\lambda_0} = \frac{p(r-1)}{pr + (1-p)} \tag{2.15}$$

for the *population attributable risk* (AR), first described by Levin (1953). This represents the proportion of cases occurring in the total population which can be explained by the risk factor. Walter (1975) has investigated some of the statistical properties of this measure.

Example: To illustrate these calculations. Table 2.12 gives the distribution of cases and controls by amount smoked for the Rothman and Keller (1972) data on oral cancer considered in § 2.6. Assuming that the controls are representative, 81% of the population at risk smokes. Weighting the relative risks for each smoking category by the proportion of smokers in that category, we find an overall relative risk of 4.1 for smokers *versus* non-smokers, the same figure obtained from simply collapsing the smoking

Table 2.12 Distribution of oral cancer cases and controls according to number of cigarettes (or equivalent) smoked per day[a]

Smoking category	None	Light 1–19	Medium 20–39	Heavy 40+	Total
Cases	26	66	248	143	483
Controls	85	97	197	68	447
RR	1.0	2.2	4.1	6.9	–
% cases explained by smoking	0	55	76	88	72
% distribution (controls)	19.0	21.7	44.1	15.2	100.0

[a] From Rothman and Keller (1972)

categories into one and calculating a single odds ratio from the resulting 2×2 table. The population attributable risk is calculated from (2.15) as

$$AR = \frac{0.81 \times 3.1}{0.81 \times 4.1 + 0.19} = 0.72.$$

Alternatively we could reason that 55% of the cancers occurring among light smokers, 76% of those among medium smokers and 86% of those among heavy smokers were in excess as compared with non-smokers. After consideration of the percentage of smokers in each category, this leads to precisely the same evaluation of the overall percentage of cases in the population attributable to smoking, namely 72%.

An important fact illustrated by this example is that the attributable risk does not depend on how the various exposure categories are defined or grouped together, as long as there is an unambiguous baseline category. Unfortunately, such a category does not exist for continuous variables such as body weight, serum cholesterol, dietary fat or fibre and degree of air pollution. For these the selection of a "lowest level" of exposure is essentially arbitrary. Yet it may have a marked effect on the attributable risk since the more extreme one makes the definition of the baseline level, the greater is the percentage of cases which will be said to be attributable to the higher levels of exposure.

If two factors are both associated with the same disease, and if their combined effect on risk is multiplicative or at least more than additive, the sum of the attributable risks associated with each of them individually may exceed 100%. The obvious interpretation of such a result is that both factors are required to produce the disease in a large proportion of the cases, which would presumably not occur if either one was absent. This phenomenon calls into question the practice of attributing a certain fraction of the cancers occurring at each site to individual environmental agents. When the disease has a multifactorial etiology, such an attribution can be rather arbitrary.

Example: Table 2.13 gives a hypothetical example of a multiplicative relationship between two risk factors which, for illustrative purposes, can be considered to be cigarette smoking and asbestos exposure among factory workers. Note the positive association between the two, such that persons exposed to asbestos are more likely to be smokers and vice versa. The lung cancer risk attributable to smoking is calculated to be 5/8 = 62.5% in the low asbestos areas, 20/27 = 74.1% in the high exposure areas. The overall attributable risk is then the average of these two figures weighted by the number of cases in the low and high asbestos areas, respectively, a figure which will vary with the distribution of asbestos exposure. In the present instance, the proportion of cases in the low asbestos area is given by

$$(1 \times 0.2 + 3 \times 0.3)/(1 \times 0.2 + 3 \times 0.3 + 6 \times 0.1 + 18 \times 0.4) = 0.1236$$

Table 2.13 Joint distribution of a hypothetical population according to two risk factors, A and B, with relative risks of lung cancer in parentheses

Factor B (e.g., asbestos exposures)	Factor A (e.g., smoking) Unexposed	Exposed	Total
Low	20% (1)	10% (6)	30%
High	30% (3)	40% (18)	70%
Total	50%	50%	100%

and the overall attributable risk is thus equal to

$$62.5 \times 0.1236 + 74.1 \times 0.8764 = 73.0\%$$

Similarly, the attributable risk for asbestos varies from 54.5% among non-smokers to 61.5% among smokers and is 60.6% overall. These hypothetical figures tell us that it might be possible to "eliminate" 70.6% of cancers by eliminating smoking, 59.4% by reducing all asbestos exposures to low levels, and 88.8% by altering both factors simultaneously. However, all these estimates depend on the degree of association between the two risk factors. Thus it is desirable to consider each of the smoking categories separately in determining the incidence attributable to asbestos, and vice versa.

Similar calculations may be performed to indicate how much of the relative difference in incidence between two populations is explained by the difference in patterns of exposure to a particular risk factor. Suppose there are K levels of exposure besides the non-exposed category and let $r_0 = 1$, r_1, ..., r_K denote the associated relative risks, which are assumed to apply equally to the two populations; let p_{1k} be the proportion of the first population exposed to level k of the risk factor, and, similarly, p_{2k} for the second population. The *crude* ratio R of overall incidence rates is then

$$R = \frac{\lambda_{20} \sum_{k=0}^{K} p_{2k} r_k}{\lambda_{10} \sum_{k=0}^{K} p_{1k} r_k} = R_0 w \qquad (2.16)$$

where λ_{10} and λ_{20} are the incidence rates for the non-exposed in populations 1 and 2, and the summation is over all values of k from 0 to K. This ratio may be decomposed into the product of two terms, the ratio of rates $R_0 = \lambda_{20}/\lambda_{10}$ which would persist if the two populations had the same patterns of exposure, and a multiplicative factor $w = \Sigma p_{2k} r_k / \Sigma p_{1k} r_k$, which indicates how much R_0 is changed by the exposure discrepancy. The ratio w has been termed the *confounding risk ratio* as it measures the degree to which the effects of one factor on incidence are confounded by the effects of another (Miettinen, 1972; Eyigou & McHugh, 1977; Schlesselman, 1978).

The difference in incidence rates between the two populations is

$$\lambda_{20} \sum_{k=0}^{K} p_{2k} r_k - \lambda_{10} \sum_{k=0}^{K} p_{1k} r_k,$$

which would be reduced to

$$\lambda_{20} \sum_{k=0}^{K} p_{1k} r_k - \lambda_{10} \sum_{k=0}^{K} p_{1k} r_k$$

if the second population had the same distribution of exposures as the first. One can therefore attribute an absolute amount $\lambda_{20} \Sigma (p_{2k} - p_{1k}) r_k$, or a proportional amount

$$\frac{\lambda_{20} \sum_{k=0}^{K} (p_{2k} - p_{1k}) r_k}{\lambda_{20} \sum_{k=0}^{K} p_{2k} r_k - \lambda_{10} \sum_{k=0}^{K} p_{1k} r_k} = \frac{R - R_0}{R - 1} = \frac{R(w-1)}{w(R-1)}, \qquad (2.17)$$

of the difference in rates to the exposure. This ratio, which might well be called the *relative attributable risk* (RAR), may be written in the form

$$\text{RAR} = \frac{AR_2 - AR_1}{1 - AR_1} \div \frac{R-1}{R} \tag{2.18}$$

where AR_1 and AR_2 are the attributable risks for populations 1 and 2. It is much less sensitive to changes in the definition of the baseline level for continuous variables than are the attributable risks themselves.

Example: Table 2.14 shows the distribution of women in Boston and Tokyo according to age at first birth, together with associated relative risks for breast cancer as estimated in an international case-control study by MacMahon et al. (1970). The data are essentially the same as shown in Table 2.7 except we now use the category "age at first birth under 20" as the baseline or referent category. Breast cancer rates for United States women are generally about $R = 5$ times those in Japan, and we assume that the same relationship holds for Boston *versus* Tokyo. In order to estimate the portion of this increase which can be attributed to the fact that more Japanese women tend to have children, and have them at younger ages, we calculate

$$w = \frac{7.5 + 27.2\,(1.2) + 23.5\,(1.56) + \ldots + 27.0\,(2.00)}{7.5 + 41.4\,(1.2) + 24.5\,(1.56) + \ldots + 18.2\,(2.00)}$$

$$= \frac{160.92}{148.82} = 1.081,$$

and

$$\text{RAR} = \frac{5\,(0.081)}{(1.081)\,4} = 0.094.$$

Thus, only 9.4% of the excess risk in Boston can be attributed to the different child-bearing customs there as compared with Japan. Even after accounting for the effects of this factor, the relative risk for Boston *versus* Tokyo would be of the order of $5 \div 1.081 = 4.63$.

Using the under age 20 category as baseline, the attributable risks may be calculated to be $AR_2 = 0.379$ for Boston and $AR_1 = 0.328$ for Tokyo. Suppose that the under age 30 category were used instead, and that the relative risks for the remaining categories were changed to $1.88/1.25 = 1.50$, $2.44/1.25 = 1.95$ and $2.00/1.25 = 1.60$, respectively. The attributable risks would then change to $AR_2 = 0.203$ for Boston and $AR_1 = 0.139$ for Tokyo. But the relative attributable risk would remain nearly constant at RAR = 0.093.

Table 2.14 Age at first birth and risk for breast cancer[a]

	Centre	Age at first birth (years)					
		<20	20–24	25–29	30–34	35+	Nulliparous
Percentage of women	Boston	7.5	27.2	23.5	10.7	4.1	27.0
in control population	Tokyo	7.5	41.4	24.5	6.2	2.2	18.2
Relative risk (all centres as in Table 2.7)		1.0	1.20	1.56	1.88	2.44	2.00

[a] From MacMahon et al. (1970)

The decomposition (2.16) was essentially provided by Cornfield et al. (1959) in the course of proving the assertions of § 2.7, *viz* that a confounding factor can explain an observed relative risk R between two populations only if the relative risk r associated with the confounder, and the ratio of the proportions exposed in each population, are both even greater than R. Consider the above formulation in the case $R = 9$, $R_0 = 1$ and $K = 1$. Let p_2 denote the proportion of exposed individuals in population 2 and let p_1 be the same for population 1. In order for the difference between these two proportions to explain completely the ninefold excess we must have $w > 9$, i.e., $(1-p_2) + rp_2 > 9\{(1-p_1) + rp_1\}$, which implies both $p_2 > 9p_1 + 8/(r-1) > 9p_1$ and $r > 9$.

We end this chapter with a brief word of caution regarding the interpretation of attributable risks, whether relative or absolute. For pedagogic reasons, language was occasionally used which seemed to imply that the elimination of a particular risk factor would result in a measured reduction in incidence. This of course supposes that the association between risk factor and disease as estimated from the observational study is in fact a causal one. Unfortunately, the only way to be absolutely certain that a causal relationship exists is to intervene actively in the system by removing the disputed factor. In the absence of such evidence, a more cautious interpretation of the attributable risk measures would be in terms of the proportion of risk *explained* by the given factor, where "explain" is used in the limited sense of statistical association. The next chapter considers in some detail the problem of drawing causal inferences from observational data such as those collected in case-control studies.

REFERENCES

Beebe, G.W., Kato, H. & Land, C.E. (1977) Mortality experience of atomic bomb survivors 1950–74. *Life Span Study Report 8*, Hiroshima, Radiation Effects Research Foundation

Berkson, J. (1958) Smoking and lung cancer: some observations on two recent reports. *J. Am. stat. Assoc., 53*, 28–38

Berry, G., Newhouse, M.L. & Turok, M. (1972) Combined effect of asbestos exposure and smoking on mortality from lung cancer in factory workers. *Lancet, ii*, 476–479

Bjarnasson, O., Day, N.E., Snaedal, G. & Tulinius, H. (1974) The effect of year of birth on the breast cancer incidence curve in Iceland. *Int. J. Cancer, 13*, 689–696

Bogovski, P. & Day, N.E. (1977) Accelerating action of tea on mouse skin carcinogenesis. *Cancer Lett., 3*, 9–13

Boice, J.D. & Monson, R.R. (1977) Breast cancer in women after repeated fluoroscopic examinations of the chest. *J. natl Cancer Inst., 59*, 823–832

Boice, J.D. & Stone, B.J. (1979) *Interaction between radiation and other breast cancer risk factors.* In: *Late Biological Effects of Ionizing Radiation, Vol. I*, Vienna, International Atomic Energy Agency, pp. 231–249

Cole, P. & MacMahon, B. (1971) Attributable risk percent in case-control studies. *Br. J. prev. soc. Med., 25*, 242–244

Cook, P., Doll, R. & Fellingham, S.A. (1969) A mathematical model for the age distribution of cancer in man. *Int. J. Cancer, 4*, 93–112

Cornfield, J. (1951) A method of estimating comparative rates from clinical data. Applications to cancer of the lung, breast and cervix. *J. natl Cancer Inst., 11*, 1269–1275

Cornfield, J., Haenszel, W., Hammond, E.C., Lilienfeld, A.M., Shimkin, M.B. & Wynder, E.L. (1959) Smoking and lung cancer: recent evidence and a discussion of some questions. *J. natl Cancer Inst., 22*, 173–203

Court Brown, W.M. & Doll, R. (1965) Mortality from cancer and other causes after radiotherapy for ankylosing spondylitis. *Br. med. J., ii,* 1327–1332

Day, N. (1976) *A new measure of age standardized incidence, the cumulative rate.* In: Waterhouse, J.A.H., Muir, C.S., Correa, P. & Powell, J., eds, *Cancer Incidence in Five Continents,* Vol. III, Lyon, International Agency for Research on Cancer *(IARC Scientific Publications No. 15),* pp. 443–452

Doll, R. (1971) The age distribution of cancer: implications for models of carcinogenesis. *J. R. stat. Soc. A, 132,* 133–166

Doll, R. & Peto, R. (1976) Mortality in relation to smoking: 20 years' observations on male British doctors. *Br. med. J., ii,* 1525–1536

Elandt-Johnson, R. (1975) Definition of rates: some remarks on their use and misuse. *Am. J. Epidemiol., 102,* 267–271

Eyigou, A. & McHugh, R. (1977) On the factorization of the crude relative risk. *Am. J. Epidemiol., 106,* 188–193

Fleiss, J.L. (1973) *Statistical Methods for Rates and Proportions.* New York, Wiley

Hammond, E.C. (1966) Smoking in relation to the death rates of one million men and women. *Natl Cancer Inst. Monogr., 19,* 127–204

Hammond, E.C., Selikoff, I.J. & Seidman, H. (1979) Asbestos exposure, cigarette smoking and death rates. *Ann. N.Y. Acad. Sci., 330,* 473–490

Koopman, J.S. (1977) Causal models and sources of interaction. *Am. J. Epidemiol., 106,* 439–444

Levin, M.L. (1953) The occurrence of lung cancer in man. *Acta Unio Int. Cancer, 9,* 531–541

Liddell, F.D.K., McDonald, J.C. & Thomas, D.C. (1977) Methods of cohort analysis: appraisal by application to asbestos mining. *J. R. stat. Soc. Ser. A, 140,* 469–491

MacGregor, P.H., Land, C.E., Choi, K., Tokuota, S., Liu, P.I., Wakabayoshi, T. & Beebe, G.W. (1977) Breast cancer incidence among atomic bomb survivors, Hiroshima and Nagasaki, 1950–69. *J. natl Cancer Inst., 59,* 799–811

MacMahon, B., Cole, P., Lin, T.M., Lowe, C.R., Mirra, A.P., Ravnihar, B., Salber, E.J., Valaoras, V.G. & Yuasa, S. (1970) Age at first birth and breast cancer risk. *Bull. World Health Org., 43,* 209–221

Miettinen, O.S. (1972) Components of the crude risk ratio. *Am. J. Epidemiol., 96,* 168–172

Mosteller, F. & Tukey, J. (1977) *Data Analysis and Regression: A Second Course in Statistics,* Reading, MA, Addison & Wesley

Prentice, R.L. & Breslow, N.E. (1978) Retrospective studies and failure time models. *Biometrika, 65,* 153–158

Rogentine, G.N., Yankee, R.A., Gart, J.J., Nam, J. & Traponi, R.J. (1972) HL-A antigens and disease. Acute lymphocytic leukemia. *J. clin. Invest., 51,* 2420–2428

Rogentine, G.N., Traponi, R.J., Yankee, R.A. & Henderson, E.S. (1973) HL-A antigens and acute lymphocytic leukemia: the nature of the HL-A2 association. *Tissue Antigens, 3,* 470–475

Rothman, K. (1976) The estimation of synergy or antagonism. *Am. J. Epidemiol., 103,* 506–511

Rothman, K.J. & Keller, A.Z. (1972) The effect of joint exposure to alcohol and tobacco on risk of cancer of the mouth and pharynx. *J. chron. Dis., 23,* 711–716

Saracci, R. (1977) Asbestos and lung cancer: an analysis of the epidemiological evidence on the asbestos-smoking interaction. *Int. J. Cancer, 20,* 323–331

Schlesselman, J.J. (1978) Assessing the effects of confounding variables. *Am. J. Epidemiol., 108,* 3–8

Selikoff, I.O. & Hammond, E.C. (1978) Asbestos associated disease in United States shipyards. *CA: A Cancer Journal for Clinicians, 28,* 87–99

Shore, R.E., Hempelmann, L.A., Kowaluk, E., Mansur, P.S., Pasternack, B.S., Albert, R.E. & Haughie, G.E. (1977) Breast neoplasms in women treated with X-rays for acute postpartum mastitis. *J. natl Cancer Inst., 59,* 813–822

Smith, P.G. (1979) *Some problems in assessing the carcinogenic risk to man of exposure to ionizing radiations.* In: Breslow, N. & Whittemore, A., eds, *Energy and Health,* Philadelphia, Society for Industrial and Applied Mathematics, pp. 61–80

Walter, S.D. (1975) The distribution of Levin's measure of attributable risk. *Biometrika, 62,* 371–374

Waterhouse, J., Muir, C., Correa, P. & Powell, J., eds (1976) *Cancer Incidence in Five Continents,* Vol. III, Lyon, International Agency for Research on Cancer *(IARC Scientific Publications No. 15)*

Wynder, E.L. & Bross, I.J. (1961) A study of etiological factors in cancer of the esophagus. *Cancer, 14,* 389–413

Wynder, E.L., Bross, I.J. & Feldman, R.M. (1957) A study of etiological factors in cancer of the mouth. *Cancer, 10,* 1300–1323

LIST OF SYMBOLS – CHAPTER 2 (in order of appearance)

l_j	length of jth time interval for rate calculation
$\lambda(t)$	instantaneous event (e.g., incidence) rate at time t
t_j	midpoint of jth time interval for rate calculation
d_j	number of events (e.g., cancer diagnoses) in j^{th} time interval
n_j	number of subjects under observation at midpoint of jth time interval
$\Lambda(t)$	cumulative event (e.g., incidence) rate at time t
$P(t)$	cumulative risk or probability of occurrence of an event (e.g., diagnosis of disease) by time t
$\approx$	approximate equality
$\tilde{\Lambda}(t)$	estimated cumulative rate
λ_{1i}	disease incidence rate in i^{th} stratum among persons exposed to risk factor
λ_{0i}	disease incidence rate in i^{th} stratum among persons not exposed to risk factor
b_i	difference in incidence rates for exposed *versus* non-exposed in i^{th} stratum
b	difference in incidence rates for exposed *versus* non-exposed in additive model
r_i	ratio of incidence rates for exposed *versus* non-exposed in i^{th} stratum
r	ratio of incidence rates for exposed *versus* non-exposed in multiplicative model; rate ratio; relative risk
β	logarithm of relative risk for exposed *versus* non-exposed

P_0	cumulative risk or probability of disease diagnosis among those not exposed to the risk factor
P_1	cumulative risk or probability of disease diagnosis among those exposed to the risk factor
$\lambda_i(t)$	average annual incidence rate for i^{th} area at age t
β_i	logarithm of relative risk of stomach cancer for country i *versus* country 1
γ	slope in fit of straight line to log-log plot of age-incidence data
r_i	relative risk of stomach cancer for country i *versus* country 1
r_{ij}	relative risk of exposure to level i of one risk factor and level j of another, with reference to the non-exposed
p	proportion of population exposed to risk factor
$Q_0 = 1-P_0$	proportion of non-exposed population which remains disease-free
$Q_1 = 1-P_1$	proportion of exposed population which remains disease-free
ψ	$P_1 Q_0/(Q_1 P_0)$; odds ratio of disease probabilities for exposed *versus* non-exposed groups
p_1	probability of exposure among diseased
p_0	probability of exposure among disease-free
AR	population attributable risk
p_{1k}	proportion of first population exposed to level k of a risk factor
p_{2k}	proportion of second population exposed to level k of a risk factor
R	crude ratio of incidence rates between two populations
λ_{10}	incidence rate for non-exposed in population 1
λ_{20}	incidence rate for non-exposed in population 2
R_0	ratio of incidence rates for non-exposed, population 2 to population 1
w	(multiplicative) confounding factor
RAR	relative attributable risk
AR_1	attributable risk for population 1
AR_2	attributable risk for population 2

3. GENERAL CONSIDERATIONS FOR THE ANALYSIS OF CASE-CONTROL STUDIES

3.1 Bias, confounding and causality

3.2 Criteria for assessing causality

3.3 Initial treatment of the data

3.4 Confounding

3.5 Interaction and effect modification

3.6 Modelling risk

3.7 Comparisons between more than two groups

3.8 Considerations affecting interpretation of the analysis

CHAPTER III

GENERAL CONSIDERATIONS FOR THE ANALYSIS
OF CASE-CONTROL STUDIES

In previous chapters we have introduced disease incidence as the basic measure of disease risk in a population. As a measure of the increased risk for a population exposed to some factor when compared with an otherwise similar population not so exposed, we have proposed the use of the proportionate increase in incidence which corresponds to the relative risk. We have described the properties of this measure, and its behaviour in cancer epidemiology, in order to demonstrate its advantages over an alternative measure of disease association, the excess risk. We have explored the logical basis for estimation of the relative risk from the results of a case-control study, from which the actual incidence rates cannot be estimated. Estimation of relative risks follows from interpreting the case-control study as the result of sampling from a large, probably fictive, cohort study from which incidence rates can hypothetically be estimated. In succeeding chapters we shall develop the statistical theory and methodology required for the analysis of case-control data. In this chapter, we shall concern ourselves with the types of conclusion that we want to draw from the data, and the steps which must be taken to ensure that these conclusions are valid. Strategies for approaching the data, the handling of different types of variables, the examination of joint association of several variables, and how the design of a study is reflected in the analysis will all be discussed.

3.1 Bias, confounding and causality

The purpose of an analysis of a case-control study is to identify those factors under study which are associated with risk for the disease. In an analysis, the basic questions to consider are the degree of association between risk for disease and the factors under study, the extent to which the observed associations may result from bias, confounding and/or chance, and the extent to which they may be described as causal. The concepts of bias and confounding are most easily understood in the context of cohort studies, and how case-control studies relate to them. Confounding is intimately connected to the concept of causality. In a cohort study, if some exposure E is associated with disease status, then the incidence of the disease varies among the strata defined by different levels of E. If these differences in incidence are caused (partially) by some other factor C, then we say that C has (partially) confounded the association between E and disease. If C is not causally related to disease, then the differences in incidence cannot be caused by C, thus C does not confound the disease/exposure association. Often the observed extraneous variables will only be surrogates for the factor causally related to disease, age and socioeconomic status being obvious examples, but we should normally consider these surrogates also as confounding variables. Confounding in a case-control study has the same basis as in a cohort study. It arises from the association in the causal network in the underlying study population and cannot normally be removed by appropriate study design alone. An essential part of the analysis is an examination of possible confounding effects and how they may be controlled. Succeeding chapters consider this problem in detail.

Bias in a case-control study, by contrast, arises from the differences in design between case-control and cohort studies. In a cohort study, information is obtained on exposures before disease status is determined, and all cases of disease arising in a given time period should be ascertained. Information on exposure from cases and controls is therefore comparable, and unbiased estimates of the incidence rates in the different subpopulations can be constructed. In case-control studies, however, information on exposure is normally obtained after disease status is established, and the cases and controls represent samples from the total. Biased estimates of incidence ratios will result if the selection processes leading to inclusion of cases and controls in the study are different (selection bias) or if exposure information is not obtained in a comparable manner from the two groups, for example because of differences in response to a questionnaire (recall bias). Bias is thus a consequence of the study design, and the design should be directed towards eliminating it. The effects of bias are often difficult to control in the analysis, although they will sometimes resemble confounding effects and can be treated accordingly (see § 3.8).

To summarize, confounding reflects the causal association between variables in the population under study, and will manifest itself similarly in both cohort and case-control studies. Bias, by contrast, is not a property of the underlying population and should not arise in cohort studies. It results from inadequacies in the design of case-control studies, either in the selection of cases or controls or from the manner in which the data are acquired.

It is not helpful to introduce the concepts of necessity or sufficiency into the discussion of causality in cancer epidemiology. Apart from occasional extremes of occupational exposure, constellations of factors have not been identified whose presence inevitably produces a cancer, or, conversely, in whose absence a tumour will inevitably not appear. Thus, we shall use the word "cause" in a probabilistic sense. By saying that a factor is a cause of a disease, we mean simply that an increase in risk results from the presence of that factor. From this viewpoint a disease can have many causes, some of which may operate synergistically. It is sometimes helpful to think in terms of a multistage model, and to consider a cause as a factor which directly increases one or more of the rates of transition from one stage to the next (Peto, 1977; Whittemore, 1977a). One factor may need the presence of another to be effective, in which case one should strictly speak of the joint occurrence as being a cause.

The most one can hope to show, even with several studies, is that an apparent association cannot be explained either by design bias or by confounding effects of other known risk factors. There are, nevertheless, several aspects of the data, even from a single study, which would make one suspect that an association is causal, which we shall now discuss (Cornfield et al., 1959; Report of the Surgeon General, 1964; Hill, 1965).

3.2 Criteria for assessing causality

Dose response

One would expect the strength of a genuine association to increase both with increasing level of exposure and with increasing duration of exposure. Demonstration of a dose response is an important indication of causality, while the lack of a dose response argues against causality.

In Chapter 2, we saw several examples of a dose response. Table 2.8 shows a smooth increase in risk for oral cancer with increasing consumption of both alcohol and tobacco, and Table 2.7 displays the increasing risk for breast cancer with increasing age at birth of first child. The latter example is not exactly one of a dose response since the dose is not defined, but the hypothesis that later age at first birth increases the risk of developing breast cancer is given strong support by the smooth trend.

The opposite situation is illustrated by the association between coffee drinking and cancer of the lower urinary tract. Table 3.1 is taken from a study by Simon, Yen and Cole (1975). Three previous studies (Cole, 1971; Fraumeni, Scotto & Dunham, 1971; Bross & Tidings, 1973) had also shown a weak association between lower urinary tract cancer and coffee drinking, but with no dose response. The authors of the 1975 paper concluded that, taking the four studies together, the association was probably not causal. The three arguments they advanced were: (1) the absence of association in some groups, (2) the general weakness of the association, and (3) the consistent absence of a dose response; the last point was considered the most telling.

A clear example of risk increasing with duration of exposure is given by studies relating use of oestrogens to palliate menopausal symptoms with an increased risk for endometrial cancer (see Table 5.1).

Table 3.1 Association between coffee drinking and tumours of the lower urinary tract[a]

Cups of coffee/day	Cases	Controls	Relative risk
<1	10	56	1.0
1–2	74	187	2.2
3–4	30	91	1.9
5+	20	48	2.3

[a] Data taken from Simon, Yen and Cole (1975)

Specificity of risk to disease subgroups

Demonstration that an association is confined to specific subcategories of disease can be persuasive evidence of causality, as indicated by the following examples.

In earlier days, when the role of cigarette smoking in the induction of lung cancer was still being established, a persuasive aspect of the data was the finding that when a non-smoker developed lung cancer, it was often the relatively rare adenocarcinoma

Table 3.2 Histological types of lung cancer found in Singapore Chinese females, 1968–73, as related to smoking history[a]

Histological type	Number	% smokers
Epidermoid carcinoma	12	83.3
Small-cell carcinoma	13	84.6
Adenocarcinoma	25	28.0
Large-cell carcinoma	8	50.0
Other types	6	50.0
Controls	156	31.4

[a] Adapted from MacLennan et al. (1977)

(Doll, 1969). This feature of the disease is shown in data from Singapore in Table 3.2 (MacLennan et al., 1977).

As a second example, the association between benzene exposure and leukaemia is restricted to particular cell types, i.e., acute non-lymphocytic (Infante, Rivisky & Wagoner, 1977; Aksoy, Erdem & Dinçol, 1974). The specificity of the association is perhaps the major reason for regarding it as causal.

The tendency for several types of cancer to aggregate in families is often difficult to interpret since family members share in part both their environment and their genes. Relative risks for first degree relatives are typically of the order of two- to threefold. The greatly increased familial risk for bilateral breast cancer especially among premenopausal women (Anderson, 1974) reduces the chance that the association is a reflection of either environmental confounding factors or bias in case ascertainment, and enhances one's belief in a genetic interpretation.

Specificity of risk to exposure subcategories

Belief in the causality of an association is also enhanced if one can demonstrate that the disease/exposure association is stronger either for different types of exposures, or for different categories of individuals. A dose response, with higher risk among the more heavily exposed, is an obvious example. Interactions can also provide insight into disease mechanisms. As an example, one can cite the risk for breast cancer following exposure to ionizing radiation: a greater risk was observed for women under age 20 at irradiation than for women irradiated at over 30 years of age (Boice & Monson, 1977; McGregor et al., 1977). Subsequent studies showed that risk was in fact greatly elevated among girls irradiated either in the two years preceding menarche or during their first pregnancy (Boice & Stone, 1978); breast tissue is proliferating rapidly at both these periods of a woman's life.

In Figure 3.1, we show the risk for lung cancer among males associated with smoking varying numbers of filter and non-filter cigarettes. There is a considerably lower risk associated with the use of filter cigarettes, indicating the importance of tars as the carcinogenic constituent of the smoke, since volatile components were not significantly reduced by filters in use at that time (Wynder & Stellman, 1979).

Fig. 3.1 Relative risk for cancer of the lung according to the number of nonfilter (NF) or filter (F) cigarettes smoked per day. Number of cases and controls shown above each bar. From Wynder and Stellman (1979).

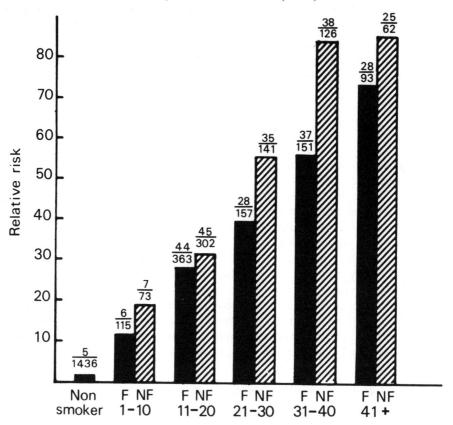

Strength of association

Demonstration of a dose response and of variation in risk according to particular exposure or disease subcategories have in common the identification of subgroups at higher risk. In general terms, the closer the association, the more likely one is to consider the association causal. One reason follows directly from a property of the relative risk described in § 2.7. If an observed association is not causal, but simply the reflection of a causal association between some other factor and disease, then this latter factor must be more strongly related to disease (in terms of relative risk) than is the former factor. The higher the risk, the less one would consider that other factors were likely to be responsible. One also has the possibility in all case-control studies that patient selection or choice of the control group may introduce bias. Bias becomes less tenable as an explanation of an observed association the stronger the association becomes. An example of this is found in the original report on the role of diethylstilboestrol administered to mothers during pregnancy in the development of vaginal adenocarcinomas in the daughters (Herbst, Ulfelder & Poskanzer, 1971). The study was based on 8 cases each with 4 matched controls; 7 out of the 8 cases had been exposed *in utero* to diethylstilboestrol, in contrast to none of the 32 controls. The magnitude of this association persuades one of its causal nature, even though recall of drug treatment some 20 years previously is a potential source of serious bias.

Temporal relation of risk to exposure

For most epithelial tumours, one expects a latent period of at least 15 years. Typically, when exposure is continuous, there is little risk until some 10–15 years after exposure starts, the relative risk then increasing to reach a plateau after 30 years or more (Whittemore, 1977b). For radiation-induced leukaemia this risk increases more quickly (Smith & Doll, 1978), and among recipients of organ transplants the risk for some lymphomas can increase strongly within a year (Hoover & Fraumeni, 1973). Although in principle both cohort and case-control studies should demonstrate the same evolution of relative risk, in practice the temporal evolution of risk following exposure has played a greater role in assessing causality in cohort studies. The reason lies in the nature of the observations. In cohort studies, it is precisely the increase in risk in the years after exposure starts that one observes. Referring back to the discussion of lung cancer risk among smokers in Chapter 2, a prospective study leads to a description of evolution of risk as shown in Figure 2.9 and Table 2.6, whereas a case-control study gives only the relative risk shown in Table 2.6, with most cases probably over age 50. The evolution of risk over time, clear from the changes in the absolute risk in Figure 2.9, is less distinct when considering only the relative risk.

More attention to this aspect of case-control study data may well prove beneficial.

Lack of alternative explanations

In the data being analysed, association between exposures of interest and disease must be shown not to be the effect of some further factor which is itself causally associated with both disease and the exposure. Treatment of potential confounding variables is discussed at length in § 3.4.

Spurious associations can also arise from biased selection of cases or controls, or from biased acquisition of information from either group. Questions of bias are usually more difficult to resolve by considerations internal to the actual data than are problems of confounding. However, if several control groups have been chosen (see § 3.7) or if the data were acquired in a manner in which disease status could not have intervened, the extent to which bias might provide an explanation of the observations is usually reduced.

Considerations external to the study

Magnitude and specificity of risk, dose response and the inability to find alternative explanations are criteria which can be satisfied at least partially by adequate treatment of the data from a single study, and analyses should be aimed in this direction. Comparison can also be made with the trends in the general population, both in terms of the exposure under study and the tumour experience. The early case-control studies of lung cancer were instigated by the parallel increase in cigarette smoking and incidence of the disease. In the paper by Jick et al. (1979) on endometrial cancer, figures are given showing the rise and fall of oestrogen use in the general population and the corresponding rise and fall in the incidence of the disease, together with data showing the high risk among long-term users and the great reduction in risk for individuals who stop taking oestrogens. Arguments offering explanations other than causality for these results would have to be unusually tortuous.

It is rare, however, for a single study to provide convincing evidence of causality. Other studies performed in different populations and using different methodologies are normally required. Demonstration of a reduction in risk after exposure has terminated is further persuasive evidence, although the absence of a reduction is no indication of lack of causality, as asbestos exposure exemplifies (Seidman, Lilis & Selikoff, 1977). Biological plausibility or the demonstration of carcinogenicity in the laboratory provide additional evidence.

General acceptance of the causal nature of an association normally would result only if these more general criteria were satisfied, with several corroborating studies and demonstrations of plausible biological pathways. Nevertheless, even if the results of a single study seldom furnish conclusive evidence of causality, the aim of the analysis should be to extract the fullest evidence for or against causality that the study can provide.

3.3 Initial treatment of the data

The first step in any analysis will be a description of the distribution among cases and among controls of the different variables included in the study. This description should include the correlations, or some other measure of association, between the exposure variables of interest. Such correlations are best computed separately for cases and controls. One would also expect to see a description of the cases and controls in terms of age, sex, and such factors as race, country of birth, hospital attended and method of diagnosis, which although not the object of the study, provide the setting for the interpretation of the later results. It must not be overlooked that the results refer to the sample studied, and generalization from these results usually depends on non-statistical arguments.

Information on exposures which are considered of importance for the cancer site under investigation will usually consist of more than a single measure. For cigarette smoking, for example, one would normally obtain information not only on the daily consumption of cigarettes, but also the age at which smoking started, and stopped if the individual no longer smokes. One may be tempted to proceed directly to a composite measure, such as cumulative exposure; such a procedure, however, may obscure important features of the disease/exposure association.

For continuing smokers, with data on cigarette consumption obtained retrospectively, one might expect lung cancer incidence to be proportional to the fourth power of duration of smoking, but related linearly to the average daily consumption of cigarettes (Doll, 1971). A man aged 60 who has smoked 20 cigarettes a day since age 40 will have one eighth the risk of a man of the same age who has smoked 10 cigarettes a day since age 20. The total cigarette consumption is the same in the two cases, but the difference in risk is eightfold. Similar differences will be seen if one considers ex-smokers. Twenty years after stopping smoking, the lung cancer risk is approximately 10% that of a man of the same age who had continued to smoke at the same daily level (Doll & Peto, 1976). Thus, if one man starts smoking at age 20 and smokes 10 cigarettes a day, and a second man smokes 20 cigarettes a day between ages 20 and 40 and then stops, by age 60 the latter will have $(20/10) \times 10\% = 20\%$ of the risk of the former. Total cigarette consumption is the same.

These examples illustrate the danger of condensing the different types of information on exposure into a single measure at the start of the analysis. Each facet of exposure should be examined separately, and only combined, if at all, at a later stage in the analysis.

The preliminary analyses associating the factors under study with disease risk will treat each factor separately. For *dichotomous variables,* a simple two-way table relating exposure to disease can be constructed. The frequency of the exposure among the controls together with an estimate of the relative risk, with corresponding confidence intervals, gives a complete summary of the data.

For *qualitative* or, as they are sometimes called, categorical variables, which can take one of a discrete set of values, direct calculation of relative risk is again straightforward. A specific level would be selected as a baseline or reference level, and risks would be calculated for the other levels relative to this baseline. Choice of the baseline level depends on whether the levels are *ordered,* such as parity or birth order, or *unordered,* as in the case of genetic phenotypes. In the latter situation, a good choice of baseline is the level which occurs most frequently. The choice is particularly important when using the estimation procedures which combine information from a series of 2×2 tables, since the estimates of relative risk between pairs of levels can vary depending on which one was selected as baseline (see § 4.5).

For ordered categorical variables, one would often choose either the highest or the lowest level, with infrequently occurring extreme levels perhaps being grouped with the next less extreme.

By choosing an extreme level as baseline, one expects to see a smooth increase (or decrease) away from unity in the relative risk associated with increasing (or decreasing) level of the factor, if the factor plays a role in disease development. In the early stages of an analysis, it is usually bad practice to group the different levels of a categorical variable before one has looked at the relevant risks associated with each level. The risks of overlooking important features of the data more than outweigh the theoretical distortion of subsequent significance levels.

Quantitative variables are those measured on some continuous scale, where the number of possible levels is limited only by the accuracy of the recording system. Variables of this type can be treated in two ways. They can be converted into ordered categorical variables by division of the scale of measurement, or they can be treated as continuous variables by postulating a specific mathematical relationship between the relative risk and the value of the variables. In preliminary analyses the former approach would usually be employed, since it provides a broad, assumption-free description of the change of risk with the changing level of the factor. The choice of mathematical relationship used in later analysis would then be guided by earlier results.

In deciding on the grouping of continuous variables, the prime objective should be to display the full range of risk associated with the variable, and also to determine the extent to which a dose response can be demonstrated. With these ends in view, the following guidelines are often of value:

1. A pure non-exposed category should be the baseline level if the numbers appear adequate (e.g., more than five to ten individuals in both case and control groups). Thus, to examine the effect of smoking, where consumption might be measured in grams of tobacco smoked per day, a clearer picture of risk is obtained by comparing different smoking categories to non-smokers than by pooling light smokers with non-smokers (Tables 6.6 and 6.8).

2. A simple dichotomy may conceal more information that it reveals. The thirtyfold range in risk for lung cancer between non-smokers and heavy cigarette smokers is greatly obscured if smoking history is dichotomized into, say, one group composed of non-smokers and smokers of less than ten cigarettes a day as opposed to another group of smokers of ten or more cigarettes a day.

3. Use of more than five or six exposure levels will only rarely give added insight to the data. The trends of risk with exposure as defined by a grouping into five levels are usually sufficient. Three levels, in fact, are often adequate, particularly when the data are too few to demonstrate a smooth increase of risk with increasing dose (Cox, 1957; Billewicz, 1965).

Example: Table 3.3 shows relative risks for breast cancer associated with age at first birth among a cohort of 31 000 Icelandic women who had visited a cervical cancer screening programme at least once by 1974 (Tulinius et al., 1978). The lowest risk group, women who gave birth before 20 years of age, is taken as the baseline level. The alternative analysis based on a dichotomy at 25 years is presented for comparison. Even as a preliminary analysis, the greater range of risk, together with the smooth trend, makes the finer categorization of age at first birth considerably more informative.

Table 3.3   Relative risk of breast cancer associated with age at first birth, after adjusting for year of birth, among 31 000 Icelandic women[a]

Age at first birth	Relative risk	
<20	1.00	1.00
20–24	1.63	
25–29	2.61	
30–34	2.53	
35+	4.12	2.05
Nulliparous	3.76	

Once the general form of the relationship between exposure level and risk has been ascertained, the change of risk can be modelled in terms of a mathematical relationship. The advantages of using mathematical models for expressing the change in risk over a range of exposure levels are economy in the number of parameters required, and a smoothing of the random fluctuations in the observed data. The advantages, in fact, are those that generally result from using a regression equation to summarize a set of points. This topic is discussed further in § 3.6 and in detail in Chapters 6 and 7.

Further analyses will investigate in a series of stages the combined action of factors of interest. First, we may wish to consider individual factors separately and to examine how the other variables modify their effect. This modification may consist of a general confounding effect, in which the association between the different exposures distorts the underlying disease exposure associations, or of interaction when the exposure risk may be heterogeneous over the different values of the other variables. Second, we may want to examine the joint effect of several exposures simultaneously.

We shall start by consideration of confounding effects.

3.4 Confounding

Confounding is the distortion of a disease/exposure association brought about by the association of other factors with both disease and exposure, the latter associations with the disease being causal. These factors are called confounding factors. One can envisage two simple types of situation. First, we might have a confounding factor that has two levels, in which disease and exposure were distributed as follows:

Confounder
- Level 1   High risk for disease / High prevalence of exposure
- Level 2   Low risk for disease / Low prevalence of exposure

As an example, the disease could be lung cancer, the exposure some occupation primarily of blue-collar workers, and the confounder cigarette smoking. At least in the United States, cigarette smoking is considerably more frequent among blue-collar workers than among managers or professional workers.

One can see in this situation that ignoring the confounder will make the association between exposure and disease risk more positive than it would otherwise be. High risk for disease and high prevalence of exposure go together, as do low risk for disease and low prevalence of exposure.

A second type of situation that might arise would be:

Confounder
- Level 1   High risk for disease / Low prevalence of exposure
- Level 2   Low risk for disease / High prevalence of exposure

One might take as an example a study relating breast cancer to use of oestrogens for menopausal symptoms, the confounder being age at menopause. Early menopause decreases breast cancer risk, but leads to greater use of replacement oestrogens (Casagrande et al., 1976). Here ignoring the confounding variable will make the association between the disease and exposure appear less positive than it should be.

We shall begin our discussion of confounding by a treatment of the statistical concepts, the occasions on which confounding is likely to occur, and to what degree, and the steps that can be taken both in design and analysis to remove the effect of confounding on observed associations. However, confounding cannot be discussed solely in statistical terms. Occasions arise in which the association of one factor with disease appears at least partially to be explained by a second factor (associated both with disease and with the first factor), but where the two factors are essentially measuring the same thing, or where the second factor is a consequence of the first. Under these circumstances, it would be inappropriate to consider the second factor as confounding the association of the first factor with disease. This problem is related to that of overmatching, which we shall consider after we have discussed the statistical aspects of confounding.

Statistical aspects of confounding: dichotomous variables

We shall start by considering two dichotomous variables, one of which we shall regard as the exposure of interest (E), the other a potential confounding variable (C).

Suppose we had obtained, when cross-tabulating disease status against exposure E, the following result based on pooling the data over levels of the confounder (C):

Exposure E

	+	−	
Case	a	b	n_1
Control	c	d	n_0
	m_1	m_0	N

As we saw in Chapter 2, the risk ratio associated with exposure to E is well approximated by the odds ratio in the above table.

$$\psi_p = ad/bc$$

where the p subscript means that ψ_p is calculated from the pooled data.

If, now, we consider that the association between E and disease may be partly a reflection of the association of C with both E and disease, than we should be concerned with the association between E and disease for fixed values of C. That is, we shall be interested in the tabulation of disease status against E obtained after stratifying the study population by variable C, as follows:

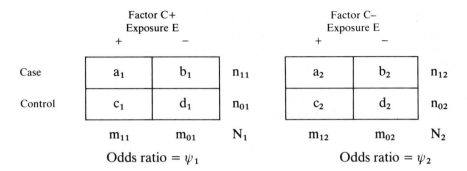

	Factor C+ Exposure E			Factor C− Exposure E		
	+	−		+	−	
Case	a_1	b_1	n_{11}	a_2	b_2	n_{12}
Control	c_1	d_1	n_{01}	c_2	d_2	n_{02}
	m_{11}	m_{01}	N_1	m_{12}	m_{02}	N_2
	Odds ratio $= \psi_1$			Odds ratio $= \psi_2$		

It is clear that the association between E and disease within each of these two 2×2 tables is independent of C since within each table C is the same for all individuals.

We shall assume in this section that $\psi_1 = \psi_2$, i.e., that the association between E and disease is the same in the two strata, and call the common value ψ. In § 3.5, we shall examine situations where this assumption does not hold. Throughout this section, we are considering the odds ratios as population values rather than sample values, so that the equality $\psi_1 = \psi_2$ refers to the underlying population.

The odds ratio ψ represents the association between E and disease after removing the confounding effect of C. Confounding occurs if, and only if, both the following conditions hold:

1. C and E are associated in the control group (which, from the assumption $\psi_1 = \psi_2$, means also in the case group).
2. Factor C is associated with disease after stratification by E.

Factor C is said to confound the association between E and disease status if, and only if, $\psi_p \neq \psi$, that is, if stratifying by C alters the association between E and disease.

These conditions are sometimes loosely expressed by saying that C is related both to exposure and to disease. It should be stressed that the association of C with E must be considered separately for diseased and disease-free persons, and that the association between C and disease must be considered separately among those exposed to E and those not exposed to E.

A distinction is usefully made between confounding effects which create a spurious association and confounding effects which mask a real association. With the former, the crude odds ratio ψ_p will be further from unity than the post-stratification odds ratio ψ. This situation is called *positive* confounding. In the latter situation, the crude odds ratio ψ_p will be closer to unity than the post-stratification odds ratio ψ. This effect is called *negative* confounding. Situations may even arise in which the crude odds ratio is on the opposite side of unity from the post-stratification odds ratio, but they are infrequent.

Confounding, as we have just seen, depends on the association of the confounding variable both with disease and with the exposure, and we can express quantitatively the degree of confounding in terms of the strength of these two associations. In § 2.9, we discussed attributable risk, and the extent to which differences in risk between two populations could be explained by some factor. The situation here is directly analogous; we are considering the degree to which the difference in risk between those exposed to

E and those not exposed to E can be explained by factor C. Equation (2.16) is then directly applicable, and we have:

$$\psi_p = \psi \times \frac{\psi_c p_1 + (1-p_1)}{\psi_c p_2 + (1-p_2)} \qquad (3.1)$$

where ψ_c is the odds ratio associating C with disease after stratification by E, p_1 is the proportion of controls among those exposed to E who are also exposed to C, and p_2 is the proportion of controls among those not exposed to E who are exposed to C (see Schlesselmann, 1978, for example). When either $\psi_c = 1$ or $p_1 = p_2$, then $\psi_p = \psi$ and there is no confounding effect, giving algebraic expression to the two conditions stated earlier in this section. Expression 3.1 generalizes the result of Cornfield given in § 2.7.

The ratio ψ_p/ψ (= w, say) is a measure of the degree of confounding and has been referred to as the *confounding risk ratio* (Miettinen, 1972). Table 3.4 gives the value of the confounding risk ratio for various degrees of association between C and disease, and for different values of p_1 and p_2. It is of interest to note that the confounding risk ratio is considerably less extreme than the association of either C with disease or C with exposure E. Confounding factors have to be strongly associated with both disease and exposure to generate spurious risk ratios greater than, say, two (see, for example, Bross, 1967). One should stress that the aim of the analysis is not to estimate the con-

Table 3.4 Confounding risk ratios associated with varying relative risk (ψ_c), frequency of occurrence of the confounding variable among controls exposed to E (p_1) and not exposed to E (p_2)

Value of p_2	$\psi_c = 2$ Value of p_1 0.1	0.3	0.5	0.8
0.1	1	1.18	1.36	1.64
0.3	0.85	1	1.15	1.38
0.5	0.75	0.87	1	1.20
0.8	0.61	0.72	0.83	1

Value of p_2	$\psi_c = 5$ Value of p_1 0.1	0.3	0.5	0.8
0.1	1	1.57	2.14	3.00
0.3	0.64	1	1.36	1.91
0.5	0.47	0.73	1	1.40
0.8	0.33	0.52	0.71	1

Value of p_2	$\psi_c = 10$ Value of p_1 0.1	0.3	0.5	0.8
0.1	1	1.95	2.80	4.32
0.3	0.51	1	1.49	2.22
0.5	0.35	0.67	1	1.49
0.8	0.23	0.45	0.67	1

founding risk ratio, but to remove the confounding effects. The purpose of Table 3.4 is simply to indicate how large these effects may be.

From (3.1), we see that ψ_p/ψ, the confounding risk ratio, is greater than unity if, and only if, either (a) C is positively associated with both E and with disease ($\psi_c > 1$ and $p_1 > p_2$) or (b) C is negatively associated with both E and with disease ($\psi_c < 1$ and $p_1 < p_2$). Consequently, if the signs of E and C are arranged to make both E and C positively associated with disease, then negative confounding will only occur if the association between E and C is negative. This result is of some value as it provides a mechanism for drawing one's attention to the concealed associations that may result from negative confounding. (Strictly speaking, E and C should be made positively associated with disease after stratification by the other variable; however, in practice, the pre- and post-stratification risk ratios will usually be on the same side of unity).

More general confounding variables

In the previous section we have considered, for a simple dichotomous confounding variable, one of the two major approaches to the treatment of confounding variables, the approach *via* stratification. The extension of this approach to variables taking several levels, or to situations where there are more than two categorical factors under consideration simultaneously, introduces no new conceptual problems. For a polytomous variable which is suspected of being a confounder, one simply stratifies individuals into groups according to the level this variable takes. When several categorical variables are all considered to be potentially confounding, one stratifies simultaneously by them all. For example, if Factor C_1 takes three levels (I, II, III) and Factor C_2 four levels (1, 2, 3, 4), and both are thought to confound the association of Factor E (which we shall take to be dichotomous) with disease, then the data have to be grouped into 12 strata, and the 2×2 tables relating Factor E to disease constructed for each as follows:

The confounding effects of C_1 and C_2 have been eliminated, and we can estimate the independent association of E with disease. Methods for constructing summary estimates of the relative risk associated with E, and summary significance tests, are given in the next chapter. Continuous variables can be incorporated into this approach by dividing up the scale of measurement and treating them as ordered categorical variables.

When the confounding variables take more than two levels, the criteria we discussed for assessing when a dichotomous variable might confound an exposure/disease association need to be slightly relaxed. For dichotomous variables, a factor confounds an association if, and only if, it is associated both with disease and exposure. The "only if" part of this criterion holds for all potentially confounding variables, but with polytomous factors we can construct examples in which a factor is related both to disease and to exposure, but does not confound the disease-exposure association (Whittemore, 1978).

There also needs to be some modification of criteria for assessing confounding when more than one confounding variable is present. In the following example, from Fisher and Patil (1974), we have two confounding variables, C_1 and C_2. Neither one alone confounds the association of E with disease, but the two jointly do confound the association. Stratifying by each of the two possible confounders, in turn, we have:

	No stratification	Stratification by C_1		Stratification by C_2	
		Factor C_1+	Factor C_1-	Factor C_2+	Factor C_2-
	Exposure E + −	Exposure E + −	Exposure E + −	Exposure E + −	Exposure E + −
Case	12 | 30	6 | 15	6 | 15	6 | 15	6 | 15
Control	4 | 22	2 | 11	2 | 11	2 | 11	2 | 11
Odds ratio	2.2	2.2	2.2	2.2	2.2

But, when we stratify by both confounders jointly we have:

	Joint stratification by C_1 and C_2			
	Factor C_1+C_2+ Exposure E + −	Factor C_1+C_2- Exposure E + −	Factor C_1-C_2+ Exposure E + −	Factor C_1-C_2- Exposure E + −
Case	1 | 10	5 | 5	5 | 5	1 | 10
Control	1 | 10	1 | 1	1 | 1	1 | 10
Odds ratio	1	1	1	1

The crude association between E and disease, unaffected by stratification by either C_1 or C_2 alone, disappears upon stratification by both confounders simultaneously. One has to distinguish between the individual confounding effects that variables may have, and the joint confounding effects when variables are considered together.

In the latter case, when considering a set of potential confounders, we can see that there is a *joint* effect only if the *joint* distribution of the confounding variables varies with E conditional on disease status, and varies with disease status conditional on E. The corresponding "if" part of this statement need not apply for a set of confounders, in analogous fashion for a single polytomous variable.

Such situations, however, can be regarded as exceptional, and are mentioned mainly for logical completeness. Normal epidemiological practice is to treat any factor related to disease and exposure as a potential confounder, and there would be few occasions on which one would investigate whether the criteria for joint confounding held (Miettinen, 1974).

Degree of stratification

With several confounding variables, or a single confounder with many values, there is the problem of how fine to make the stratification. If the data are divided into an excessive number of cells, information will be lost; but, if the stratification is too coarse then its object will not be achieved and some confounding will remain. Guidelines can be provided by considering the confounding risk ratio resulting from different levels of stratification. Suppose we have a confounding factor C which can take K levels, and after stratification by E the K levels have associated relative risks $r_1 = 1, r_2, ..., r_K$ (level 1 is baseline). We suppose that these levels occur with frequencies $p_{11}, ..., p_{1K}$, respectively, among the controls exposed to the factor of interest E, and frequencies $p_{21}, ..., p_{2K}$ among controls not exposed to E. As an extension of (3.1) following from (2.16), the confounding risk ratio, which we shall write as w, is the ratio of the odds ratio ψ_p associated with E before stratification by C to the odds ratio ψ after stratification by C, and is given by:

$$w = \frac{\psi_p}{\psi} = \frac{\sum\limits_{k=1}^{K} p_{1k} r_k}{\sum\limits_{k=1}^{K} p_{2k} r_k} \tag{3.2}$$

Now suppose the K levels of C are grouped into a smaller number of levels, say J. Since the p_{1k} and p_{2k} are not the same, the risk among one set of pooled levels relative to the risk among the lowest set of pooled levels may differ between those exposed to E and those not exposed to E. Thus, pooling levels of C may have generated an interaction between C and E. This effect, however, will usually be small, and we shall consider the relative risks in those not exposed to E as summarizing the relative risks in the pooled levels of C. The frequency of occurrence of the J pooled levels of C we shall denote by p^*_{1j} among those exposed to E and by p^*_{2j} among those not exposed to E, $j = 1, ..., J$. The relative risk in the jth pooled level (among those not exposed to E) we shall write as $r^*_j, j = 1, ..., J$, with $r^*_j = 1$. The confounding risk ratio for the pooled levels of C, w^*, say, is then given by:

$$w^* = \frac{\sum\limits_{j=1}^{J} r_j^* p_{1j}^*}{\sum\limits_{j=1}^{J} r_j^* p_{2j}^*} \tag{3.3}$$

Comparison of w^* with w enables one to assess the extent to which the grouped levels of C remove the full confounding effect. The ratio w/w^* is a measure of the residual confounding effect.

The relationship between w^* and w can be examined more closely. The K levels of C have been classed into J groups. Within each group of levels, if the risk ratios and the ratios (p_{1k}/p_{2k}) are not identical, there will be a residual confounding effect and a corresponding residual confounding risk ratio, which for the jth group we will write as w^*_j $(j = 1, \ldots, J)$.

We can then express the overall confounding risk ratio w in terms of the w^*_j as:

$$w = \frac{\sum\limits_{j=1}^{J} w_j^* r_j^* p_{1j}^*}{\sum\limits_{j=1}^{J} r_j^* p_{2j}^*}$$

which gives, from (3.3)

$$\frac{w}{w^*} = \frac{\sum\limits_{j=1}^{J} w_j^* r_j^* p_{1j}^*}{\sum\limits_{j=1}^{J} r_j^* p_{1j}^*} \tag{3.4}$$

The overall measure of residual confounding (w/w^*) is the weighted average over the J groups of the residual confounding risk ratio within each of the grouped levels of C. Computation of the different w^*_j will identify those groups for which finer stratification may be necessary.

As an example, we might consider a study of lung cancer in which interest was focused on an exposure E, other than smoking, and cigarette smoking is to be treated as a confounder. Table 3.5 gives the confounding risk ratio for various possible groupings of cigarette consumption. Data from Doll and Peto (1978) are used for the risk ratios, and the distribution of cigarette consumption among British doctors is used as the distribution among those not exposed to E, i.e., as the values of p_{2k}. The smoking distribution p_{1k} represents a heavy smoking population, an industrially exposed group, for example.

This example has some interesting features. One can see that the grouping 0, 1–9, 10–19, 20–29, 30–40 leaves an inappreciable residual confounding effect and that the grouping 0, 1–19, 20–40 leaves a residual confounding risk ratio of 1.16 at most. A considerable residual confounding effect remains if non-smokers are grouped even with those smoking 1–4 cigarettes a day, underlining the importance of keeping an unexposed group, as stressed in § 3.3. This residual effect makes only a minor contribution to the total confounding effect, as most weight is attached to the heavy smokers (see equation 3.4), but if one is interested in light smokers, this effect is obviously important.

Table 3.5 Residual confounding effects after various degrees of stratification by cigarette consumption

Average daily cigarette consumption	Risk ratio[a]	p_{2i}^a %	p_{1i} %	Grouping, with residual confounding risk ratio within each group						
				I	II	III	IV	V	VI	VII
0	1	38	10	1.0	1.0			1.0		
1–4	5.6	3	2	0.97		1.39	1.39			1.31
5–9	3.2	8	7		1.05				1.57	
10–14	9.4	10	9	1.01		1.01				
15–19	11.3	10	12				1.01			
20–24	23.2	15	15	1.01		1.01	1.01	1.28	1.37	
25–29	24.9	7	15		1.16					1.34
30–34	38.2	5	15	1.02		1.02	1.02		1.16	
35–40	50.7	4	15							
Confounding risk ratio = 1.93				1.91	1.68	1.86	1.51	1.41	1.61	1.44

[a] Data adapted from Doll and Peto (1978)

When stratifying by several confounding variables simultaneously, the joint confounding risk ratio will often be more extreme than either one singly. In fact, if the confounding variables are mutually independent, the joint confounding risk ratio will be the product of the individual confounding risk ratios. If the levels of the different confounding variables are grouped, then the overall residual confounding risk ratio is the product of the individual residual risk ratios. For example, suppose we had two independent confounding variables like that in Table 3.5. The joint confounding risk ratio would be $(1.93)^2 = 3.72$. If both variables are grouped as in column II, the individual residual confounding risk ratios are $1.93/1.68 = 1.15$, whereas the joint residual confounding risk ratio is $(1.15)^2 = 1.32$. Thus for the same level of stratification, the residual confounding effect tends to increase with the number of confounding variables. An increasing penalty is paid if one yields to the temptation to coarsen the stratification as the confounding variables increase in number. The control of confounding by stratification clearly runs into trouble as the number of confounding variables increases, unless one has very large samples. What is required is a method, after a relatively fine stratification of each variable, of combining different strata into roughly homogeneous groups. Various *ad hoc* methods have been proposed, such as the sweep and smear technique (Bunker et al., 1969) or the confounder score index (Miettinen, 1976), but these methods can give incorrect answers (Scott, 1978; Pike, Anderson & Day, 1979), and the unified approach *via* logistic regression is recommended (see Chapters 6 and 7).

Effect of study design on confounding effects

An extreme but not unusual example of positive confounding would be data such as the following:

	Factor C+ Exposure E		Factor C− Exposure E		Pooled levels of C Exposure E	
	+	−	+	−	+	−
Case	90	10	1	9	91	19
Control	9	1	10	90	19	91
Odds ratio	1		1		22.9	

From these tables it can be seen that the cell entries when C is positive differ markedly from the cell entries when C is negative. This lack of balance has two consequences. First, the unequal ratio of cases to controls and the unequal proportion of those exposed to E, in the two post-stratification tables, lead to strong positive confounding. Second, as a reflection of the confounding the minimum cell entries in the two tables obtained after stratification are both much smaller (both equal to one, in fact) than half the minimum cell entry in the pooled table (equal to 19). Thus one can expect the estimate of the odds ratio to be considerably less precise than an estimate obtained from more balanced tables. Both effects can be mitigated by equalizing the ratio of cases to controls in those exposed and those not exposed to a confounder C, in which case we say the design is balanced for Factor C. The results could be represented as follows:

	Factor C+ Exposure E			Factor C− Exposure E			Pooled levels of C Exposure E		
	+	−		+	−		+	−	
Case	a_1	b_1	n_1	a_2	b_2	n_2	a_1+a_2	b_1+b_2	n_1+n_2
Control	c_1	d_1	mn_1	c_2	d_2	mn_2	c_1+c_2	d_1+d_2	$m(n_1+n_2)$
Odds ratio	ψ			ψ			ψ_p		

Balancing or even equalizing cases and controls in each stratum does not eliminate confounding, as the following example illustrates:

	Factor C+ Exposure E		Factor C− Exposure E		Pooled levels of C Exposure E	
	+	−	+	−	+	−
Case	50	50	90	10	140	60
Control	10	90	50	50	60	140
Odds ratio	9		9		5.44	

However, using expression (3.1) and the balance in the design one can show that the odds ratio in the pooled table, ψ_p, lies between unity and ψ, that is we have:

$$1 < \psi_p < \psi, \text{ if } \psi > 1$$

or

$$1 > \psi_p > \psi, \text{ if } \psi < 1.$$

Thus, in contrast to the unbalanced situation, where the confounding effects can be either positive or negative and where the pooled odds ratio can be the opposite side of unity from the within-stratum odds ratio, *with a balanced design the expected pooled odds ratio is both on the same side of and closer to unity than the expected within-stratum odds ratio.* An unstratified analysis will bias the odds ratio towards unity, unless the confounding and exposure variables are (conditional on disease status) independent, but not change the side of unity on which the odds ratio lies.

Obviously the odds ratio of C with disease bears no relation to the true association. *If a factor has been balanced, the data so generated give no information on the association of that factor with disease.* Interaction can still be estimated, however, as is discussed in § 3.5.

Balance, as described above, where the control series is chosen to ensure equal frequency of cases and controls in different strata, is sometimes referred to as frequency matching. On other occasions, where for each case a set of controls is chosen to have the same, or nearly the same, values of prescribed covariates, we speak of individual matching. In later chapters matching refers specifically to individual matching.

Incorporation of matching factors in the analysis

The purpose of matching, as we have just seen, is to control confounding and increase the information per observation in the post-stratification analysis. Most studies, and certainly those of cancer, would match for age and sex, since both could confound the effect of most other factors. A large number of studies match on additional variables, often to the point where each case may be associated with a set of controls in an individual stratum. One purpose of this matching, as we have mentioned, is to improve the precision of the estimates of the relevant relative risks obtained from a stratified analysis. Some matching factors, such as place of residence or membership of a sibship, represent a complex of factors. Then, the purpose of the matching is to eliminate the confounding effect of a range of only vaguely specified variables, since the matching provides a stratification by these variables which would otherwise be difficult to perform because of their indeterminate nature. In these circumstances, matching can be an important way of eliminating bias in the risk estimate. The result given for a dichotomous matching variable can be extended without difficulty to any complexity of matching variables. The expected odds ratio resulting from an analysis incorporating the matching is always more extreme than the expected odds ratio obtained ignoring the matching (Seigel & Greenhouse, 1973).

Now, the purpose of matching implies that the matching factors must *a priori* be considered as ones for which stratification would be necessary, that is, as confounding variables. It would follow *that variables which have been used for matching in the design should be incorporated in the analysis as confounding variables.* Until recently, there were limitations on the type of analysis that could be done which fully incorporated the matching. However, the analytical methods now available do not suffer from these limitations.

The extent to which the analysis should incorporate the matching variables will depend on how the variables are used for matching. If matching is performed only on age and sex then a stratified analysis rather than one which retains individual matching may be more appropriate. Individual matching in the analysis is only necessary if matching in the design was genuinely at the individual level. However, preservation of individual matching, even if artificial, can sometimes have computational advantages and often means little loss of information (see § 7.6).

Overmatching

It might be inferred from our discussion that the post-stratification analysis is always the one of interest, that if we can find a variable which appears to alter the association between disease and the exposure then we should treat that variable as a confounder, but this approach ignores the biological meaning of the variables in question and their position in the sequence of events which leads to disease.

A diagrammatic representation of (positive) confounding might be as follows:

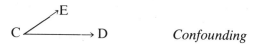

$$C \nearrow^{E} \longrightarrow D \qquad Confounding$$

In many situations, however, such a figure does not correspond to the true state of affairs. Two such situations merit particular attention. The first is when an apparent confounding variable in fact results from the exposure it appears to confound. We could represent this occurrence diagrammatically as

$$E \longrightarrow C \longrightarrow D \qquad Overmatching$$

where C is part of the overall pathway

$$E \longrightarrow \ldots \longrightarrow D.$$

Chronic cough, smoking, and lung cancer can be cited as an example. One would expect the pattern of cigarette smoking among those with chronic cough to be closer to the smoking pattern of lung cancer cases than to that of the general population. The result of stratifying by the presence of chronic cough before diagnosis of lung cancer might almost eliminate the lung cancer-smoking association. The real association between smoking and lung cancer is obscured by the intervention of an intermediate stage in the disease process. A similar example is given by cancer of the endometrium, use of oestrogens and uterine bleeding. If use of oestrogens by postmenopausal women induces uterine bleeding, itself associated with endometrial cancer, then one might expect stratification by a previous history of uterine bleeding to reduce the association between endometrial cancer and oestrogens. If history of chronic cough or a history of uterine bleeding were used as stratifying factors in the respective analyses, or as a matching factor in the design, then one would call the resulting reductions in the

strength of the disease/exposure association examples of
examples, the overmatching consists of using as a confou
presence is caused by the exposure.

A second way in which overmatching may occur is w'
confounder represent the same underlying cause of th
such a situation as:

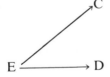

Composite v

C and E now represent different aspects of the same composite factor
to disease. For example, C and E might both be aspects of dietary fibre, or altern...
measures of socioeconomic status. From the diagram it is clear that both should have
equal status as associates of disease. One might, somewhat arbitrarily, decide to take
one of the two, or even attempt to form a composite variable using regression methods.
It would clearly be inappropriate to consider one as confounding the effect of the
other, or to consider the association of one with disease after stratification by the other.

In both the above situations, overmatching will lead to biased estimates of the relative
risk of interest.

A third way in which overmatching may occur is through excessive stratification. The
standard errors of post-stratification estimates of relative risk tend to be larger than
the standard errors of pre-stratification estimates (see § 7.0). Stratification by factors
which are not genuine confounding variables will therefore increase the variability of
the estimates without eliminating any bias, and can be regarded as a type of overmatching. It is commonly seen when data are stratified by a variable known to be
associated with exposure but not in itself independently related to disease. It does not
give rise to bias. If one recalls the section of Chapter 1 relating to overmatching in the
design of a study, one can see close parallels between the different manifestations of
overmatching in the design and the analysis of a study.

We may represent diagrammatically the situation in which a variable is related to
exposure but not to disease as:

$$E \longrightarrow D \qquad \nearrow C$$

No confounding

C is not a genuine confounding variable. Simply by chance, however, substantial
confounding may appear to occur, as the result of random sampling. This eventuality
will arise more often the more strongly E and C are associated. It may be difficult to
decide whether such an event has occurred, and this will normally require consideration
of how C and disease could, logically or biologically, be related. If several studies
have been performed, such confounding may appear as an inconsistency in the results,
with different factors appearing to have confounding effects in different studies. Good
evidence may be available from previous studies that C is not causally related to disease,
in which case it should not be incorporated as a confounder. If, nevertheless, it appears

ong confounding effect, the design of the study should be carefully exam-
ure that it is not acting as a surrogate for some other potential confounder,
rticular that it is not acting through selection bias (see § 3.7).
that the situation

$$E \xrightarrow{\quad C \quad} D$$

may lead to genuine confounding when the variables are measured with error. Consider as an example:

	Factor C+ Exposure E		Factor C− Exposure E		Pooled levels of C Exposure E	
	+	−	+	−	+	−
Case	90	1	10	9	100	10
Control	9	10	1	90	10	100
Odds ratio	100		100		100	

Suppose now that E is misclassified 10% of the time, yielding a variable which we shall denote by E*. The tables become, approximately:

	Factor C+ Exposure E*		Factor C− Exposure E*		Pooled levels of C Exposure E*	
	+	−	+	−	+	−
Case	81	10	10	9	91	19
Control	9	10	10	81	19	91
Odds ratio	9		9		22.9	

The post-stratification odds ratio relating E* to disease is much less than that relating E to disease but in addition a confounding effect has arisen, with a confounding risk ratio of 22.9/9 = 2.54. The odds ratio relating C to disease, after stratification by E*, is 9 rather than 1. The reason is clear: both E* and C are correlates of E, and both are related to disease only through E. Only if E is exactly known does knowledge of C contribute nothing extra to assessment of disease risk.

It is clear from our discussion of confounding that it is not an issue which can be settled on statistical grounds. One has to consider the nature of the variables concerned, and of their relationships with each other and with disease.

Variables to be included as confounding variables

We have considered the conditions under which an observed association may be the result of a confounding effect, and when overmatching might occur, and have discussed the criteria for deciding which factors to incorporate in the analysis as confounding factors when confronting the data from a particular study. Normally there will be two basic aims: first, to remove from the disease/exposure associations of interest all the confounding effects present in the study data set, whether positive or negative; second, to ensure that genuine associations are not reduced by overmatching.

To satisfy the first aim, questions of statistical significance are irrelevant. Given that a confounding factor has to be associated both with disease and with exposure, one might contemplate testing whether both associations are significant in the available data. If their association were not significant, then one might discard the factor as a potential confounder. *This approach is incorrect* (Dales & Ury, 1978), and it can lead to substantial confounding effects remaining in the association, as the following example shows:

Stratification by potential confounder

	Factor C+ Exposure E		Factor C− Exposure E		Pooled levels of C Exposure E	
	+	−	+	−	+	−
Case	80	40	5	5	85	45
Control	8	4	40	40	48	44
Odds ratio	1		1		1.73 ($\chi^2 = 3.91$)	

The association between E and C, after cross-classification by disease status, does not achieve significance at the 5% level: $\chi^2 = 1.63$ using the Mantel-Haenszel χ^2 given by equation (4.23). Thus, in the data C and E are not significantly associated, but an appreciable and statistically significant (at least in the formal sense) association between E and disease exists before stratification by C, which vanishes upon stratification.

With this example in mind, and recalling the initial discussion of overmatching, we can propose three criteria for treating a variable as a confounding variable in the analysis.

1. If a variable C is known from other studies to be related to disease, and if this association is not subsidiary to a possible exposure/disease association, then C should be treated as a confounding variable. The significance of the association between C and disease in the data at hand is of no relevance. Irrespective of the association between E and C in the general population, if there is an association between E and C in the study sample then part of the association between E and disease in the study sample will be a reflection of the causal association between C and disease. The contribution of C to the E-disease association must be eliminated before proceeding to further considerations of a possible causal role for E in disease development. Age and sex will almost always be confounding variables, and should be treated as such.

2. If a variable C is related to disease, but this association is subsidiary to the association between E and disease, by which we mean that either C is caused by E or forms a part of the chain of events by which disease develops from E, then C should not be considered as a confounder of the disease/exposure association.

3. If a factor is thought important enough to be incorporated in the design of the study as a matching or balancing factor, then it should be treated as a confounding variable in the analysis.

In the situation when E and C are known to be related, and if in the data C is also related to disease, then there will be an apparent confounding effect. In this situation, unlike the previous one, it is less clear what the interpretation should be in terms of causality. Incorporating C as a confounding variable implies that one is giving the C-disease association precedence over the E-disease association, which one would not always want to do, as for example when C and E are different measures of the same composite factor. The possibility must be considered that selection bias has operated with respect to C in the choice of either cases or controls or in the manner of acquiring information. Control of this bias may be possible by treating it as if it were a confounding effect. This is discussed in § 3.7.

3.5 Interaction and effect modification

In our discussion of the joint effect of different factors, and specifically in the context of confounding, we have assumed that the odds ratio associating one factor to disease is unaltered by variation in the value of other factors. This simple assumption can only be an approximation, although as we saw in Chapter 2, on many occasions the approximation is fairly close. On other occasions, appreciable variations in the odds ratio were noted, and these variations themselves were of biological importance.

If the odds ratios associating factor A and disease vary with the level of a second factor B, then it is common epidemiological parlance to describe B as an effect modifier. The term is not a particularly happy one, however. A departure from a multiplicative model might arise, for example, if two factors operated in the same way at the cellular level and their joint effect were additive, which would make little sense biologically to describe as effect modification. We prefer to use the term 'interaction', in keeping with usual statistical terminology.

The main reasons for studying interactions are first because they may modify the definition of high risk groups, and second because they may provide insight into disease mechanisms. Interaction implies that in certain subgroups the relative risk associated with exposure is higher than in the rest of the population. Both the specificity of risk for these subgroups, and the fact that the level of exposure-associated risk will be higher than the general risk in the population would tend to increase one's belief in the causal nature of the association, as was discussed earlier in the chapter. The aim should not be to eliminate interactions by suitable transformations, but rather to understand their nature; this point is well made by Rothman (1974).

One should note that using a variable as a matching factor in the design, so that its individual effect on risk cannot be studied, does not alter the interactive effects that the factor may have with other exposures. A simple example will illustrate the point.

	Factor B+ Factor A			Factor B− Factor A		
	+	−		+	−	
Case	50	50	100	25	25	50
Control	5	5	10	20	80	100
Odds ratio		1			4	

Suppose now that the ratio of controls to cases were the same for each level of B. The results would then be, for example:

	Factor B+ Factor A			Factor B− Factor A		
	+	−		+	−	
Case	50	50	100	25	25	50
Control	50	50	100	10	40	50
Odds ratio		1			4	

Thus, the two odds ratios relating factor A to disease for the two levels of B are un-altered, but the odds ratio relating B to disease is greatly modified. Matching does not alter interaction effects between variables used for matching and those not so used.

Analysis of interaction effects

The first step is to investigate if appreciable interactions are present. In the simplest situation, one may just wish to test whether the relative risks in two groups, defined perhaps by age or some other dichotomized variable, are the same; the type of test proposed in Chapter 4 would be appropriate. In more complex situations, two approaches are possible. First, the observed distribution of the exposure variables among the cases and controls can be compared with the distribution under the multiplicative model (see § 2.6). Patterns in the departures of observed from expected may indicate the superiority of an alternative model for the joint action. With two or three variables which can be stratified into a few categories each, the presentation is simple, as shown in Table 3.6 for data relating oral cancer risk to use of tobacco and alcohol (from Wynder, Bross & Feldman, 1957; see also Rothman, 1976). The expected values, obtained using unconditional maximum likelihood methods (Chapter 6, particularly § 6.6) enable one to examine the adequacy of the overall fit of the multiplicative model. In Table 3.6, the fit is good. A feature of Table 3.6 is that apparently substantial differences in the odds ratios can arise from fairly small differences between observed and expected numbers of cases and controls in a cell. The cell corresponding to < 1 units of alcohol/day and 34+ cigarettes/day is an example.

Table 3.6 Risk for oral cancer associated with alcohol and tobacco[a]

A. Observed and expected number of cases in each smoking and drinking category, with the observed number of controls

Alcohol (average consumption in units/day)	Tobacco (cigarettes/day) ≤15			16–20			21–34			34+		
	Obs. Cont.	Obs. Cases	Exp. Cases	Obs. Cont.	Obs. Cases	Exp. Cases	Obs. Cont.	Obs. Cases	Exp. Cases	Obs. Cont.	Obs. Cases	Exp. Cases
<1	31	16	18.84	19	25	22.54	13	12	13.67	3	13	10.96
1–2	8	7	6.07	18	19	19.10	5	5	5.51	5	10	10.32
3–6	8	20	18.47	16	40	42.14	5	24	22.54	4	19	19.84
6+	2	10	9.62	5	30	30.22	4	35	34.28	4	40	40.88

B. Observed and expected relative risks in each smoking and drinking category

Alcohol (average consumption in units/day)	Tobacco (cigarettes/day) ≤15		16–20		21–34		34+	
	Obs.	Exp.	Obs.	Exp.	Obs.	Exp.	Obs.	Exp.
<1	1.00	1.00	2.55	1.57	1.79	1.80	8.41	3.24
1–2	1.70	1.00	2.05	1.57	1.94	1.80	3.88	3.24
3–6	4.85	2.85	4.85	4.47	9.31	5.10	9.21	9.23
6+	9.70	6.03	11.64	9.47	16.98	10.85	19.37	19.53

[a] From Wynder, Bross and Feldman (1957)

If significant or appreciable interaction terms are present, one would then attempt to understand the nature of their effect. First, examination of the discrepancies between the observed numbers and those expected under the no-interaction model may indicate that the interaction corresponds to unsystematic but excessive variation. It is a common feature of epidemiological data to show variation slightly higher than that theoretically expected on the basis of random sampling considerations. Since the excess variation probably arises from minor unpredictable irregularities in data collection, one would suspect that it is due mainly to chance, augmented perhaps by variation of extraneous factors.

A second interpretation of the departures from a multiplicative model may be that the variables interact in a different way. An obvious alternative would be to try to fit an additive model for the relative risks. The data on occupational exposure, cigarette smoking and bladder cancer from Boston (Cole, 1973) suggest a better fit for an additive model, as do data on use of oestrogens at the menopause, obesity and risk for endometrial cancer (Mack et al., 1976).

A third interpretation is that specific groups, as defined by the interactive factors, are at higher risk due either to greater susceptibility or to greater exposure. An example of greater susceptibility with age at exposure is provided by the variation in risk for breast cancer due to irradiation (Boice & Stone, 1978). An example of differences in exposure is given by the risk for cancer of the lung and nasal sinuses among nickel refinery workers in South Wales (Doll, Mathews & Morgan, 1977). The risk appears confined to those first employed before 1930. Changes in the operation of the refinery at that time could, quite plausibly, have removed the carcinogenic agents, and the change in risk assists in identifying what those agents may have been.

3.6 Modelling risk

The use of stratification and cross-tabulation to investigate the joint effect on risk of two variables, in terms of how the two factors mutually confound each other and interact, is reasonably straightforward. However, even with two variables, as the number of values each variable can take increases, the control of confounding by means of stratification can lead to substantial losses of information, and tests for interaction will lack power. As the complexity of the problem increases, the approach *via* stratification becomes not only unwieldy but increasingly wasteful of information. The different effects associated with different levels of a variable will not normally be unrelated, and can be expected to change smoothly. For example, for a quantitative variable, risk will usually vary in a manner which can be described by a simple family of curves. It would be rare to need more than second degree terms, after perhaps some initial transformation of the scale.

Similarly, interactive effects between several variables will not normally vary in a structureless way, and general experience has been that most situations are well described by some simple structure of the interactions. These considerations lead to the use of regression methods, in which the risk associated with each variable is expressed as some explicit function, and interaction effects are described in terms of the specific parameters of interest. Chapters 6 and 7 are devoted to the development of these methods, which will not be further discussed here except to outline briefly their advantages. These can be summarized as follows:

1. One can study the joint effect of several exposures simultaneously. The stratification approach we considered earlier places the emphasis on one specific exposure. Study of the combined risk associated with several exposures is an important complement of the single exposure analysis.
2. When the number of levels of the confounding variables increases, one can remove their effect as fully as by fine stratification but with less loss of information.
3. One can test for specific interaction effects of interest with the considerable increase in power this provides. One also obtains a parametric description of the interaction.
4. The risk associated with different levels of a quantitative variable can be expressed in simple and descriptive terms.

In studies where controls are individually matched to cases, these advantages are accentuated, as Chapters 5 and 7 make apparent. But regression methods should not replace analyses based on cross-tabulation, rather they should complement and extend them, as we illustrate in Chapter 6.

3.7 Comparisons between more than two groups

So far, we have considered methods of analysis appropriate for comparisons between one case group and one control group. Situations occur, however, when comparisons among more than two groups are required. One may want to test whether the relative risk for some factor is the same over different subcategories of disease, for example, different histological types of lung cancer or different subsites of the oesophagus or the large bowel. Or one may want to test whether the results obtained using different control groups can be taken as equivalent, or whether observed differences are easily explained as chance phenomena. The approach most commonly taken is an informal one, in which one calls attention to appreciable differences in risk when comparisons are made between different pairs of groups, but one does not attempt a formal test of significance.

The methods presented in Chapters 6 and 7 can be extended to the comparison of more than two groups. In particular, if the study design incorporated individual matching, then a dummy variable, indicating disease subcategory could be introduced and interaction examined between this dummy variable and the exposure of interest. However, investigating heterogeneity of disease subcategory or of type of control group by introducing interaction terms is only appropriate if, for each stratum, every individual belongs to one disease subcategory or one control group. If within a stratum more than two groups are represented, then the underlying probability structure needs extension. One cannot simply write

$$pr(\text{control}) = 1 - pr(\text{case}).$$

One has to generalize this expression to

$$\sum_i pr(\text{case, disease category i}) + \sum_j pr(\text{control, type j}) = 1$$

Mantel (1966) and Prentice and Breslow (1978) have indicated how a generalized logistic function, appropriate to this situation, can be formed and how the various estimation and hypothesis-testing procedures can be derived. The only difficulty in practical use is that the number of parameters can become unwieldy.

One would anticipate that the generalized logistic model will be used more in the future than it has been in the past, at least in the context of epidemiological studies. But, in this monograph we will not consider its development any further, since computer programmes are not readily available to put the techniques in operation, and no important matter of principle is involved. Extensions of the regression models of Chapters 6 and 7 are conceptually simple, and with some labour could be made operational.

3.8 Considerations affecting interpretation of the analysis

The interpretation of a study will depend not only on the numerical results of various analyses, but also on more general considerations of how the study was conducted, the nature of the factors under investigation and the consistency with other studies done in the same field. We conclude this chapter by a brief discussion of some of these aspects.

Bias

Bias is a property of the design of a study and was discussed in Chapter 1. Various features can be incorporated in the design which permit at least partial assessment of the extent of possible bias; these features are selection of different types of control groups, different series of cases, or different ways of obtaining similar information.

One can include in the study, for example, cases of cancers at different sites, to demonstrate whether the observed effects are specific for the site of interest. An example of this procedure is given by Cook-Mozaffari et al. (1979) in a study of oesophageal cancer in Iran. Frequent practice is to use both a hospital and a population series of controls. If recall and selection bias are present then they should be different in the two groups, and the divergence between the results should indicate the extent of the biasing effect.

The effects of design bias can sometimes be controlled in the analysis in the same way as one controls for confounding. Thus suppose that, whether by selection bias or differential recall, the relative representation of some factor in the case and control groups is different from the relative representation in the study population, and that this factor is related to the exposure of interest. Then, even if the factor does not confound the exposure/disease association in the underlying population, an apparent confounding effect will be seen in the data at hand which can be controlled in the same way as other confounding effects. Care must be taken to ensure that overmatching does not result. Stratification or adjustment by a factor leads to an increase in the variance of the estimates of parameters of interest and routine adjustment by factors for which there is no reason to suspect bias will lead to a loss of information.

More generally, the effects of bias will often be the creation of apparent confounding effects, but little information may be available on the specific variable involved. As in § 3.4, one can assess the strength of association that must exist between these hidden confounding variables and both disease risk and the exposure of interest for the observed association to be due to bias. Biases have to be strong to generate relative risks greater than twofold.

Missing data

Sufficient control should normally be exercised over the conduct of a study to ensure that few, if any, of the data that one intended to collect are missing. Sometimes, however, source documents such as hospital records may be lost or otherwise missing, or respondents may be unable to supply the information required or be unwilling to answer certain questions. The essential point when faced with missing data is to be aware that the occurrence is usually not a random event. The probability that data are missing will be associated with the exposures one is studying, or with disease status or both. If information on some variable is unavailable for any more than a small percentage of individuals, then inferences about that variable will be of doubtful value.

Common practice is to eliminate from analyses including a certain variable all individuals for whom information on that variable is missing. In a matched pair design, the individual matched to an eliminated individual will also be eliminated. Since the individuals eliminated will often form a selected group, their elimination can lead to a biased estimate of relative risk. An attempt can be made to estimate the degree of bias involved. One approach is to replace missing values by the two extreme values, thus bracketing the true results. An alternative, for categorical variables, is to create an additional category for missing data. The relative risk for this category will give an indication of the degree of bias.

If one can be sure that no bias relates to the absence of data, for example, the accidental loss of biological samples, then one might consider using some of the powerful techniques that have recently been developed for data missing at random (Demster, Laird & Rubin, 1977). These techniques have the advantage that an individual's entire record is not discarded just because a single datum is missing.

Errors of classification

Errors in classifying disease status and in measuring the exposure variables may both be appreciable. For the former, it has long been realized that a certain proportion of the controls may be at an early stage of disease and should have been diagnosed as cases. Under most circumstances, one might expect this proportion and hence the effect to be small, but when the disease under study is particularly common, the effect may become appreciable. The consequence is the same as when misdiagnosed cases are included in the disease group. Both errors lead to underestimates of the relative risk.

Errors of measurement in the exposure variables have been considered by several authors (Bross, 1954; Newell, 1963; Goldberg, 1975; Barron, 1977). Here the effect is also to reduce the apparent risk, unless the errors are linked in some unusual manner to confounding variables. For a dichotomous exposure variable, with a probability Φ of misclassifying an exposed case or control and a probability ϑ of misclassifying a non-exposed person, we have:

$$\text{True odds ratio } \psi = p_1(1-p_0)/p_0(1-p_1)$$

but

$$\text{Observed odds ratio} = \frac{(p_1 + \vartheta/d) \{(1-p_0) + \Phi/d\}}{(p_0 + \vartheta/d) \{(1-p_1) + \Phi/d\}}$$

where p_1 is the true probability of exposure among cases, p_0 the exposure probability for controls, and $d = 1 - \Phi - \vartheta$.

For example, if $p_0 = 0.3$ and $p_1 = 0.1$, with the true relative risk $\psi = 3.9$, then misclassification rates of 10% ($\Phi = \vartheta = 0.1$) will reduce the relative risk to 2.4, and misclassification of 20% reduces the relative risk to 1.7. It should be remembered that sometimes one is not measuring precisely the factor of interest, and that for this reason assessments of the importance of a factor may be too modest. Dietary items would be clear examples; current epidemiological methods are certainly inadequate for estimating retrospectively the intake of dietary fibre or animal fat. Demonstration of an effect for either of these items in a case-control study would be virtually all one could expect, and estimates of relative risk, or attributable risk, are likely to be serious understatements of the real effect. As another example, weak associations (i.e., relative risks of 1.5 or 2) between HLA antigens and disease, particularly locus A or B antigens, are often interpreted as indicating the existence of genes at other loci of the HLA region which are strongly associated with disease.

The problem of multiple comparisons

The results of studies are often presented as if the only variables included in the study were those which *a posteriori* showed association with disease. One has to distinguish between factors which are clearly part of the main hypothesis motivating the study, and those which were included in the study for less obvious reasons. Disease associations demonstrated for the former can be interpreted without consideration of multiple comparisons, but for the latter one or two factors out of a hundred in the study are expected to be significant at the 1% level (this issue is well discussed in the paper by Mantel and Haenszel, 1959). The area where this consideration is most explicitly acknowledged is in the study of genetic polymorphisms and disease, perhaps because non-confirmatory repeat studies are relatively easy to perform. In studies of HLA antigens, for example, it is now required practice to correct nominal significance levels obtained from the 2×2 tables for each antigen by the number of antigens tested (i.e., comparisons). This correction may in fact be over-conservative, especially if interest is mainly directed at the more common antigens, but correction procedures based on, say, a full Bayesian analysis would probably be too complex. A test of association not requiring correction for the number of antigens, based on the multivariate estimates of gene frequencies, has been proposed in this context (Rogentine et al., 1972).

In other areas, when a study has investigated many factors, a few of which achieve nominal significance in the analysis, the interpretation must be cautious, and further studies would be needed to confirm the association. A good example is given by the first report of an association between use of reserpine and risk for breast cancer (Boston Collaborative Drug Surveillance Program, 1974). This study emanated from the Boston Drug Surveillance Program, and the reported association was one out of several hundred possible comparisons (i.e., perhaps 20 tumour sites and 10 or 15 different drugs). As the result on its own was thus uninterpretable, publication was delayed until two further studies had been performed (Armstrong, Stevens & Doll, 1974; Heinonen et al., 1974).

It must always be recognized that no study can be regarded in isolation; the results of each must be viewed in the light of all other relevant information.

REFERENCES

Aksoy, M., Erdem, S. & Dinçol, G. (1974) Leukemia in shoe workers exposed chronically to benzene. *Blood, 44,* 837–841

Anderson, D.E. (1974) Genetic study of breast cancer: identification of a high risk group. *Cancer, 34,* 1090–1097

Armstrong, B., Stevens, N. & Doll, R. (1974) Retrospective study of the association between use of Rauwolfia derivatives and breast cancer in English women. *Lancet, ii,* 672–675

Barron, B.A. (1977) The effects of misclassification on the estimation of relative risk. *Biometrics, 33,* 414–418

Billewicz, W.Z. (1965) The efficiency of matched samples: an empirical investigation. *Biometrics, 21,* 623–643

Boice, J.D. & Monson, R. (1977) Breast cancer in women after repeated fluoroscopic examinations of the chest. *J. natl Cancer Inst., 59,* 823–832

Boice, J.D. & Stone, B.J. (1978) *Interaction between radiation and other breast cancer risk factors.* In: *Late Biological Effects of Ionizing Radiation,* Vol. I, Vienna, International Atomic Energy Agency, pp. 231–249

Boston Collaborative Drug Surveillance Program (1974) Reserpine and breast cancer. *Lancet, ii,* 669–671

Bross, I. (1954) Misclassification in 2×2 tables. *Biometrics, 10,* 478–486

Bross I.J. (1967) Pertinency of an extraneous variable. *J. chron. Dis., 20,* 487–497

Bross, I. & Tidings, J. (1973) Another look at coffee drinking and cancer of the urinary bladder. *Prev. Med., 2,* 445–451

Bunker, J.P., Forrest, W.H., Mosteller, F. & Vandám, L.D., eds (1969) *The National Halothane Study,* Washington DC, US Government Printing Office

Casagrande, J., Gerkins, V., Henderson, B.E., Mack, T. & Pike, M.C. (1976) Exogenous estrogens and breast cancer in women with natural menopause. *J. natl Cancer Inst., 56,* 839–841

Cole, P. (1971) Coffee drinking and cancer of the lower urinary tract. *Lancet, i,* 1335–1337

Cole, P. (1973) *A population-based study of bladder cancer.* In: Doll, R. & Vodopija, I., eds, *Host Environment Interactions in the Etiology of Cancer in Man,* Lyon, International Agency for Research on Cancer *(IARC Scientific Publications No. 7),* pp. 83–87

Cook-Mozaffari, P.J., Azordegan, F., Day, N.E., Ressicaud, A., Sabai, C. & Aramesh, B. (1979) Oesophageal cancer studies in the Caspian littoral of Iran: results of a case-control study. *Br. J. Cancer, 39,* 293–309

Cornfield, J., Haenszel, W., Hammond, E.C., Lilienfeld, A.M., Shimkin, M.B. & Wynder, E.L. (1959) Smoking and lung cancer: recent evidence and a discussion of some questions. *J. natl Cancer Inst., 22,* 173–203

Cox, D.R. (1957) A note on grouping. *J. Am. stat. Assoc., 52,* 543–547

Dales, L.G. & Ury, H.K. (1978) An improper use of statistical significance testing in studying covariables. *Int. J. Epidemiol., 7,* 373–377

Demster, A.P., Laird, N.M. & Rubin, D.B. (1977) Maximum likelihood from incomplete data via the EM algorithm (with discussion). *J. R. stat. Soc. B., 39,* 1–38

Doll, R. (1969) *Preface.* In: Kreyberg, L., ed., *Aetiology of Lung Cancer,* Oslo, Universitetsforlaget, pp. 9–10

Doll, R. (1971) The age distribution of cancer. Implication for models of carcinogenesis. *J. R. stat. Soc. A, 134,* 133–155

Doll, R. & Peto, R. (1976) Mortality in relation to smoking: 20 years' observation on male British doctors. *Br. med. J., ii,* 1525–1536

Doll, R. & Peto, R. (1978) Cigarette smoking and bronchial carcinoma: dose and time relationships among regular smokers and life long non-smokers. *J. Epidemiol. Community Health, 32,* 303–313

Doll, R., Mathews, J.D. & Morgan, L.G. (1977) Cancer of the lung and nasal sinuses in nickel workers: a reassessment of the period of risk. *Br. J. ind. Med., 34,* 102–105

Fisher, L. & Patil, K. (1974) Matching and unrelatedness. *Am. J. Epidemiol., 100,* 347–349

Fraumeni, J.F., Scotto, J. & Dunham, L.J. (1971) Coffee drinking and bladder cancer. *Lancet, ii,* 1204

Goldberg, J. (1975) The effect of misclassification on the bias in the difference between two proportions and the relative odds in the fourfold table. *J. Am. stat. Assoc., 70,* 561–567

Heinonen, O.P., Shapiro, S., Tuominen, L. & Turunen, M.I. (1974) Reserpine use in relation to breast cancer. *Lancet, ii,* 675–677

Herbst, A.L., Ulfelder, H. & Poskanzer, D.C. (1971) Adenocarcinoma of the vagina. *New Engl. J. Med., 284,* 878–881

Hill, A.B. (1965) The environment and health: association or causation. *Proc. R. Soc. Med., 58,* 295–300

Hoover, R. & Fraumeni, J.F. (1973) Risk of cancer in renal transplant recipients. *Lancet, ii,* 55–57

Infante, P.F., Rivisky, R.A. & Wagoner, J.F. (1977) Leukaemia in benzene workers. *Lancet, ii,* 76–78

Jick, H., Watkins, R.M., Hunter, J.R., Dinan, B.J., Madsen, S., Rothman, K.J. & Walker, A.M. (1979) Replacement estrogens and endometrial cancer. *New Engl. J. Med., 300,* 218–222

Mack, T., Pike, M.C., Henderson, B.E., Pfeffer, R.I., Gerkins, V.R., Arthur, M. & Brown, S.E. (1976) Estrogens and endometrial cancer in a retirement community. *New Engl. J. Med., 294,* 1262–1267

MacLennan, R., Da Costa, J., Day, N.E., Law, C.H., Ng, Y.K. & Shanmugaratnam, K. (1977) Risk factors for lung cancer in Singapore Chinese, a population with high female incidence rates. *Int. J. Cancer, 20,* 854–860

Mantel, N. (1966) Models for complex contingency tables and polychotomous dosage response curves. *Biometrics, 22,* 83–95

Mantel, N. & Haenszel, W. (1959) Statistical aspects of the analysis of data from the retrospective study of disease. *J. natl Cancer Inst., 22,* 719–748

McGregor, D.H., Land, C.E., Choi, K., Tokuoka, S., Liu, P.I., Wakabayashi, T. & Beebe, G.W. (1977) Breast cancer incidence among atomic bomb survivors, Hiroshima and Nagasaki, 1950–69. *J. natl Cancer Inst., 59,* 799–811

Miettinen, O.S. (1972) Components of the crude risk ratio. *Am. J. Epidemiol., 96,* 168–172

Miettinen, O.S. (1974) Confounding and effect modification. *Am. J. Epidemiol., 100,* 350–353

Miettinen, O.S. (1976) Stratification by a multivariate confounder score. *Am. J. Epidemiol., 104,* 609–620

Newell, D.J. (1963) Misclassification in 2 × 2 tables. *Biometrics, 19,* 187–188

Peto, R. (1977) *Epidemiology, multi-stage models and short-term mutagenicity tests.* In: Hiatt, H.H., Watson, J.D. & Winston, J.A., eds, *Origins of Human Cancer,* Cold Spring Harbor, NY, Cold Spring Harbor Publications, pp. 1403–1428

Pike, M.C., Anderson, J. & Day, N. (1979) Some insight into Miettinen's multivariate confounder score approach to case-control study analysis. *J. Epidemiol. Community Health, 33,* 104–106

Prentice, R. & Breslow, N.E. (1978) Retrospective studies and failure time models. *Biometrika, 65,* 153–158

Report of the Surgeon General (1964) *Smoking and Health,* Washington DC, US Government Printing Office *(DHEW Publication No. 1103)*

Rogentine, G.N., Yankee, R.A., Gart, J.J., Nam, J. & Traponi, R.J. (1972) HLA antigens and disease: acute lymphocytic leukemia. *J. clin. Invest., 51,* 2420–2428

Rothman, K.J. (1974) Synergy and antagonism in cause-effect relationships. *Am. J. Epidemiol., 99,* 385–388

Rothman, K.J. (1976) The estimation of synergy or antagonism. *Am. J. Epidemiol., 103,* 506–511

Schlesselman, J.J. (1978) Assessing effects of confounding variables. *Am. J. Epidemiol., 108,* 3–8

Scott, R.C. (1978) The bias problem in sweep-and-smear analysis. *J. Am. stat. Assoc., 73,* 714–718

Seidmann, H., Lilis, R. & Selikoff, I.J. (1977) *Short-term asbestos exposure and delayed cancer risk.* In: Nieburgs, H.E., ed., *Prevention and Detection of Cancer,* Part 1: *Prevention,* Vol. I: *Etiology,* New York, Marcel Dekker, Inc., pp. 943–960

Seigel, D.G. & Greenhouse, S.W. (1973) Validity in estimating relative risk in case-control studies. *J. chron. Dis., 26,* 219–226

Simon, D., Yen, S. & Cole, P. (1975) Coffee drinking and cancer of the lower urinary tract. *J. natl Cancer Inst., 54,* 587–593

Smith, P.G. & Doll, R. (1978) *Age- and time-dependent changes in the rates of radiation-induced cancers in patients with ankylosing spondylitis following a single course of x-ray treatment.* In: *Late Biological Effects of Ionizing Radiation,* Vol. I, Vienna, International Atomic Energy Agency, pp. 205–218

Tulinius, H., Day, N.E., Johannesson, G., Bjarnason, O. & Gonzalez, M. (1978) Reproductive factors and risk for breast cancer in Iceland. *Int. J. Cancer, 21,* 724–730

Whittemore, A.S. (1977a) *Epidemiologic implications of the multi-stage theory of carcinogenesis.* In: Whittemore, A.S., ed., *Environmental Health Quantitative Methods,* Philadelphia, SIAM, pp. 73–87

Whittemore, A.S. (1977b) The age distribution of human cancers for carcinogenic exposures of varying intensity. *Am. J. Epidemiol., 106,* 518–532

Whittemore, A.S. (1978) The collapsibility of multi-dimensional contingency tables. *J. R. stat. Soc. B, 40,* 328–340

Wynder, E.L. & Stellman, S.D. (1979) Impact of long-term filter cigarette usage on lung and larynx cancer risk: a case-control study. *J. natl Cancer Inst., 62,* 471–479

Wynder, E.L., Bross, I.J. & Feldman, R.M. (1957) A study of the etiological factors in cancer of the mouth. *Cancer, 10,* 1300–1323

LIST OF SYMBOLS – CHAPTER 3 (in order of appearance)

E	Exposure
C	Confounder
a	Number of exposed cases
b	Number of non-exposed cases
c	Number of exposed controls
d	Number of non-exposed controls

n_1	Number of cases
n_0	Number of controls
m_1	Number exposed
m_0	Number non-exposed
N	Total number
$\psi_p = ad/bc$	Pooled odds ratio relating E and disease
a_1	Number of exposed cases at 1st level of C
a_2	Number of exposed cases at 2nd level of C

(similarly for b, c, d, n_1, n_0, m_1, m_0, N)

$$\psi_1 = \frac{a_1 d_1}{b_1 c_1} = \quad \text{odds ratio relating E and disease at level 1, factor C}$$

$$\psi_2 = \frac{a_2 d_2}{b_2 c_2} = \quad \text{odds ratio relating E and disease at level 2, factor C}$$

ψ	common value of ψ_1 and ψ_2, assuming they are equal; within stratum odds ratio
ψ_c	odds ratio relating C and disease after stratification by E
p_1	proportion of exposed controls who are at level 1(+) of C
p_2	proportion of non-exposed controls who are at level 1(+) of C
$w = \psi_p/\psi$	confounding risk ratio
r_k	relative risk associated with level k of a confounder C
p_{1k}	proportion of exposed controls who are at level k of factor C
p_{2k}	proportion of non-exposed controls who are at level k of factor C
r^*_j	relative risk associated with j^{th} combination of levels of a confounder C
p^*_{1j}	proportion of exposed controls having the jth combination of levels of factor C
p^*_{2j}	proportion of non-exposed controls having the jth combination of levels of factor C
w^*	confounding risk ratio when K levels of factor C are grouped into J combinations (see equation 3.3)
M	ratio of controls to cases in a balanced design
Φ	probability that an exposed case or control is mistakenly classified as non-exposed
ϑ	probability that a non-exposed case or control is mistakenly classified as exposed
p_1	exposure probability for cases
p_0	exposure probability for controls

4. CLASSICAL METHODS OF ANALYSIS OF GROUPED DATA

4.1 The Ille-et-Vilaine study of oesophageal cancer

4.2 Exact statistical inference for a single 2×2 table

4.3 Approximate statistical inference for a 2×2 table

4.4 Combination of results from a series of 2×2 tables; control of confounding

4.5 Exposure at several levels: the $2 \times K$ table

4.6 Joint effects of several risk factors

CHAPTER IV

CLASSICAL METHODS OF ANALYSIS OF GROUPED DATA

This chapter presents the traditional methods of analysis of case-control studies based on a grouping or cross-classification of the data. The main outlines of this approach, which has proved extremely useful for practising epidemiologists, are contained in the now classic paper by Mantel and Haenszel (1959). Most of the required calculations are elementary and easily performed on a pocket calculator, especially one that is equipped with log, exponential and square-root keys. Rothman and Boice (1979) have recently published a set of programmes for such a calculator which facilitates many of the analyses presented below.

The statistical procedures introduced in this chapter are appropriate for study designs in which stratification or "group-matching" is used to balance the case and control samples *vis-à-vis* the confounding variables. The following chapter develops these same methods of analysis for use with designs in which there is individual matching of cases to controls. While our treatment of this material attempts to give the reader some appreciation of its logical foundations, the emphasis is on methodological aspects rather than statistical theory. Some of the more technical details are labelled as such and can be passed over on a first reading. These are developed fully in the excellent review papers by Gart (1971, 1979) on statistical inferences connected with the odds ratio. Fleiss (1973) presents an elementary and very readable account of many of the same topics. Properties of the binomial, normal and other statistical distributions mentioned in this chapter may be found in any introductory text, for example Armitage (1971).

4.1 The Ille-et-Vilaine study of oesophageal cancer

Throughout this chapter we will illustrate the various statistical procedures developed by applying them to a set of data collected by Tuyns et al. (1977) in the French department of Ille-et-Vilaine (Brittany). Cases in this study were 200 males diagnosed with oesophageal cancer in one of the regional hospitals between January 1972 and April 1974. Controls were a sample of 778 adult males drawn from electoral lists in each commune, of whom 775 provided sufficient data for analysis. Both types of subject were administered a detailed dietary interview which contained questions about their consumption of tobacco and of various alcoholic beverages in addition to those about foods. The analyses below refer exclusively to the role of the two factors, alcohol and tobacco, in defining risk categories for oesophageal cancer.

Table 4.1 summarizes the relevant data. Since no attempt had been made to stratify the control sample, there is a tendency for the controls to be younger than the cases,

Table 4.1   Distribution of risk factors for cases and controls: Ille-et-Vilaine study of oesophageal cancer[a]

	Cases	Controls
Age (years)		
25–34	1	115
35–44	9	190
45–54	46	167
55–64	76	166
65–74	55	106
75+	13	31
Mean	60.0	50.2
S.D	9.2	14.3
Alcohol (g/day)		
0–39	29	386
40–79	75	280
80–119	51	87
120+	45	22
Mean	84.9	44.4
S.D	48.4	31.9
Tobacco (g/day)		
0–9	78	447
10–19	58	178
20–29	33	99
30+	31	51
Mean	16.7	10.5
S.D	12.9	11.9

[a] Data taken from Tuyns et al. (1977)

Table 4.2   Correlations between risk variables in the control sample: Ille-et-Vilaine study of oesophageal cancer[a]

	Age	Tobacco	Alcohol
Age	1.0	−0.02	−0.02
Tobacco		1.0	0.15
Alcohol			1.0

[a] Data taken from Tuyns et al. (1977)

a feature which has to be accounted for in the analysis. Cases evidently have a history of heavier consumption of both alcohol and tobacco than do members of the general population. Correlations among these risk variables in the population controls indicate that there are no systematic linear trends of increased or decreased consumption with age, and that the two risk variables are themselves only weakly associated (Table 4.2).

To take an initial look at the relationship between alcohol and risk using traditional epidemiological methods, we might dichotomize alcohol consumption, using as a cut-off point the value (80 g/day) closest to the median for the cases, as there are many more controls. This yields the basic 2×2 table:

Average daily alcohol consumption

	80+ g	0–79 g	Total
Cases	96	104	200
Controls	109	666	775
Total	205	770	975

Of course such a simple dichotomization into "exposed" and "unexposed" categories can obscure important information about a risk variable, particularly concerning dose-response (§ 3.2). Summarizing the entire set of data in a single table ignores the possible confounding effects of age and tobacco (§ 3.4); these two deficiencies are momentarily ignored.

From the data in this or any similar 2×2 table one wants to estimate the relative risk and also to assess the degree of uncertainty inherent in that estimate. We need to know at what level of significance we can exclude the null hypothesis that the true relative risk ψ is equal to unity, and we need to determine a range of values for ψ which are consistent with the observed data. Appropriate methods for making such tests and estimates are presented in the next two sections.

4.2 Exact statistical inference for a single 2×2 table[1]

When a single stratum of study subjects is classified by two levels of exposure to a particular risk factor, as in the preceding example, the data may be summarized in the ubiquitous 2×2 table:

	Exposed	Unexposed	
Diseased	a	b	n_1
Disease-free	c	d	n_0
	m_1	m_0	N

(4.1)

A full understanding of the methods of analysis of such data, and their rationale, requires that the reader be acquainted with some of the fundamental principles of statistical inference. We thus use this simplest possible problem as an opportunity to review the basic concepts which underlie our formulae for statistical tests, estimates and confidence intervals.

Inferential statistics and analyses, as opposed to simple data summaries, attempt not only to describe the results of a study in as precise a fashion as possible but also to assess the degree of uncertainty inherent in the conclusions. The starting point for

---

[1] Parts of this section are somewhat technical and specialized; they may be skimmed over at first reading.

such analyses is a *statistical model* for the observed data which contains one or more *unknown parameters*. Two such models for the 2×2 table were introduced implicitly in the discussion in § 2.8. According to the first, which can be called the cohort model, the marginal totals of m_1 exposed and m_0 unexposed persons are regarded as fixed numbers determined by the sample size requirements of the study design. There are two unknown parameters, the probabilities P_1 and P_0 of developing the disease during the study period. Since subjects are assumed to be sampled at random from the exposed and unexposed subpopulations, the *sampling distribution* of the data is thus the product of two *binomial* distributions with parameters (P_1, m_1) and (P_0, m_0). In the second model, which is more appropriate for case-control studies, the marginal totals n_1 and n_0 are regarded as fixed by design. The distribution of the data is again a product of two binomials, but this time the parameters are (p_1, n_1) and (p_0, n_0) where p_1 and p_0 are the exposure probabilities for cases and controls.

According to § 2.8 the key parameter for case-control studies is the odds ratio ψ, partly because it takes on the same value whether calculated from the exposure or the disease probabilities. The fact that the probability distributions of the full data depend on two parameters, either (P_1, P_0) or (p_1, p_0), complicates the drawing of conclusions about the one parameter in which we are interested. Hypotheses that specify particular values for the odds ratio, for example, the hypothesis $H_0 : \psi = 1$ of no association between exposure and disease, do not completely determine the distribution of the data. Statistics which could be used to test this hypothesis depend in distribution on *nuisance* parameters, in this case the baseline disease or exposure probabilities. Inferences are much simpler if we can find another probability distribution, using perhaps only part of the data, which depends exclusively on the single parameter of interest.

A distribution which satisfies this requirement is the *conditional distribution of the data assuming all the marginal totals are fixed*. Cox (1970) and Cox and Hinkley (1974) discuss several abstract principles which support the use of this distribution. Its most important property from our viewpoint is that the (conditional) probability of observing a given set of data is the same whether one regards those data as having arisen from a case-control or a cohort study. In other words, the particular sampling scheme which was used does not affect our inferences about ψ. Regardless of which of the two product binomial models one starts with, the probability of observing the data (4.1) conditional on all the marginal totals n_1, n_0, m_1, m_0 remaining fixed is

$$\mathrm{pr}(a \mid n_1, n_0, m_1, m_0; \psi) = \frac{\binom{n_1}{a}\binom{n_0}{m_1-a} \psi^a}{\sum_u \binom{n_1}{u}\binom{n_0}{m_1-u} \psi^u} \qquad (4.2)$$

Here $\binom{n}{u}$ denotes the *binomial coefficient*

$$\binom{n}{u} = \frac{n(n-1)(n-2)\ldots(n-u+1)}{u(u-1)(u-2)\ldots(1)}$$

which arises in the binomial sampling distribution. The summation in the denominator is understood to range over all values u for the number of exposed cases (a) which are possible given the configuration of marginal totals, namely $0, m_1 - n_0 \leqq u \leqq m_1, n_1$.

Two aspects of the conditional probability formula (4.2) are worthy of note. First, we have expressed the distribution solely in terms of the number a of exposed cases. This is adequate since knowledge of a, together with the marginal totals, determines the entire 2×2 table. Expressing the distribution in terms of any of the other entries (b, c or d) leads to the same formula either for ψ or for ψ^{-1}. Second, the formula remains the same upon interchanging the roles of n and m, which confirms that it arises from either cohort or case-control sampling schemes.

As an example, consider the data

2	1	3
3	1	4
5	2	7

(4.3)

The possible values for a determined by the margins are a = 1, 2 and 3, corresponding to the two tables

1	2	3
4	0	4
5	2	7

and

3	0	3
2	2	4
5	2	7

in addition to that shown in (4.3). Thus the probability (4.2) for a = 2 may be written

$$
\frac{\binom{3}{2}\binom{4}{3}\psi^2}{\binom{3}{1}\binom{4}{4}\psi + \binom{3}{2}\binom{4}{3}\psi^2 + \binom{3}{3}\binom{4}{2}\psi^3}
$$

$$
= \frac{\dfrac{3 \times 2}{2 \times 1} \times \dfrac{4 \times 3 \times 2}{3 \times 2 \times 1}\psi^2}{\dfrac{3}{1} \times \dfrac{4 \times 3 \times 2 \times 1}{4 \times 3 \times 2 \times 1}\psi + \dfrac{3 \times 2}{2 \times 1} \times \dfrac{4 \times 3 \times 2}{3 \times 2 \times 1}\psi^2 + \dfrac{3 \times 2 \times 1}{3 \times 2 \times 1} \times \dfrac{4 \times 3}{2 \times 1}\psi^3}
$$

$$
= \frac{12\psi^2}{3\psi + 12\psi^2 + 6\psi^3} = \frac{4\psi}{1 + 4\psi + 2\psi^2} .
$$

Similarly, the probabilities of the values a = 1 and a = 3 are $1/(1 + 4\psi + 2\psi^2)$ and $2\psi^2/(1 + 4\psi + 2\psi^2)$, respectively.

Estimation of ψ

The distribution (4.2) for $\psi \neq 1$ is known in the probability literature as the *non-central hypergeometric distribution*. When $\psi = 1$ the formula becomes considerably simpler and may be written

$$\text{pr}(a \mid n_1, n_0, m_1, m_0; \psi = 1) = \frac{\binom{n_1}{a}\binom{n_0}{m_1 - a}}{\binom{n_1 + n_0}{m_1}}, \tag{4.4}$$

which is the (central) hypergeometric distribution. So called *exact* inferences about the odds ratio ψ are based directly on these conditional distributions. The *conditional maximum likelihood estimate* $\hat{\psi}_{\text{cond}}$, i.e., the value which maximizes (4.2), is given by the solution to the equation

$$a = E(a \mid n_1, n_0, m_1, m_0; \psi), \tag{4.5}$$

where E denotes the expectation of the discrete distribution. For example, with the data (4.3) one must solve

$$2 = \frac{1 + 8\psi + 6\psi^2}{1 + 4\psi + 2\psi^2},$$

a quadratic equation with roots $\pm\sqrt{\frac{1}{2}}$, of which the positive solution is the one required. Note that this estimate, $\hat{\psi}_{\text{cond}} = \sqrt{\frac{1}{2}} = 0.707$, differs slightly from the *empirical odds ratio* $\frac{ad}{bc} = \frac{2}{3} = 0.667$. Unfortunately, if the data are at all extensive, (4.5) defines a polynomial equation of high degree which can only be solved by numerical methods.

Tests of significance

Tests of the hypothesis that ψ takes on a particular value, say $H:\psi = \psi_0$, are obtained in terms of *tail probabilities* of the distribution (4.2). Suppose, for example, that $\psi_0 = 10$. The conditional probabilities associated with each of the three possible values for a are then:

a	$\text{pr}(a \mid 3,4,5,2; \psi = 10)$
1	$\dfrac{1}{1 + 40 + 200} = 0.004$
2	$\dfrac{40}{1 + 40 + 200} = 0.166$
3	$\dfrac{200}{1 + 40 + 200} = 0.830$

Having observed the data (4.3), in which a = 2, the *lower* tail probability, $p_L = 0.004 +$ $0.166 = 0.17$, measures the degree of evidence against the hypothesis $H:\psi = 10$ in favour of the alternative hypothesis that $\psi<10$. While the data certainly suggest that $\psi<10$, the fact that p_L exceeds the conventional significance levels of 0.01 or 0.05 means that the evidence against H is weak. Much stronger evidence would be provided if a = 1, in which case the *p-value* or *attained significance level* is 0.004.

More generally, the lower tail probability based on the distribution (4.2) is defined by

$$p_L = \sum_{u \leq a} \mathrm{pr}(u \mid n_1, n_0, m_1, m_0; \psi_0) \tag{4.6}$$

and measures the degree of evidence against the hypothesis $H:\psi = \psi_0$ in favour of $\psi<\psi_0$. Similarly, the upper tail probability

$$p_U = \sum_{u \geq a} \mathrm{pr}(u \mid n_1, n_0, m_1, m_0; \psi_0) \tag{4.7}$$

measures the degree of evidence against H and in favour of $\psi>\psi_0$. In both cases the summation is over values of u consistent with the observed marginal totals, with u less than or equal to the observed a in (4.6) and greater than or equal to a in (4.7). If no alternative hypothesis has been specified in advance of the analysis, meaning we concede the possibility of a putative "risk factor" having either a protective or deleterious effect, it is common practice to report twice the minimum value of p_L and p_U as the attained significance level of a *two-sided* test[1].

The hypothesis most often tested is the *null* hypothesis $H_0:\psi = 1$, meaning no association between risk factor and disease. In this case the tail probabilities may be computed relatively simply from the (central) hypergeometric distribution (4.4). The resulting test is known as *Fisher's exact test*. For the data in (4.3) the exact upper p-value is thus

$$\left\{ \binom{3}{2}\binom{4}{3} + \binom{3}{3}\binom{4}{2} \right\} \div \binom{7}{5} = 18/21 = 0.86,$$

while the lower p-value is

$$\left\{ \binom{3}{1}\binom{4}{4} + \binom{3}{2}\binom{4}{3} \right\} \div \binom{7}{5} = 15/21 = 0.71,$$

neither of them, of course, being significant.

Confidence intervals

Confidence intervals for ψ are obtained by a type of testing in reverse. Included in the two-sided interval with a specified *confidence coefficient* of $100(1-\alpha)\%$ are all values ψ_0 which are *consistent with the data* in the sense that the two-sided p-value

---

[1] An alternative procedure for computing two-sided p-values is to add $p_{min} = \min(p_L, p_U)$ to the probability in the opposite tail of the distribution obtained by including as many values of the statistic as possible without exceeding p_{min}. This yields a somewhat lower two-sided p-value than simply doubling p_{min}, especially if the discrete probability distribution is concentrated on only a few values.

for the test of $H: \psi = \psi_0$ exceeds α. In other words, the confidence interval contains those ψ_0 such that both p_L and p_U exceed $\alpha/2$, where p_L and p_U depend on ψ_0 as in (4.6) and (4.7). In practice, the interval is determined by two endpoints, a *lower confidence limit* ψ_L and an *upper confidence limit* ψ_U. The upper limit satisfies the equation

$$\alpha/2 = \sum_{u \leq a} \mathrm{pr}(u \,|\, n_1, n_0, m_1, m_0; \psi_U) \qquad (4.8)$$

while the lower limit satisfies

$$\alpha/2 = \sum_{u \geq a} \mathrm{pr}(u \,|\, n_1, n_0, m_1, m_0; \psi_L). \qquad (4.9)$$

Thus the exact upper $100(1-\alpha)\% = 80\%$ confidence limit for the data (4.3) is obtained from the equation

$$\alpha/2 = 0.10 = \frac{1 + 4\psi}{1 + 4\psi + 2\psi^2},$$

with solution $\psi_U = 18.25$, while the lower limit solves

$$\alpha/2 = 0.10 = \frac{4\psi + 2\psi^2}{1 + 4\psi + 2\psi^2},$$

with solution $\psi_L = 0.0274$. Since there are so few data in this example, most reasonable values of ψ are consistent with them and the interval is consequently very wide.

Although such exact calculations are feasible with small 2×2 tables like (4.3), as soon as the data become more extensive they are not. The equations for conditional maximum likelihood estimation and confidence limits all require numerical methods of solution which are not possible with pocket calculators. Thomas (1971) provides an algorithm which enables the calculations to be carried out on a high-speed computer, but extensive data will render even this approach impracticable. Fortunately, with such data, the exact methods are not necessary. We next show how approximations may be obtained for the estimates, tests and confidence intervals described in this section which are more than accurate enough for most practical situations. Occasionally the exact methods, and particularly Fisher's exact test, are useful for resolving any doubts caused by the small numbers which might arise, for example, when dealing with a very rare exposure. The exact procedures are also important when dealing with matched or finely stratified samples, as we shall see in Chapters 5 and 7.

4.3 Approximate statistical inference for a 2×2 table

The starting point for approximate methods of statistical inference is the *normal approximation* to the conditional distribution. When all four cell frequencies are large, the probabilities (4.2) are approximately equal to those of a continuous normal distribution whose mean $A = A(\psi)$ is the value which a must take on in order to give an empirical or calculated odds ratio of ψ (Hannan & Harkness, 1963). In other words, to find the *asymptotic mean* we must find a number A such that when A replaces a, and the remaining table entries are filled in by subtraction

A	B = n_1–A	n_1
C = m_1–A	D = n_0–m_1 + A	n_0

$$m_1 \qquad\qquad m_0 \qquad\qquad N$$

$$\text{(4.10)}$$

we have

$$\frac{AD}{BC} = \frac{A(n_0-m_1+A)}{(n_1-A)(m_1-A)} = \psi. \tag{4.11}$$

This is a quadratic equation, only one of whose roots yields a possible value for A in the sense that A, B, C and D are all positive. Under the special null hypothesis $H_0 : \psi = 1$, the equation simplifies and we calculate

$$A(1) = \frac{m_1 n_1}{N}, \tag{4.12}$$

which is also the mean of the exact distribution (4.4). The quantities A, B, C and D in (4.10) are known as *fitted values* for the data under the hypothesized ψ.

Once A is found and the table is completed as in (4.10), the *variance* Var = Var($a;\psi$) of the approximating normal distribution is defined in terms of the reciprocals of the fitted values

$$\text{Var} = \left[\frac{1}{A} + \frac{1}{B} + \frac{1}{C} + \frac{1}{D}\right]^{-1}. \tag{4.13}$$

When $\psi = 1$ this reduces to

$$\text{Var}(a;\psi = 1) = \frac{n_1 n_0 m_1 m_0}{N^3},$$

whereas the variance of the corresponding exact distribution is slightly larger

$$\text{Var}(a;\psi = 1) = \frac{n_1 n_0 m_1 m_0}{N^2(N-1)}. \tag{4.14}$$

Using the approximating normal distribution in place of (4.2) leads to computationally feasible solutions to the problems outlined earlier.

Estimation

The asymptotic maximum likelihood estimate is obtained by substituting the asymptotic mean A(ψ) for the right-hand side of (4.5) and solving for ψ. This yields

$$\hat{\psi} = \frac{ad}{bc},$$

the observed or empirical odds ratio, whose use in (4.11) leads to A($\hat{\psi}$) = a as required. It is reassuring that these somewhat abstract considerations have led to the obvious estimate in this simple case; in other more complicated situations the correct or "best" estimate is not at all obvious but may nevertheless be deduced from analogous considerations. The empirical odds ratio is also the *unconditional* maximum likelihood estimate based on the two parameter product binomial distribution mentioned earlier.

Tests of significance

Large sample hypothesis tests are obtained *via* normal approximations to the tail probabilities (4.6) and (4.7) of the discrete conditional distribution. Figure 4.1 illustrates this process schematically. The approximating continuous distribution is first chosen to have the same mean and variance as the discrete one. Probabilities for the continuous distribution are represented by areas under the smooth curve, and for the discrete distribution by the areas of the rectangles centred over each possible value. Thus the exact probability in the right tail associated with the observed value 8 consists of the sum of the areas of the rectangles over 8, 9 and 10. It is clear from the diagram that this is best approximated by taking the area under the continuous curve from $7^{1}/_{2}$ to infinity. If we did not subtract $^{1}/_{2}$ from the observed value but instead took the area under the normal curve from 8 to infinity as an approximate p-value, we would underestimate the actual tail probability of the discrete distribution. More generally, if the values of the discrete distribution are spaced a constant distance Δ units apart, it would be appropriate *to reduce the observed value by* $^{1}/_{2}\,\Delta$ before referring it to a continuous distribution for approximation of an upper tail probability. Similarly, in the lower tail, the observed value would be increased by $^{1}/_{2}\,\Delta$. Such an adjustment of the test statistic is known as the *continuity correction*.

Since the hypergeometric distribution takes on integral values, for the problem at hand $\Delta = 1$. Thus the approximating tail probabilities may be written

and

$$p_U \approx 1 - \Phi\left(\frac{a-A-{}^{1}/_{2}}{\sqrt{\mathrm{Var}}}\right)$$

$$p_L \approx \Phi\left(\frac{a-A+{}^{1}/_{2}}{\sqrt{\mathrm{Var}}}\right)$$

(4.15)

where A and Var are the null mean and variance defined in (4.12) and (4.14), and Φ is the cumulative of the standard normal distribution. For a one-tailed test we generally report the upper tail probability, provided that the alternative hypothesis $\psi > 1$ has been specified before the study or it was the only one plausible. Similarly, for a one-tailed test against $\psi < 1$ we report p_L; however, for a two-tailed test, appropriate when the direction of the alternative cannot be specified in advance, we report twice the minimum value of p_L and p_U.

A convenient way of carrying out these calculations is in terms of the *corrected chi-square statistic*[1]:

$$\chi^2 = \frac{(|a-A|-{}^{1}/_{2})^2}{\mathrm{Var}} = \frac{(|ad-bc|-{}^{1}/_{2}N)^2\,(N-1)}{n_0 n_1 m_0 m_1}.$$

(4.16)

---

[1] N-1 is often replaced by N in this expression.

Fig. 4.1 Normal approximation to discrete probability distribution. Note that the discrete probabilities for the values 8, 9 and 10 are better approximated by the area under the normal curve to the right of $7^1/_2$ than by the area under the normal curve to the right of 8.

ZZZZZZ = normal distribution from $7^1/_2$ to infinity

NNNNNN = discrete probabilities for the values 8, 9, and 10.

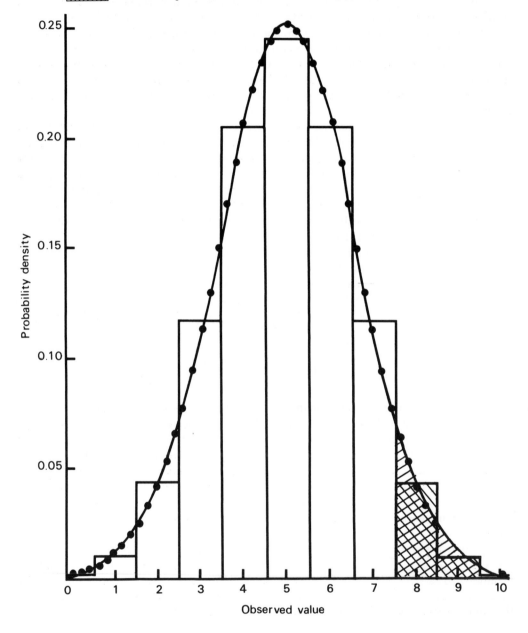

Referring this statistic to tables of percentiles of the chi-square distribution with one degree of freedom yields the approximate *two-sided* significance level, which may be halved to obtain the corresponding single-tail test.

There is no doubt that the $^{1}/_{2}$ continuity correction in (4.15) and (4.16) results in a closer approximation to the p-values obtained from the exact test discussed in the last section (Mantel & Greenhouse, 1968). Since the conditional distribution involves only the odds ratio as a parameter, and thus permits the derivation of point estimates, confidence intervals and significance tests in a unified manner, we feel it is the most appropriate one for assessing the evidence from any given set of data, and we therefore recommend the $^{1}/_{2}$ correction. This point, however, is somewhat controversial. Some authors argue that the exact test is inappropriate and show that more powerful tests can be constructed (for example, Liddell, 1978). These tests are not based on the conditional distribution, and their significance values are influenced by nuisance parameters.

It is important to recognize that when the sample is small we cannot rely on the asymptotic normal distribution to provide a reasonable approximation to the exact test. A general "rule of thumb" is that the approximations to significance levels in the neighbourhood of 0.05 or larger are reasonably good, providing that the *expected* frequencies for all four cells in the 2×2 tables are at least 5 under the null hypothesis (Armitage, 1971). These expectations may need to be considerably larger if p-values less than 0.05 are to be well approximated. For smaller samples, or when in doubt, recourse should be made to Fisher's exact test.

Cornfield's limits

Cornfield (1956) suggested that confidence intervals for the relative risk be obtained by approximating the discrete probabilities in (4.8) and (4.9). This leads to the equations

$$a - A(\psi_L) - {}^{1}/_{2} = Z_{\alpha/2}\sqrt{\mathrm{Var}(a; \psi_L)}$$

and

$$a - A(\psi_U) + {}^{1}/_{2} = -Z_{\alpha/2}\sqrt{\mathrm{Var}(a; \psi_U)}$$

(4.17)

for the lower and upper limit, respectively. Here $Z_{\alpha/2}$ is the $100(1-\alpha/2)$ percentile of the standard normal distribution (e.g., $Z_{.025} = 1.96$), while $A(\psi)$ and $\mathrm{Var}(a; \psi)$ are defined by (4.11) and (4.13). Cornfield's limits provide the best approximation to the exact limits (4.8) and (4.9), and come closest to achieving the nominal specifications (e.g., 95% confidence) of any of the confidence limits considered in this section (Gart & Thomas, 1972). Unfortunately the equations (4.17) are quartic equations which must be solved using iterative numerical methods. While tedious to obtain by hand, their solution has been programmed for a high-speed computer (Thomas, 1971).

The rule of thumb used to judge the adequacy of the normal approximation to the exact test may be extended for use with these approximate confidence intervals (Mantel & Fleiss, 1980). For 95% confidence limits, one simply establishes that the ranges $A(\psi_L) \pm 2\sqrt{\mathrm{Var}(a; \psi_L)}$ and $A(\psi_U) \pm 2\sqrt{\mathrm{Var}(a; \psi_U)}$ are both contained within the range of possible values for a. More accurate confidence limits are of course obtained if the mean and variance of the exact conditional distribution are substituted in (4.17) for A and Var; however, this requires solution of polynomial equations of an even higher order.

Logit confidence limits

A more easily calculated set of confidence limits may be derived from the normal approximation to the distribution of log $\hat{\psi}$ (Woolf, 1955). This has mean log ψ and a large sample variance which may be estimated by the sum of the reciprocals of the cell entries

$$\text{Var}(\log \hat{\psi}) = \frac{1}{a} + \frac{1}{b} + \frac{1}{c} + \frac{1}{d}. \qquad (4.18)$$

Consequently, approximate $100(1-\alpha)\%$ confidence limits for log ψ are

$$\log \psi_U, \log \psi_L = \log \hat{\psi} \pm Z_{\alpha/2}\sqrt{\text{Var}(\log \hat{\psi})} \qquad (4.19)$$

which may be exponentiated to yield ψ_L and ψ_U. Gart and Thomas (1972) find that such limits are generally too narrow, especially when calculated from small samples. Since log $\hat{\psi}$ is the difference between two logit transformations (see Chapter 5), the limits obtained in this fashion are known as *logit limits*.

Test-based confidence limits

Miettinen (1976) has provided an even simpler and rather ingenious method for constructing confidence limits using only the point estimate and χ^2 test statistic. Instead of using (4.18), he solves

$$\frac{\log^2(\hat{\psi})}{\text{Var}(\log \hat{\psi})} = \chi^2,$$

for the variance of $\log(\hat{\psi})$, arguing that both left and right side provide roughly equivalent statistics for testing the null hypothesis $\psi = 1$. This technique is of even greater value in complex situations where significance tests may be fairly simple to calculate but precise estimates for the variance require more effort.

Substituting the test-based variance estimate into (4.19) yields the approximate limits

$$\psi_L, \psi_U = \hat{\psi}^{(1 \pm Z_{\alpha/2}/\chi)}, \qquad (4.20)$$

where $\hat{\psi}$ is raised to the power $(1 \pm Z_{\alpha/2}/\chi)$. Whether ψ_L corresponds to the $-$ sign in this expression and ψ_U to the $+$ sign, or vice versa, will depend on the relative magnitude of $Z_{\alpha/2}$ and χ. The χ^2 statistic (4.16), however, should be calculated *without the continuity correction* especially when $\hat{\psi}$ is close to unity, since otherwise the variance may be overestimated and the limits too wide. In those rare cases where $\hat{\psi}$ is exactly equal to unity, the uncorrected χ^2 is equal to zero and the test-based limits are consequently undefined.

Halperin (1977) pointed out that the test-based variance estimate is strictly valid only if $\psi = 1$. When case and control sample sizes are equal ($n_1 = n_0$) the variance for other values of ψ is systematically underestimated by this approach, the true average probability is less than the nominal $100(1-\alpha)\%$, and the resulting confidence limits are too narrow (Gart, 1979). If there are large differences in the numbers of cases and controls, the true variance of log $\hat{\psi}$ may sometimes be overestimated and the resulting limits will be too wide. Nevertheless the test-based limits may be advocated on the basis of their simplicity since they yield numerical results which are often in reasonable agreement with the other procedures and of sufficient accuracy for many practical purposes, at least when the estimated relative risk is not too extreme. They also provide convenient initial values from which to start the iterative solution of the equations for the more accurate limits, if these are desired.

Example: We illustrate these calculations with data from the 2×2 table shown in § 4.1. The (unconditional) maximum likelihood estimate of the relative risk is:

$$\hat{\psi} = \frac{96 \times 666}{104 \times 109} = 5.64,$$

while the corrected χ^2 test statistic is

$$\chi^2 = \frac{(|196 \times 666 - 104 \times 109| - \frac{1}{2}\, 975)^2\, 974}{200 \times 775 \times 770 \times 205} = 108.11$$

corresponding to a two-sided significance level of $p<0.0001$. The uncorrected χ^2 is slightly larger at 110.14. We use this latter value for determining the test-based 95% confidence intervals. These are

$$\psi_U, \psi_L = 5.64^{\,(1 \pm 1.96/\sqrt{110.14})} = 4.08, 7.79.$$

To calculate the logit limits we need

$$\text{Var}(\log \hat{\psi}) = \frac{1}{96} + \frac{1}{104} + \frac{1}{109} + \frac{1}{666} = 0.0307,$$

leading to limits for log ψ of log $5.65 \pm 1.96 \times \sqrt{0.0307} = 1.730 \pm 0.343$, i.e., $\psi_L = 4.00$ and $\psi_U = 7.95$. By way of contrast, the Cornfield limits (4.17) yield $\psi_L = 3.94$ and $\psi_U = 8.07$.

For these data the logit limits are wider than the test-based limits, reflecting the fact that the estimated odds ratio is far from unity and the test-based variance is therefore too small. Both the logit and the test-based limits are too narrow in comparison with Cornfield's limits, but the magnitude of the discrepancy is not terribly great from a practical viewpoint. To gauge the accuracy of the normal approximation used to derive the Cornfield limits, following the procedure suggested by Mantel and Fleiss, we need to calculate the means and variances of the number of exposed cases under each of the two limits. The means are obtained as the solution for $A = A(\psi)$ in the quadratic equations (4.11)

$$\frac{A(775 - 205 + A)}{(200 - A)(205 - A)} = \psi$$

for $\psi = \psi_L$ and ψ_U, namely:

$$A(\psi_L) = A(3.94) = 84.22$$

corresponding to fitted frequencies of

84.22	115.78	200
120.78	654.22	775
205	770	

and variance of

$$Var(a; \psi' = 3.94) = \left[\frac{1}{84.22} + \frac{1}{115.78} + \frac{1}{120.78} + \frac{1}{654.22} \right]^{-1} = 32.98;$$

and

$$A(\psi'_U) = A(8.07) = 107.48$$

with fitted frequencies

107.48	92.52	200
97.52	677.48	775
205	770	

and variance of

$$Var(a; \psi' = 8.07) = \left[\frac{1}{107.48} + \frac{1}{92.52} + \frac{1}{97.52} + \frac{1}{677.48} \right]^{-1} = 31.40.$$

It is instructive to verify that the empirical odds ratios calculated from the fitted frequencies satisfy

$$\frac{84.22 \times 654.22}{115.78 \times 120.78} = 3.94 = \psi'_L$$

and

$$\frac{107.48 \times 677.48}{97.52 \times 92.52} = 8.07 = \psi'_U,$$

respectively. The actual range of possible values for a is max(0,205–775) to min(200,205), i.e., (0,200). This is much broader than the intervals including two standard deviations on both sides of the fitted means $84.22 \pm 2\sqrt{32.98} = (72.7, 95.7)$ and $107.48 \pm 2\sqrt{31.40} = (96.3, 118.7)$. Hence there is little doubt about the accuracy of the normal approximation for these data.

4.4 Combination of results from a series of 2×2 tables; control of confounding

The previous two sections dealt with a special situation which rarely occurs in practice. We have devoted so much attention to it in order to introduce, in a simplified setting, the basic concepts needed to solve more realistic problems, such as those posed by the presence of nuisance or confounding factors. Historically one of the most important methods for control of confounding has been to divide the sample into a series of strata which were internally homogeneous with respect to the confounding factors. Separate relative risks calculated *within* each stratum are free of bias arising from confounding (§ 3.4).

In such situations one first needs to know whether the association between exposure and disease is reasonably constant from stratum to stratum. If so, a summary measure of relative risk is required together with associated confidence intervals and tests of significance. If not, it is important to describe how the relative risk varies according to changes in the levels of the factors used for stratum formation. In this chapter we emphasize the calculation of summary measures of relative risk and tests of the hypothesis that it remains constant from stratum to stratum. Statistical models which are particularly suited to evaluating and describing *variations* in relative risk are introduced in Chapters 6 and 7.

Example continued: Since incidence rates of most cancers rise sharply with age, this must always be considered as a potential confounding factor. We have already noted that the Ille-et-Vilaine cases were on average about ten years older than controls (Table 4.1). If age were also related to alcohol consumption, this would indicate that confounding existed in the data and we would expect to see the age-adjusted relative risk change accordingly. We know from Table 4.2, however, that age and alcohol are not strongly correlated, so that in this case the confounding effect may be minimal. Nevertheless we introduce age-stratification in order to illustrate the basic process.

Dividing the population into six 10-year age intervals yields the following series of 2×2 tables, whose sum is the single 2×2 table considered earlier (§ 4.1):

Age (years)		Daily alcohol consumption 80+ g	0–79 g	Odds ratio
25–34	Case	1	0	∞
	Control	9	106	
35–44	Case	4	5	5.05
	Control	26	164	
45–54	Case	25	21	5.67
	Control	29	138	
55–64	Case	42	34	6.36
	Control	27	139	
65–74	Case	19	36	2.58
	Control	18	88	
75+	Case	5	8	∞
	Control	0	31	

Some 0 cells occur in the youngest and oldest age groups, which have either a small number of cases or a small number of exposed. While these two tables do not by themselves provide much useful information about the relative risk, the data from them may nevertheless be combined with the data from other tables to obtain an overall estimate. There appears to be reasonable agreement between the estimated relative risks for the other four age groups, with the possible exception of that for the 65–74-year-olds.

A full analysis of such a series of 2×2 tables comprises: (1) a test of the null hypothesis that $\psi = 1$ in all tables; (2) point and interval estimation of ψ assumed to be common to all tables; and (3) a test of the homogeneity or no-interaction hypothesis that ψ is constant across tables. Of course if this latter hypothesis is rejected, the results from (1) and (2) are of little interest. In this situation it is more important to try to understand and describe the sources of variation in the relative risk than simply to provide a summary measure.

The entries in the ith of a series of I 2×2 tables may be identified as follows:

	Exposed	Unexposed	
Cases	a_i	b_i	n_{1i}
Controls	c_i	d_i	n_{0i}
	m_{1i}	m_{0i}	N_i

(4.21)

Conditional on fixed values for the marginal totals n_{1i}, n_{0i}, m_{0i} in each table, the probability distribution of the data consists of a product of I non-central hypergeometric terms of the form (4.2). A completely general formulation places no restriction on the odds ratios ψ_i in each table, but in most of the following we shall be working under the hypothesis that they are equal, $\psi_i = \psi$.

Summary chi-square: test of the null hypothesis

Under the hypothesis of no association, the expectation and variance of the number of exposed cases a_i in the ith table are:

$$A_i(1) = \frac{n_{1i}m_{1i}}{N_i},$$

and

(4.22)

$$\mathrm{Var}(a_i; \psi = 1) = \frac{n_{1i}n_{0i}m_{1i}m_{0i}}{N_i^2(N_i-1)},$$

respectively (see equations 4.12 and 4.14). If the odds ratio is the same in each table, we would expect the a_i to be generally either larger ($\psi > 1$) or smaller ($\psi < 1$) than their mean values when $\psi = 1$. Hence an appropriate test is to compare the total $\Sigma_i a_i$ of the exposed cases with its expected value under the null hypothesis, dividing the difference by its standard deviation. The test statistic, corrected for the discrete nature of the data, may be written

$$\chi^2 = \frac{\left(\left| \sum_{i=1}^{I} a_i - \sum_{i=1}^{I} A_i(1) \right| - \frac{1}{2} \right)^2}{\sum_{i=1}^{I} \mathrm{Var}(a_i; \psi = 1)}.$$

(4.23)

This summary test was developed by Cochran (1954) and by Mantel and Haenszel (1959), with the latter suggesting use of the exact variances (4.22). Referring χ^2 to tables of the chi-square distribution with one degree of freedom provides two-sided significance levels for evaluating the null hypothesis; these may be halved for a one-tail test.

Mantel and Fleiss (1980) suggest an extension of the "rule of 5" for evaluating the adequacy of the approximation to the exact p-value obtained from the summary chi-square statistic. They first calculate the maximum and minimum values that the total number of the exposed cases Σa_i may take subject to fixed marginals in each of the contributing 2×2 tables. These are $\Sigma \min(m_{1i}, n_{1i})$ for the maximum and $\Sigma \max(0, m_{1i} - n_{0i})$ for the minimum, respectively. Provided that the calculated mean value under the null hypothesis $\Sigma A_i(1)$ is at least five units away from both these extremes, the exact and approximate p-values should agree reasonably well for p's in the range of 0.05 and above. Similar considerations apply when evaluating the accuracy of the normal approximation in setting confidence limits (see equation 4.27 below). Here the mean values $\Sigma A_i(\psi)$ calculated at the confidence limits ψ_L and ψ_U for the odds ratio should both be at least $2\sqrt{\Sigma_i \text{Var}(a_i; \psi)}$ units away from the minimum and maximum values.

Logit estimate of the common odds ratio[1]

Woolf (1955) proposed that a combined estimate of the log relative risk be calculated simply as a weighted average of the logarithms of the observed odds ratios in each table. The best weights are inversely proportional to the estimated variances shown in (4.18). Thus the logit estimate $\hat{\psi}_1$ is defined by

$$\log \hat{\psi}_1 = \frac{\Sigma w_i \log \left(\dfrac{a_i d_i}{b_i c_i} \right)}{\Sigma w_i} \tag{4.24}$$

$$\text{where } w_i = \left\{ \frac{1}{a_i} + \frac{1}{b_i} + \frac{1}{c_i} + \frac{1}{d_i} \right\}^{-1}.$$

The variance of such an estimate is given by the reciprocal of the sum of the weights, namely

$$\text{Var}(\log \hat{\psi}_1) = \left(\Sigma w_i \right)^{-1}.$$

While the logit estimate behaves well in large samples, where all cell frequencies in all strata are of reasonable size, it runs into difficulty when the data are thin. For one thing, if any of the entries in a given table are 0, the log odds ratio and weight for that table are not even defined. The usual remedy for this problem is to add $^1/_2$ to each entry before calculating the individual odds ratios and weights (Gart & Zweifel, 1967; Cox, 1970). However the estimate calculated in this fashion is subject to unacceptable bias when combining information from large numbers of strata, each containing only a few cases or controls (Gart, 1970; McKinlay, 1978); thus it is not recommended for general use.

---

[1] This and the following subsections may be omitted at a first reading as they discuss, for the sake of completeness, estimates of the common odds ratio which are not used in the sequel.

Maximum likelihood estimate

The maximum likelihood estimate (MLE) of the common odds ratio is found by equating totals of the observed and expected numbers of exposed cases:

$$\sum_{i=1}^{I} a_i = \sum_{i=1}^{I} E(a_i \mid n_{1i}, n_{0i}, m_{1i}, m_{0i}; \psi).$$ (4.25)

For the exact or conditional MLE the expectations $E(a_i)$ are calculated under the non-central hypergeometric distributions (4.2), which means solution of a high degree polynomial equation. While the computational burden is thus sufficient to rule out use of this estimate for routine problems, a computer programme is available for special circumstances (Thomas, 1975). Calculation of the variance of the conditional MLE requires the variance of the conditional distribution and access to another computer programme (Zelen, 1971; Breslow, 1976).

For the unconditional MLE, based on the distribution of all the data without assuming fixed margins for each 2×2 table, the expectations $E(a_i)$ in (4.25) are those of the approximating normal distributions. Thus the estimation procedure requires finding fitted frequencies for all the cells, as in (4.10), such that the total of the observed and fitted numbers of exposed cases agree (Fienberg, 1977). While iterative calculations are also required here, they are generally less arduous than for the exact estimate and do not become any more complicated when the numbers in each cell are increased. As discussed in § 6.5, general purpose computer programmes for fitting logistic regression or log linear models may be used to find the unconditional MLE and estimates of its variance.

When there are many strata, each containing small numbers of cases and controls, the unconditional MLE is biased in the sense of giving values for ψ which are systematically more extreme (further from unity) than the true odds ratio. Numerical results on the magnitude of this bias in some special situations are given in Chapter 7. While the conditional MLE is not subject to this particular problem, it may be computationally burdensome even when there is ready access to an electronic computer. Hence none of the estimates considered so far are sufficiently simple or free of bias to be recommended for general use by the non-specialist.

The Mantel-Haenszel (M-H) estimate

Mantel and Haenszel (1959) proposed as a summary relative risk estimate the statistic

$$\hat{\psi}_{mh} = \frac{\sum_{i=1}^{I} a_i d_i / N_i}{\sum_{i=1}^{I} b_i c_i / N_i},$$ (4.26)

which can be recognized as a weighted average of the individual odds ratios $\hat{\psi}_i = (a_i d_i) / (b_i c_i)$, with weights $b_i c_i / N_i$ which approximate the inverse variances of the individual estimates when ψ is near 1.

The Mantel-Haenszel (M–H) formula is not affected by zero cell entries and will give a consistent estimate of the common odds ratio even with large numbers of small strata. When the data in each stratum are more extensive it yields results which are in good agreement with the MLEs (Gart, 1971; McKinlay, 1978). In view of its computational simplicity, it thus appears to be the ideal choice for the statistician or epidemiologist working with a pocket calculator on tabulated data. Its only major drawback is the lack of a robust variance estimate to accompany it.

Approximate confidence intervals

Exact confidence limits for this problem are discussed by Gart (1971) and have been programmed by Thomas (1975). Since their calculation is quite involved, however, we limit our discussion to the three types of approximate limits considered for the single 2×2 table. Following the same line of reasoning used to derive the Cornfield limits (4.17), normal approximations to the exact upper and lower $100(1-\alpha)\%$ confidence bounds are obtained as the solution of

$$\frac{\sum\limits_{i=1}^{1} a_i - \sum\limits_{i=1}^{1} A_i(\psi_U) + \frac{1}{2}}{\sqrt{\sum\limits_{i=1}^{1} \text{Var}(a_i; \psi_U)}} = -Z_{\alpha/2}$$

and   (4.27)

$$\frac{\sum\limits_{i=1}^{1} a_i - \sum\limits_{i=1}^{1} A_i(\psi_L) - \frac{1}{2}}{\sqrt{\sum\limits_{i=1}^{1} \text{Var}(a_i; \psi_L)}} = Z_{\alpha/2},$$

respectively. Since $A_i(\psi)$ and $\text{Var}(a_i; \psi)$ are defined as in (4.11) and (4.13), the calculation requires iterative solution of a series of quadratic equations (Thomas, 1975). The approximation is improved by use of the exact means and variances in place of the asymptotic ones. Though this requires even more calculation, use of the exact (conditional) moments is especially important when the number of strata is large and the data thin.

The logit limits are more easily obtained with a pocket calculator. These are defined by

$$\log \psi_U, \log \psi_L = \log \hat{\psi}_1 \pm Z_{\alpha/2} \Big/ \sqrt{\sum_{i=1}^{1} w_i},$$ (4.28)

where $\hat{\psi}_1$ is the logit estimate and the w_i are the associated weights (4.24). Problems can be anticipated with their use in those same situations where the logit estimate has difficulties, namely when stratification becomes so fine that individual cell frequencies are small.

Miettinen's test-based limits require only a point estimate and test statistic. We recommend use of the M-H estimate for this purpose, and also use of the *uncorrected* version of χ^2. Thus

$$\psi_U, \psi_L = \hat{\psi}_{mh}^{(1 \pm Z_{\alpha/2}/\chi)}.$$ (4.29)

For reasons discussed in the previous section, these test-based limits become less accurate when the estimated relative risk is far from unity. They should not, however, be subject to the same tendency to increasing bias with increasing stratification as is the case with the logit limits.

Test for homogeneity of the odds ratio

All the procedures discussed so far in this section have been developed under the hypothesis that the odds ratio is constant across strata. If this were not the case, and a particular stratum had an odds ratio which was much larger than average, then we would expect the observed number of exposed cases a_i for that stratum to be larger than the expected number $A_i(\hat{\psi})$ based on the overall fitted odds ratio. Similarly, if the stratum odds ratio were small, we would expect a_i to be smaller than $A_i(\hat{\psi})$. Thus a reasonable test for the adequacy of the assumption of a common odds ratio is to sum up the squared deviations of observed and fitted values, each standardized by its variance:

$$\sum_{i=1}^{I} \frac{\{a_i - A_i(\hat{\psi})\}^2}{\text{Var}(a_i; \hat{\psi})} . \tag{4.30}$$

If the homogeneity assumption is valid, and the size of the sample is large relative to the number of strata, this statistic follows an approximate chi-square distribution on I-1 degrees of freedom. While this is true regardless of which estimate $\hat{\psi}$ is inserted, use of the unconditional MLE has the advantage of making the total deviation $\Sigma_i\{a_i - A_i(\hat{\psi})\}$ zero. The statistic (4.30) is then a special case of the chi-square goodness of fit statistic for logistic models (§ 6.5); however, the M-H estimate also gives quite satisfactory results.

Unfortunately the global statistic (4.30) is not as useful as it may seem at first sight. If the number of strata is large and the data thinly spread out, the distribution of the statistic may not approximate the nominal chi-square even under the hypothesis of homogeneity. This is precisely the situation where the unconditional MLE breaks down. More importantly, even where it is valid the statistic may lack power against alternatives of interest. Suppose, for example, that the I strata correspond to values x_i of some continuous variable such as age and that the observed odds ratios systematically increase or decrease with advancing age. Such a pattern is completely ignored by the global test statistic, which is unaffected by the order of the strata. In such situations one should compute instead

$$\frac{\left[\sum_{i=1}^{I} x_i\{a_i - A_i(\hat{\psi})\}\right]^2}{\sum_{i=1}^{I} x_i^2 \text{Var}(a_i; \hat{\psi}) - \left[\sum_{i=1}^{I} x_i \text{Var}(a_i; \hat{\psi})\right]^2 \Big/ \sum_{i=1}^{I} \text{Var}(a_i; \hat{\psi})} , \tag{4.31}$$

referring its value to tables of chi-square with one degree of freedom for a test of trend in ψ_i with x_i. If the x's are equally spaced, a continuity correction should be applied to the numerator of this statistic before squaring. Additional tests for trends in relative risk with one or several variables are easily carried out in the context of the modelling approach. (In fact [4.31] is the "score" statistic for testing $\beta = 0$ in the model log $\psi_i = \alpha + \beta x_i$. [See § 6.4, especially equation 6.18, and also § 6.12.])

In a similar context, suppose the I strata can be divided into H groups of size $I = I_1 + I_2 + \ldots + I_H$, and that we suspect the odds ratios are homogeneous within groups but not between them. Then, in place of the statistic (4.30) for testing overall homogeneity, we would be better advised to use

$$\sum_{h=1}^{H} \frac{\left[\sum_{i \epsilon I_h} a_i - A_i(\hat{\psi})\right]^2}{\sum_{i \epsilon I_h} \text{Var}(a_i; \hat{\psi})}, \tag{4.32}$$

where the notation $\underset{i \epsilon I_h}{\Sigma}$ denotes summation over the strata in the hth group. This statistic will be chi-square with only H-1 degrees of freedom under the homogeneity hypothesis, and has better power under the indicated alternative.

An alternative statistic for testing homogeneity, using the logit approach, is to take a weighted sum of the squared deviations between the separate estimates of log relative risk in each table and the overall logit estimate log $\hat{\psi}_1$. This may be written

$$\sum_{i=1}^{I} w_i \log^2 \hat{\psi}_i - \left\{\sum_{i=1}^{I} w_i \log \hat{\psi}_i\right\}^2 \Big/ \sum_{i=1}^{I} w_i, \tag{4.33}$$

where the $\hat{\psi}_i$ denote the individual odds ratios and w_i the weights (4.24), both calculated after addition of $^1/_2$ to each cell entry. While this statistic should yield similar values to (4.30) when all the individual frequencies are large, it is even more subject to instability with thin data and is therefore not recommended for general practice.

Some other tests of homogeneity of the odds ratio which have been proposed are incorrect and should not be used (Halperin et al., 1977; Mantel, Brown & Byar, 1977). As an example we should mention the test obtained by adding the individual χ^2 statistics (4.16) for each table and subtracting the summary χ^2 statistic (4.23) (Zelen, 1971). This does not have an approximate chi-square distribution under the hypothesis of homogeneity unless all the odds ratios are equal to unity.

Example continued: Table 4.3 illustrates these calculations for the data for six age groups relating alcohol to oesophageal cancer introduced at the beginning of the section. The summary χ^2 statistic (4.23) for testing $\psi = 1$ is obtained from the totals in columns (2), (3) and (4) as

$$\chi^2 = \frac{(|96-48.890|-^1/_2)^2}{26.106} = 83.22,$$

which yields an equivalent normal deviate of $\chi = 9.122$, p<0.0001. This is a slightly lower value than that obtained without stratification for age. Following the suggestion of Mantel and Fleiss (1980) for evaluating the adequacy of the normal approximation, we note that the minimum possible value for Σa_i consistent with the observed marginal totals is 0, while the maximum is 167, and that both extremes are sufficiently distant from the null mean of 48.890 to permit accurate approximation of p-values well below 0.05.

The logit estimate of the common odds ratio is calculated from the totals in columns (5) and (6) as

$$\log \hat{\psi}_1 = \frac{45.609}{28.261.} = 1.614$$

i.e.,

$$\hat{\psi}_1 = \exp(1.614) = 5.022.$$

Similarly, from columns(7) and (8) we obtain the M-H estimate

$$\hat{\psi}_{mh} = \frac{58.439}{11.330} = 5.158.$$

By way of contrast, the conditional and asymptotic (unconditional) maximum likelihood estimates for this problem are $\hat{\psi}_{cond} = 5.251$ and $\hat{\psi}_{ml} = 5.312$, respectively. These numerical results confirm the tendency for the $^1/_2$ correction used with the logit estimate to result in some bias towards unity, and the opposite tendency for the estimate based on unconditional maximum likelihood. However, since the cell frequencies are of reasonably good size, except for the most extreme age groups, these tendencies are not large and all four estimates agree fairly well.

In practice one would report the estimated odds ratio with two or three significant digits, e.g., 5.2 or 5.16 for $\hat{\psi}_{mh}$. We have used more decimals here simply in order to illustrate the magnitude of the differences between the various estimates.

Ninety-five percent logit confidence limits, starting from the logit estimate, are

$$\log \psi_U, \psi_L = 1.614 \pm 1.96/\sqrt{28.261}$$

i.e.,
$$\psi_L = \exp(1.614 - 0.369) = 3.47$$

$$\psi_U = \exp(1.614 + 0.369) = 7.26.$$

However, since we know the logit point estimate is too small, these are perhaps best centered around $\log \hat{\psi}_{mh}$ instead, yielding

$$\psi_L = 5.158 \times \exp(-0.369) = 3.57$$
$$\psi_U = 5.158 \times \exp(0.369) = 7.46.$$

Test-based limits centred about the M-H estimate are computed from (4.29) as

$$\psi_L = 5.158^{(1-1.96/9.220)} = 3.64$$

$$\psi_U = 5.158^{(1+1.96/9.220)} = 7.31,$$

where $\chi = 9.220 = \sqrt{85.01}$ is the uncorrected test statistic, rather than the corrected value of 9.122. These limits are noticeably narrower than the logit limits. By way of contrast the Cornfield (4.27) limits $\psi_L = 3.60$ and $\psi_U = 7.84$, while yielding a broader interval (on the log scale) than either the logit or test-based limits, show the same tendency towards inflated values as does the unconditional maximum likelihood estimate. Thus, while all methods of calculation provide roughly the same value for the lower limit, namely 3.6, the upper limit varies between about 7.3 and 7.8.

In order to carry out the test for homogeneity we need first to find fitted values (4.11) for all the cell frequencies under the estimated common odds ratio. Using the (unconditional) MLE $\hat{\psi}_{ml} = 5.312$, we solve for A in the first table via

$$\frac{A(105 + A)}{(10-A)(1-A)} = 5.312,$$

which gives $A(5.312) = 0.328$. Fitted values for the remaining cells are calculated by subtraction, so as to yield a table with precisely the same marginal totals as the observed one, viz:

0.328	0.672	1
9.672	105.328	115
10	106	116

The variance estimate (4.13) is then

$$\text{Var}(a_i; \psi = 5.312) = \left(\frac{1}{0.328} + \frac{1}{0.672} + \frac{1}{9.672} + \frac{1}{105.328}\right)^{-1} = 0.215.$$

Table 4.3 Combination of data from a series of 2×2 tables

(1) Stratum (age in years)	(2) Data			(3)(4) Test of null hypothesis[a]		(5)(6) Logit estimate[b]		(7)(8) Mantel-Haenszel estimate		(9)(10) Test of homogeneity[c]	
	a	b	n_1								
	c	d	n_0								
	m_1	m_2	N	A(1)	V(1)	$\log \hat{\psi}$	w	$\dfrac{ad}{N}$	$\dfrac{bc}{N}$	$A(\hat{\psi})$	$V(\hat{\psi})$
25–34	1	0	1	0.086	0.079	3.515	0.360	0.914	0.0	0.328	0.215
	9	106	115								
	10	106	116								
35–44	4	5	9	1.357	1.106	1.625	2.233	3.296	0.653	4.104	2.030
	26	164	190								
	30	169	199								
45–54	25	21	46	11.662	6.858	1.717	7.884	16.197	2.859	24.500	7.782
	29	138	167								
	54	159	213								
55–64	42	34	76	21.668	10.670	1.832	10.412	24.124	3.793	40.135	10.557
	27	139	166								
	69	173	242								
65–74	19	36	55	12.640	6.449	0.938	6.943	10.385	4.025	23.740	6.238
	18	88	106								
	37	124	161								
75+	5	8	13	1.477	0.944	3.708	0.429	3.523	0.0	3.203	0.996
	0	31	31								
	5	39	44								
Totals (except as noted)	96	104	200	48.890	26.106	45.609[d]	28.261	58.439	11.330	96.000	27.819
	109	666	775								
	205	770	975								

[a] Mean A(1) and variance V(1) of a under $\psi = 1$ from (4.12) and (4.14)
[b] Log relative risk estimates and weights from (4.24); $^1/_2$ added to each cell
[c] Mean and variance from (4.11) and (4.13) for $\hat{\psi} = \hat{\psi}_{ml}$, the unconditional MLE (4.25)
[d] Sum of $\log \hat{\psi}$ weighted by w

These values are listed at the head of columns (9) and (10) of Table 4.3; subsequent entries are calculated in precisely the same fashion for the other 2×2 tables. Thus the homogeneity chi-square (4.30) becomes

$$\frac{(1-0.328)^2}{0.215} + \frac{(4-4.104)^2}{2.030} + \ldots + \frac{(5-3.203)^2}{0.996} = 9.32$$

which when referred to tables of chi-square on $I-1=5$ degrees of freedom yields $p = 0.10$.

Notice that the total of the fitted values $A(\hat{\psi})$ in column (9) of Table 4.3 is precisely equal to the observed total, namely 96. In fact this relation is the defining characteristic of the unconditional MLE (see equation 4.25). If the fitted values are obtained instead from the M-H estimate, $\hat{\psi}_{mh} = 5.158$, they total 95.16 and give a value 9.28 to the homogeneity chi-square, very close to that already obtained. Thus it is perfectly feasible to carry out the test for homogeneity without having recourse to an *iteratively* computed estimate.

The alternative logit test statistic for homogeneity (4.33) is calculated as $0.360(3.515)^2 + 2.233(1.625)^2 + \ldots + 0.429(3.708)^2 - (45.609)^2/28.261 = 6.93$ ($p=0.23$). The reason this takes a smaller value is that for the extreme age categories, which contribute the most to the homogeneity chi-square, the addition of $1/2$ to the cell frequencies brings the odds ratios closer to the overall estimate.

Neither version of the formal test thus provides much evidence of heterogeneity. However, since the test lacks power it is important to continue the analysis by searching for patterns in the deviations between observed and fitted values which could indicate some sort of trend in the odds ratios. Certainly there is no obvious linear trend with age. This may be confirmed by assigning "dose" levels of $x_1 = 1$, $x_2 = 2$, ..., $x_6 = 6$ to the six age categories and computing the single degree of freedom chi-square for trend (4.31). We first need the intermediate quantities

$$\Sigma x_i\{a_i - A_i(\hat{\psi})\} = 1(1-0.328) + 2(4-4.104) + \ldots + 6(5-3.203) = -3.454$$

$$\Sigma x_i \text{Var} (a_i; \hat{\psi}) = 1 \times 0.215 + 2 \times 2.030 + \ldots + 6 \times 0.996 = 107.02$$

$$\Sigma x_i^2 \text{Var}(a_i; \hat{\psi}) = 1 \times 0.215 + 4 \times 2.030 + \ldots + 36 \times 0.996 = 439.09$$

from which we may calculate the test statistic

$$\frac{(-3.454 + 1/2)^2}{439.09 - \frac{(107.02)^2}{27.819}} = 0.32.$$

When referred to tables of chi-square on one degree of freedom, this gives $p = 0.58$, i.e., no evidence for a trend.

4.5 Exposure at several levels: the $2 \times K$ table

The simple dichotomization of a risk variable in a 2×2 table with disease status will often obscure the full range of the association between exposure and risk. Qualitative exposure variables may occur naturally at several discrete levels, and more information can be obtained from quantitative variables if their values are grouped into four or five ordered levels rather than only two. Furthermore, this is the only way one can demonstrate the dose-response relationship which is so critical to the interpretation of an association as causal (§ 3.2). Hence there is a need for methods of analysis of several exposure levels analogous to those already considered for two levels.

Unstratified analysis

Suppose that there are $K > 2$ levels of exposure and that the subjects have been classified in a single $2 \times K$ table relating exposure to disease:

	Exposure level				
	1	2	...	K	Totals
Cases	a_1	a_2	...	a_K	n_1
Controls	c_1	c_2	...	c_K	n_0
Totals	m_1	m_2	...	m_K	N

$$(4.34)$$

The usual approach to data analysis in this situation is to choose one exposure level, say level 1, as a baseline against which to compare each of the other levels using the methods already given for 2×2 tables. In this way one obtains relative risks $r_1 = 1$, $r_2, r_3, \ldots, r_K$ for each level, confidence intervals for these relative risks, and tests of the hypothesis that they are individually equal to unity.

To aid the interpretation of the results of such a series of individual tests, some of which may reach significance and others not, it is helpful to have available an overall test of the null hypothesis that the K relative risks r_k are all simultaneously equal to unity, i.e., that there is no effect of exposure on disease. Under this hypothesis, and conditional on the marginal totals $n_1, n_0, m_1, \ldots, m_K$, the numbers of cases exposed at the kth level have the expectations

$$e_k = E(a_k) = \frac{m_k n_1}{N},$$ (4.35)

variances

$$\text{Var}(a_k) = \frac{m_k(N - m_k)n_1 n_0}{N^2(N-1)}$$ (4.36)

and covariances $(k \neq h)$

$$\text{Cov}(a_k, a_h) = -\frac{m_k m_h n_1 n_0}{N^2(N-1)}$$ (4.37)

of the *K-dimensional hypergeometric distribution*. The test statistic itself is the usual one for testing the homogeneity of K proportions (Armitage, 1971), namely

$$\left(\frac{N-1}{N}\right) \sum_{k=1}^{K} (a_k - e_k)^2 \left\{\frac{1}{e_k} + \frac{1}{m_k - e_k}\right\} = (N-1)\left(\frac{1}{n_1} + \frac{1}{n_0}\right) \sum_{k=1}^{K} \frac{(a_k - e_k)^2}{m_k},$$ (4.38)

which may be referred to tables of chi-square on K–1 degrees of freedom[1].

When the levels of the exposure variable have no natural order, as for a genetic polymorphism, this approach can be taken no further. However, for quantitative or ordered qualitative variables the overall chi-square wastes important information. A more sensitive way of detecting alternative hypotheses is to test for a *trend* in

---

[1] The leading term $\left(\frac{N-1}{N}\right)$ is often ignored.

disease risk with increasing levels of exposure. Suppose that there are "doses" x_k associated with the various levels of exposure, where we may simply take $x_k = k$ for an ordered variable. An appropriate statistic for testing trend is to consider the regression of the deviations (a_k-e_k) on x_k (Armitage, 1955; Mantel, 1963). When squared and divided by its variance this becomes

$$\frac{N^2(N-1)\left\{\sum_{k=1}^{K} x_k(a_k-e_k)\right\}^2}{n_1 n_0 \left\{N \sum_{k=1}^{K} x_k^2 m_k - \left(\sum_{k=1}^{K} x_k m_k\right)^2\right\}}, \qquad (4.39)$$

which should be referred to tables of chi-square on one degree of freedom. If the x_k are spaced one unit apart, as in the case of $x_k = k$, an appropriate correction for continuity is to reduce the *absolute value* of the numerator term $\Sigma x_k(a_k-e_k)$ by $1/2$ before squaring. Estimation of the quantitative trend parameter is best discussed in terms of the modelling approach of Chapter 6.

Adjustment by stratification

Confounding variables may be incorporated in the analysis of $2 \times K$ tables by stratification of the data just as described in § 4.4 for a 2×2 table. The frequencies of cases and controls classified by exposures for the ith of I strata are simply expressed by the addition of subscripts to the entries in (4.34):

Stratum i	Exposure level				Totals
	1	2	...	K	
Cases	a_{1i}	a_{2i}	...	a_{Ki}	n_{1i}
Controls	c_{1i}	c_{2i}	...	c_{Ki}	n_{0i}
Totals	m_{1i}	m_{2i}	...	m_{Ki}	N_i

(4.40)

Methods for analysis of a series of 2×2 tables may be used to estimate the adjusted relative risk for each level of exposure relative to the designated baseline level, to put confidence limits around this estimate, to test the significance of its departure from unity, and to test whether it varies from stratum to stratum. A peculiarity which results from this procedure when there is more than one $2 \times K$ table is that the estimated relative risks may not be consistent with each other. More precisely, if r_{21} is the summary estimate of the odds ratio comparing level 2 with level 1, and r_{31} the summary measure for level 3 compared with level 1, their ratio r_{31}/r_{21} is not algebraically identical to the summary odds ratio r_{32} comparing level 3 with level 2. This problem does not arise with a single table, since it is true for this case that

$$r_{31}/r_{21} = \frac{a_3 c_1/a_1 c_3}{a_2 c_1/a_1 c_2} = \frac{a_3 c_2}{a_2 c_3} = r_{32}.$$

Nor will it arise with a series of tables in which the relative risks comparing each pair of levels are the same from table to table. Therefore, inconsistency can be regarded as a particular manifestation of the problem of interaction (see § 5.5). Recourse must be made to the methods in Chapters 6 and 7 in order to have adjusted estimates of relative risk which display such consistency, and for general tests of interaction. Otherwise one is well advised to use as baseline category the one which contains the most information, i.e., the k such that the sum of the reciprocals of the numbers of cases and controls,

$$\sum_{i=1}^{I} \left\{ \frac{1}{a_{ki}} + \frac{1}{c_{ki}} \right\},$$

is a minimum.

The generalization to stratified data of the statistic (4.38), which tests the global null hypothesis, is somewhat more complicated as it involves matrix manipulations (Mantel & Haenszel, 1959). Let us denote by e_i the K–1 dimensional vector of expectations $e_i = E(a_i) = E(a_{1i}, \ldots, a_{K-1,i})$ of numbers of cases exposed to each of the first K–1 levels in the ith stratum, and by V_i the corresponding K–1 × K–1 dimensional covariance matrix. These are calculated as in formulae (4.35), (4.36), and (4.37) with the addition of i subscripts to all terms. Let $e. = \Sigma e_i$, $V. = \Sigma V_i$, and $a. = \Sigma a_i$ denote the sums of these quantities cumulated over the I strata. Then the global null hypothesis that there is no effect of exposure on disease, after adjustment by stratification, may be tested by referring the statistic

$$(a.-e.)^T \, V.^{-1}(a.-e.) \tag{4.41}$$

to tables of chi-square with K–1 degrees of freedom. This reduces to (4.38) if I = 1, i.e., there is only a single stratum.

Calculation of this statistic requires matrix inversion, and while perfectly feasible to perform by hand for small values of K (say K=3 and 4), it becomes more difficult for larger values. Various approximate statistics have therefore been suggested (Armitage, 1966). One *conservative* approximation, which always yields values less than or equal to those of (4.41), is given by

$$\sum_{k=1}^{K} \frac{(a_{k.}-e_{k.})^2}{\sum_{i=1}^{I} \frac{n_{0i}e_{ki}}{N_i-1}}. \tag{4.42}$$

Unfortunately, the difference between (4.42) and (4.41) increases as the distributions of exposures among the combined case-control sample in each stratum become more disparate, which is one situation in which stratification may be important to reduce bias (Crowley & Breslow, 1975).

The statistic for the adjusted test of trend which generalizes (4.39) is more easily obtained as

$$\frac{\left\{ \sum_{k=1}^{K} x_k(a_{k.}-e_{k.}) \right\}^2}{\sum_{i=1}^{I} \frac{n_{0i}}{N_i-1} \left\{ \sum_{k=1}^{K} x_k^2 e_{ki} - \frac{1}{n_{1i}} \left(\sum_{k=1}^{K} x_k e_{ki} \right)^2 \right\}}. \tag{4.43}$$

Here the numerator term represents the regression of the x's on the differences between the total observed and expected frequencies, while the denominator is its variance under the null hypothesis (Mantel, 1963). This statistic also should be referred to tables of chi-square with one degree of freedom, and a continuity correction applied to the numerator if the x_k values are equally spaced.

Example continued: As an illustration of the analysis of the effects of a risk factor taking on several levels, Table 4.4 presents data from Ille-et-Vilaine with alcohol consumption broken down into four levels rather than the two shown in § 4.1. Relative risks are calculated for each level of consumption against a baseline of 0–39 g/day as the empirical odds ratio for the corresponding 2×2 table. Each of these is individually highly significant as judged from the χ^2 test statistics, all of which exceed the critical value of 15.1 for significance at the $p = 0.0001$ level. Moreover, there is a clear increase in risk with increasing consumption. The confidence limits shown are those of Cornfield. It is perhaps worth remarking that the test-based limits are in better agreement with those for the lower levels (e.g., 2.29–5.57 for 40–79 g/day) than for the higher ones (16.22–45.92 for 120+ g/day), as would be expected in such a situation with a trend of risk.

While there is no doubt regarding the statistical significance of the observed differences in risk, and in particular the trend with increasing consumption, we nevertheless compute the chi-square test statistics (4.38) and (4.39) for purposes of illustration. The first step is the calculation of the table of expected values under the null hypothesis,

Table 4.4   Distribution of alcohol consumption for cases and controls: relative risks and confidence limits for each level, with and without adjustment for age

	Alcohol consumption (g/day)				Totals
	0–39	40–79	80–119	120+	
Cases	29	75	51	45	200
Controls	386	280	87	22	775
Totals	415	355	138	67	975
Unadjusted analysis					
RR ($\hat{\psi}$)	1.0	3.57	7.80	27.23	
χ^2	–	31.54	72.77	156.14	
95% confidence limit	–	2.21–5.77	4.54–13.46	13.8–54.18	

Global test of H_0: $\chi_3^2 = 158.8$ Test for trend: $\chi_1^2 = 151.9$

Adjusted for age					
RR ($\hat{\psi}_{mh}$)	1.0	4.27	8.02	28.57	
RR ($\hat{\psi}_{ml}$)	1.0	4.26	8.02	37.82	
χ^2	–	36.00	57.15	135.49	
95% confidence limit	–	2.56–7.13	4.37–14.82	16.69–87.73	
Test for homogeneity (χ_5^3)		6.59	6.69	10.33	

Global test of H_0: $\chi_3^2 = 141.4$ Test for trend: $\chi_1^2 = 134.0$

	Alcohol consumption (g/day)				
	0–39	40–79	80–119	120+	Totals
Cases	85.13	72.82	28.31	13.74	200.00
Controls	329.87	282.18	109.69	53.26	775.00
Totals	415.00	355.00	138.00	67.00	975.00

where the first row consists of the expected values e_k for cases and the second consists of the expected values m_k-e_k for controls. Thus, for example,

$$e_1 = \frac{415 \times 200}{975} = 85.13$$

and $m_1-e_1 = 415-85.13 = 329.87$. Note that the row and column totals of the observed and expected values agree. We then have from (4.38)

$$\frac{974}{975} \left\{ (29-85.13)^2 \left(\frac{1}{85.13} + \frac{1}{329.87} \right) + \ldots + (45-13.74)^2 \left(\frac{1}{13.74} + \frac{1}{53.26} \right) \right\} = 158.8,$$

which would normally be referred to tables of chi-square with three degrees of freedom.

Table 4.5   Distribution of alcohol consumption for cases and controls: in six age strata

Age (years)		Alcohol consumption (g/day)				Total
		0–39	40–79	80–119	120+	
25–34						
	Cases	0	0	0	1	1
	Controls	61	45	5	4	115
	Total	61	45	5	5	116
35–44						
	Cases	1	4	0	4	9
	Controls	88	76	20	6	190
	Total	89	80	20	10	199
45–54						
	Cases	1	20	12	13	46
	Controls	77	61	27	2	167
	Total	78	81	39	15	213
55–64						
	Cases	12	22	24	18	76
	Controls	77	62	19	8	166
	Total	89	84	43	26	242
65–74						
	Cases	11	25	13	6	55
	Controls	60	28	16	2	106
	Total	71	53	29	8	161
75+						
	Cases	4	4	2	3	13
	Controls	23	8	0	0	31
	Total	27	12	2	3	44

In calculating the chi-square for trend (4.39) we assign "doses" of $x_1 = 0$, $x_2 = 1$, $x_3 = 2$, and $x_4 = 3$ to the four consumption levels, this assignment being justified on the grounds that the levels are more or less equally spaced. This yields

$$\frac{975^2 \times 974\ \{0(29-85.13)+\ldots+3(45-13.74)-\frac{1}{2}\}^2}{200 \times 775\ \{975(0 \times 415+\ldots+9 \times 67)-(0 \times 415+\ldots+3 \times 67)^2\}} = 151.9.$$

Hence most of the heterogeneity represented in the three degrees of freedom chi-square is "explained" by the linear increase in risk with dose.

In order to adjust these results for the possible confounding effects of age, we again stratify the population into six strata as shown in Table 4.5. Adjusted estimates of relative risk (Table 4.4) are obtained from the series of six 2×2 tables comparing each level with baseline, using the techniques already described in § 4.3. Since there was little correlation between age and alcohol consumption in the sample, and hence little confounding, the adjusted and unadjusted estimates do not differ much. If we calculate directly the relative risks for 120+ g/day *versus* 40–79 g/day using the series of six corresponding 2×2 tables we find a M-H summary odds ratio of $\hat{\psi}_{mh} = 8.71$ and MLE of $\hat{\psi}_{ml} = 9.63$. Neither of these agrees with the ratio of estimates for those two levels relative to 0–39 g/day shown in the table, i.e., $28.57/4.27 = 6.69$ and $37.82/4.26 = 8.88$, respectively. As mentioned earlier, the only way to achieve exact consistency among the summary measures is to build it into a modelling approach (Chapters 6 and 7).

The tendency of the unconditional MLE towards inflated values with thin data is evident for the 120 g/day category; in this case the conditional MLE is $\hat{\psi}_{cond} = 34.90$. Adjustment results in slightly less significant chi-squares and wider confidence limits, in accordance with the idea that "unnecessary" stratification leads to a slight loss of information or efficiency (§ 7.6). There is some evidence that the

Table 4.6   Expectations and covariances under the null hypothesis for the data in Table 4.5

Age (years)	Expected number of cases by level of alcohol (g/day)				Covariance matrix[a]		
	0–39	40–79	80–119	120+	0–39	40–79	80–119
25–34	0.53	0.39	0.04	0.04	0.25	−0.20	−0.02
					−0.20	0.24	−0.02
					−0.02	−0.02	0.04
35–44	4.03	3.62	0.90	0.45	2.14	−1.55	−0.39
					−1.55	2.08	−0.35
					−0.39	−0.35	0.78
45–54	16.85	17.49	8.42	3.24	8.41	−5.05	−2.43
					−5.05	8.54	−2.52
					−2.43	−2.52	5.42
55–64	27.95	26.38	13.50	8.17	12.17	−6.68	−3.42
					−6.68	11.86	−3.23
					−3.42	−3.23	7.65
65–74	24.25	18.11	9.91	2.73	8.98	−5.29	−2.89
					−5.29	8.05	−2.16
					−2.89	−2.16	5.38
75+	7.98	3.55	0.59	0.89	2.22	−1.57	−0.26
					−1.57	1.86	−0.12
					−0.26	−0.12	0.41
Totals	81.59	69.54	33.36	15.52	34.17	−20.34	−9.41
					−20.34	32.63	−8.40
					−9.41	−8.40	19.68

[a] The final row and column of this matrix, corresponding to the fourth level of 120+ g/day, are not shown as they are not needed for the subsequent calculations. They could be obtained from the fact that the sum of the matrix elements over any row or column is zero.

relative risk for the highest consumption level may vary with age, but the chi-square of 10.33 on five degrees of freedom does not quite attain nominal significance at $p = 0.05$, and considerable doubt exists as to the true significance level because of the small numbers in some tables. There is no evident trend in the relative risk with increasing age.

Expected values and covariances for the exposure frequencies of the cases *within* each stratum, calculated according to formulae (4.35)–(4.37), are presented in Table 4.6. For example, in the second stratum we have

$$\text{Var}(a_{12}) = \frac{89 \times (199-89) \times 9 \times 190}{199 \times 199 \times 198} = 2.14$$

and

$$\text{Cov}(a_{12}, a_{22}) = -\frac{89 \times 80 \times 9 \times 190}{199 \times 199 \times 198} = -1.55.$$

The cumulated vector of expected exposures **e.** and covariance matrix **V.** are shown at the bottom of the table.

The adjusted global test (4.41) of the null hypothesis is calculated from the total observed values shown in Table 4.4 and the totals shown at the bottom of Table 4.6 as

$$(29-81.59,\ 75-69.54,\ 51-33.36) \begin{bmatrix} 0.108 & 0.091 & 0.091 \\ 0.091 & 0.111 & 0.091 \\ 0.091 & 0.091 & 0.133 \end{bmatrix} \begin{pmatrix} 29-81.59 \\ 75-69.54 \\ 51-33.36 \end{pmatrix} = 141.4,$$

where the 3×3 matrix is the inverse of the cumulated covariance matrix. To find the conservative approximation to this we compute from (4.42)

$$\frac{(29-81.59)^2}{\frac{1}{115}(0.53) + \frac{190}{198}(4.03) + \ldots + \frac{31}{43}(7.98)}$$

$$+ \quad \frac{(75-69.54)^2}{\frac{1}{115}(0.39) + \frac{190}{198}(3.62) + \ldots + \frac{31}{43}(3.55)}$$

$$\vdots$$

$$+ \quad \frac{(45-15.52)^2}{\frac{1}{115}(0.04) + \frac{190}{198}(0.45) + \ldots + \frac{31}{43}(0.89)}$$

$$= \quad 139.0.$$

In calculating the adjusted single degree of freedom test for trend (4.43), we first find the denominator terms

$$\sum x_k^2 e_{k1} = 0(0.53) + 1(0.39) + 4(0.04) + 9(0.04) = 0.91$$

$$\frac{(\sum x_k e_{k1})^2}{n_{11}} = \frac{\{0(0.53) + 1(0.39) + 2(0.04) + 3(0.04)\}^2}{1} = 0.35$$

$$\vdots \qquad\qquad \vdots$$

$$\sum x_k^2 e_{k6} = 0(7.98) + 1(3.55) + 4(0.59) + 9(0.89) = 13.92$$

$$\frac{(\sum x_k e_{k6})^2}{n_{16}} = \frac{\{0(7.98) + 1(3.55) + 2(0.59) + 3(0.89)\}^2}{13} = 4.21$$

and then use these in

$$\frac{\{0(29-81.59)+1(75-69.54)+\ldots+3(45-15.52)-\frac{1}{2}\}^2}{\frac{1}{115}(0.91-0.35)+\frac{190}{198}(11.27-5.09)+\ldots+\frac{31}{43}(13.92-4.21)} = 134.0.$$

The test statistics are little affected by the adjustment process in this particular example, and the trend continues to account for the major portion of the variation[1].

Table 4.7 presents a summary of the results for tobacco analogous to those for alcohol shown in Table 4.4. While there is a clear association between an increased dose and increased risk, the relationship is not as strong as with alcohol nor does the linear trend component account for as much of it. In this case adjustment for age appears to increase the strength of the association, especially for the highest exposure category.

Table 4.7   Distribution of tobacco consumption for cases and controls: relative risks and confidence limits for each level, with and without adjustment for age

| | Tobacco consumption (g/day) | | | | |
	0–9	10–19	20–29	30+	Total
Cases	78	58	33	31	200
Controls	447	178	99	51	775
Total	525	236	132	82	975
Unadjusted analysis					
RR ($\hat{\psi}$)	1.0	1.87	1.91	3.48	
χ^2		9.81	7.01	23.78	
95% confidence limit		1.25–2.78	1.17–3.11	2.03–5.96	

Global test of H_0: $\chi_3^2 = 29.3$ Test for trend: $\chi_1^2 = 26.9$

Adjusted for age					
RR ($\hat{\psi}_{mh}$)	1.0	1.83	1.98	6.53	
RR ($\hat{\psi}_{ml}$)	1.0	1.85	1.99	6.60	
χ^2		8.29	6.76	37.09	
95% confidence limit		1.21–2.82	1.18–3.37	3.33–13.14	

Global test of H_0: $\chi_3^2 = 39.3$ Test for trend: $\chi_1^2 = 34.2$

4.6 Joint effects of several risk factors

By defining each exposure category as a particular combination of factor levels, these same basic techniques can be used to explore the joint effects of two or more factors on disease risk. Relative risks are obtained using as baseline the category corresponding to the combination of baseline levels of each individual factor. Summary estimates of relative risk for one factor, adjusted for the effects of the others, are

---

[1] N.B. Since the intermediate results shown here are given only to two significant figures, whereas the exact values were used for calculation, some slight numerical discrepancies may be apparent when the reader works through these calculations himself.

obtained by including the latter among the stratification variables. Rather than attempt a discussion in general terms, details of this approach are best illustrated by a continuation of our analysis of the Ille-et-Vilaine data.

Example continued: The joint distribution of alcohol and tobacco consumption among cases and controls is shown in Table 4.8. Using the 0–9 g/day tobacco and 0–39 g/day alcohol categories as baseline, relative risks for each of the 15 remaining categories were obtained after stratification of the population into six age groups (Table 4.9). One of the difficulties of this method is that, as the data become more thinly spread out, an increasing fraction of the 2×2 tables from which the relative risks are calculated have at least one zero for a marginal total. This means that more and more data are effectively excluded from analysis since such tables make absolutely no contribution to any of the summary relative risk estimates or test statistics considered earlier. For example, only three out of the six tables contrasting the 30+ g/day tobacco, 120+ g/day alcohol exposure with the baseline level, namely those for the 45–54, 55–64 and 65–74 year age groups, were actually used to calculate the summary risk measure of 240.63. The remainder had at least one zero in a marginal total. This may explain the notable difference between the age-adjusted estimate and the crude relative risk estimate of $(10 \times 252)/(3 \times 9) = 93.33$. It is nevertheless apparent that people in this category of high alcohol/high tobacco consumption are at exceptional risk.

Table 4.9 shows a clear trend of increased risk with increased alcohol consumption within each tobacco category and likewise a trend with tobacco for each alcohol level. As neither of these variables accounts for the effects of the other, we say that they operate *independently* in producing their effects. Evidence for the lack of confounding in this instance comes from comparing the relative risks for alcohol which are simultaneously adjusted for age and tobacco (margin of Table 4.9) with those adjusted for age only Table 4.4). There is good agreement except perhaps for the highest level, where tobacco adjustment reduces the Mantel-Haenszel estimate from 28.6 to 22.8. Likewise the tobacco risks adjusted for alcohol and age do not depart greatly from those adjusted for age only (Table 4.7). Of course in other situations there may be risk factors which are partially confounded, some of their effect being due to the association with the other factor and some independent of it; and if there is complete confounding the effects of one may disappear after adjustment for the other.

Table 4.8 Joint classification of cases and controls by consumption of alcohol and tobacco

| Alcohol (g/day) | Tobacco (g/day) | | | | | | | |
| | 0–9 | | 10–19 | | 20–29 | | 30+ | |
	Cases	Controls	Cases	Controls	Cases	Controls	Cases	Controls
0–39	9	252	10	74	5	35	5	23
40–79	34	145	17	68	15	47	9	20
80–119	19	42	19	30	6	10	7	5
120+	16	8	12	6	7	5	10	3

Table 4.9 Age-adjusted relative risks for joint exposure to alcohol and tobacco

| Alcohol (g/day) | Tobacco (g/day) | | | | Adjusted for tobacco |
	0–9	10–19	20–29	30+	
0–39	1.0	3.90	4.17	9.44	1.0
40–79	8.18	8.63	10.57	52.47	4.05
80–119	12.94	13.88	17.97	155.62	7.49
120+	51.45	67.21	108.66	240.63	22.80
Adjusted for alcohol	1.0	1.51	1.56	8.10	

Computation of each of the simultaneously adjusted estimates shown in the margins of Table 4.9 involved the summarization of 24 2×2 tables, although many of these are omitted from the calculation because of zero marginals (for example, only 12 tables were used in the estimation of the relative risk of 8.10 for the highest tobacco level). Implicit in this calculation is the assumption that the odds ratios are constant over those tables being summarized, i.e., that the relative risks for tobacco do not depend on alcohol or age, while those for alcohol are independent of tobacco. Thus the relative risks shown in the margin of Table 4.9 are those obtained under the *multiplicative* hypothesis that the joint effect of alcohol and tobacco on incidence is the product of their individual effects (§ 2.6). *Smoothed* estimates of the relative risks for the combined categories under the multiplicative model are obtained by multiplying together the summary relative risks for each factor adjusting for the other. Thus the smoothed estimate for the 40–79 g/day alcohol, 10–19 g/day tobacco category is $1.51 \times 4.05 = 6.12$, compared with the individual cell estimate of 8.63.

Although we have shown that the method of stratification can be used to study the joint effects of two or more risk factors, it is not, in fact, well suited to this task. Computations become burdensome to perform by hand because so many strata must be created. Spreading the data out thinly may result in the loss of a large part of it from analysis. Hence, such multivariate analyses are best carried out using the regression models of Chapters 6 and 7, which permit a more economic, systematic and quantitative description of the effects of the several factors and their interactions.

REFERENCES

Armitage, P. (1955) Test for linear trend in proportions and frequencies. *Biometrics, 11*, 375–386

Armitage, P. (1966) The chi-square test for heterogeneity of proportions, after adjustment for stratification, *J. R. Stat. Soc. B., 28*, 150–163

Armitage, P. (1971) *Statistical Methods in Medical Research,* Oxford, Blackwell Scientific Publications

Breslow, N. (1976) Regression analysis of the log odds ratio: a method for retrospective studies. *Biometrics, 32*, 409–416

Cochran, W.G. (1954) Some methods for strengthening the common χ^2 tests. *Biometrics, 10*, 417–451

Cornfield, J. (1956) *A statistical problem arising from retrospective studies.* In: Neyman, J., ed., *Proceedings of the Third Berkeley Symposium, IV,* Berkeley, University of California Press, pp. 133–148

Cox, D.R. (1970) *The Analysis of Binary Data,* London, Methuen

Cox, D.R. & Hinkley, D.V. (1974) *Theoretical Statistics,* London, Chapman & Hall

Crowley, J. & Breslow, N. (1975) Remarks on the conservatism of $\Sigma(0-E)^2/E$ in survival data. *Biometrics, 31*, 957–961

Fienberg, S.E. (1977) *The Analysis of Cross-Classified Categorical Data,* Cambridge, Mass., MIT Press

Fleiss, J.L. (1973) *Statistical Methods for Rates and Proportions,* New York, Wiley

Gart, J.J. (1970) Point and interval estimation of the common odds ratio in the combination of 2×2 tables with fixed marginals. *Biometrics, 26*, 409–416

Gart, J.J. (1971) The comparison of proportions: a review of significance tests, confidence intervals, and adjustments for stratification. *Rev. Int. Stat. Inst., 39*, 148–169

Gart, J.J. (1979) Statistical analyses of the relative risk. *Environ. Health Perspect.,* *32,* 157–167

Gart, J.J. & Thomas, D.G. (1972) Numerical results on approximate confidence limits for the odds ratio, *J. R. Stat. Soc. B., 34,* 441–447

Gart, J.J. & Zweifel, J.R. (1967) On the bias of the logit and its variance, with application to quantal bioassay. *Biometrika, 54,* 181–187

Halperin, M. (1977) Letter to the Editor. *Am. J. Epidemiol., 105,* 496–498

Halperin, M., Ware, J.H., Byar, D.P., Mantel, N., Brown, C.C., Koziol, J., Gail, M. & Green, S.B. (1977) Testing for interaction in an $I \times J \times K$ contingency table. *Biometrika, 64,* 271–275

Hannan, J. & Harkness, W.L. (1963) Normal approximation to the distribution of two independent binomials, conditional on fixed sum. *Ann. Math. Stat., 34,* 1593–1595

Liddell, D. (1978) Practical tests of the 2×2 contingency tables. *Statistician, 25,* 295–304

Mantel, N. (1963) Chi-square tests with one degree of freedom: extensions of the Mantel-Haenszel procedure. *J. Am. Stat. Assoc., 58,* 690–700

Mantel, N. & Fleiss, J.L. (1980) Minimum requirements for the Mantel-Haenszel one-degree of freedom chi-square test and a related rapid procedure. *Am. J. Epidemiol.* (in press)

Mantel, N. & Greenhouse, S.W. (1968) What is the continuity correction? *Am. Stat. 22,* 27–30

Mantel, N. & Haenszel, W. (1959) Statistical aspects of the analysis of data from retrospective studies of disease. *J. natl Cancer Inst., 22,* 719–748

Mantel, N., Brown, C. & Byar, D.P. (1977) Tests for homogeneity of effect in an epidemiologic investigation. *Am. J. Epidemiol., 106,* 125–129

McKinlay, S.M. (1978) The effect of non-zero second-order interaction on combined estimators of the odds ratio. *Biometrika, 65,* 191–202

Miettinen, O.S. (1976) Estimability and estimation in case-referent studies. *Am. J. Epidemiol., 103,* 226–235

Rothman, K. & Boice, J. (1979) *Epidemiologic analysis with a programmable calculator (NIH Publication No. 79–1649),* Washington DC, US Government Printing Office

Thomas, D.G. (1971) Exact confidence limits for an odds ratio in a 2×2 table. *Appl. Stat., 20,* 105–110

Thomas, D.G. (1975) Exact and asymptotic methods for the combination of 2×2 tables. *Comput. Biomed. Res., 8,* 423–446

Tuyns, A.J., Péquignot, G. & Jensen, O.M. (1977) Le cancer de l'oesophage en Ille-et-Vilaine en fonction des niveaux de consommation d'alcool et de tabac. *Bull. Cancer, 64,* 45–60

Woolf, B. (1955) On estimating the relationship between blood group and disease. *Ann. Human Genet., 19,* 251–253

Zelen, M. (1971) The analysis of several 2×2 contigency tables. *Biometrika, 58,* 129–137

LIST OF SYMBOLS – CHAPTER 4 (in order of appearance)

ψ	odds ratio (approximate relative risk)
a	number of exposed cases
b	number of unexposed cases
c	number of exposed controls
d	number of unexposed controls
n_1	number of cases (subtotal)
n_0	number of controls (subtotal)
m_1	number of exposed (subtotal)
m_0	number of unexposed (subtotal)
N	total number of cases and controls
P_1	probability of disease development for exposed
P_0	probability of disease development for unexposed
p_1	probability of exposure for a case
p_0	probability of exposure for a control
H_0	the null hypothesis that exposure has no effect on risk ($\psi = 1$)
$\binom{n}{u}$	binomial coefficient (see p. 125); there are $\binom{n}{u}$ ways of choosing u objects from n objects
pr ( )	the probability of an event ( )
pr (|)	the probability of one event conditional on another
$\hat{\psi}_{cond}$	conditional maximum likelihood estimate of the common odds ratio
E (|)	expectation of one random variable conditional on the values of another
H	a statistical hypothesis regarding the value of some parameter, for example $\psi = \psi_0$
p_L	lower tail probability or p-value
p_U	upper tail probability or p-value
ψ_L	lower confidence limit on the odds ratio
ψ_U	upper confidence limit on the odds ratio
α	size of a statistical test, predetermined significance level such that if the p-value falls below α one rejects the hypothesis
$A = A(\psi)$	expected number (asymptotic) of exposed cases when marginal totals of the 2×2 table are fixed, when the true odds ratio is ψ; fitted value for number of exposed cases when the true odds ratio is ψ
B, C, D	fitted values for remaining entries in the 2×2 table
$Var = Var(a; \psi)$	variance (asymptotic) of the number a of exposed cases when the marginal totals of the 2×2 table are fixed and the true odds ratio is ψ
$\hat{\psi}$	an estimate of the odds ratio
Δ	distance between adjacent observations of a discrete distribution (assumed constant)
Φ	cumulative distribution function of the standard normal distribution, e.g., $\Phi(-1.96) = 0.025$, $\Phi(1.96) = 0.975$
$\|x\|$	absolute value of a number x; the positive part of x; $\|3\| = \|-3\| = 3$

$Z_{\alpha/2}$	the $100(1-\alpha/2)$ percentile of the standard normal distribution: $\Phi(Z_{\alpha/2}) = 1-\alpha/2$
log	the natural logarithm; log to the base e
χ^2	a statistic which has (asymptotically) a chi-square distribution under the null hypothesis
χ	the square root of a χ^2 statistic
i	subscript added to denote the ith stratum, e.g., a_i = number of exposed cases in the ith stratum, ψ_i odds ratio in i^{th} stratum, etc.
$\hat{\psi}_1$	"logit" estimate of the common odds ratio in a series of 2×2 tables
w_i	weights associated with the logit estimate in the ith stratum
$\hat{\psi}_{ml}$	(unconditional) maximum likelihood estimate (MLE) of the odds ratio
$\hat{\psi}_{mh}$	Mantel-Haenszel (M-H) estimate of the common odds ratio in a series of 2×2 tables
a_k	number of cases exposed to level k of a polytomous factor
c_k	number of controls exposed to level k of a polytomous factor
m_k	number of subjects (cases + controls) exposed to level k of a polytomous factor
e_k	expected number of cases exposed to level k under the null hypothesis and assuming fixed marginals in a $2 \times K$ table
Cov(x,y)	covariance between two variables x and y
Var(x)	variance of a variable x
$\mathbf{e}_i$	vector of expected values of the numbers of cases exposed to the first $K-1$ levels of a polytomous factor in the ith stratum
$\mathbf{V}_i$	variance-covariance matrix of the numbers of cases exposed to the first $K-1$ levels of a polytomous risk factor in the ith stratum
.	denotes summation over the subscript which it replaces; e.g., for the doubly subscripted array $\{a_{ki}\}$, $a_{k.} = \Sigma_i a_{ki} = a_{k1} + \ldots + a_{kI}$
χ^2_ν	a statistic which has (asymptotically) a chi-square distribution with ν degrees of freedom under the null hypothesis

5. CLASSICAL METHODS OF ANALYSIS OF MATCHED DATA

5.1 Los Angeles retirement community study of endometrial cancer

5.2 Matched pairs: dichotomous exposures

5.3 1:M matching: dichotomous exposures

5.4 Dichotomous exposure: variable number of controls

5.5 Multiple exposure levels: single control

5.6 More complex situations

CHAPTER V

CLASSICAL METHODS OF ANALYSIS OF MATCHED DATA

As a technique for the control of confounding, stratification may be introduced either at the design stage of a study or during the analysis of results. An advantage of using it in design, keeping a constant ratio of controls to cases in each stratum, is that one avoids the inefficiencies resulting from having some strata with a gross imbalance of cases and controls. In the Ille-et-Vilaine study, for example, the 115 controls ascertained between 25 and 34 years of age are effectively lost from the analysis, or make only a minimal contribution to it, because there is only a single case with which to compare them (Table 4.1). Of course such gains in efficiency are only achieved if the analysis takes proper account of the stratification, which must be done in general anyway in order to avoid biased estimates of the relative risk (§ 3.4).

The ultimate form of a stratified design occurs when each case is individually matched to a set of controls, usually one or two but sometimes more, chosen to have similar values for certain of the important confounding variables. Some choices of control population intrinsically imply a matched design and analysis, as with neighbourhood or familial controls. If the exposure levels of the risk factor to be analysed are dichotomous or polytomous, the tests and estimates developed in the last chapter may be employed directly by considering each matched pair or set to be a separate stratum. Of course those "asymptotic" techniques which lead to trouble with sparse data should be avoided, while some of the "exact" procedures which were not considered feasible with general strata are quite tractable and useful with matched data. In this chapter we take advantage of the special structure imposed by the matching, so as to express many of the previously discussed tests and estimates in simple and succinct form.

5.1 Los Angeles retirement community study of endometrial cancer

An example which we shall use to illustrate the methods for matched data analysis is the study of the effect of exogenous oestrogens on the risk of endometrial cancer reported by Mack et al. (1976). These investigators identified 63 cases of endometrial cancer occurring in a retirement community near Los Angeles, California (USA) from 1971 to 1975. Each case was matched to four control women who were alive and living in the community at the time the case was diagnosed, who were born within one year of the case, who had the same marital status and who had entered the community at approximately the same time. In addition, controls were chosen from among women who had not had a hysterectomy prior to the time the case was diagnosed, and who were therefore still at risk for the disease.

Information on the history of use of several specific types of medicines, including oestrogens, anti-hypertensives, sedatives and tranquilizers, was abstracted from the medical record of each case and control. Other abstracted data relate to pregnancy history, mention of certain diseases, and obesity. Table 5.1 summarizeş the distribution of cases and controls according to some of the key variables. Note the almost perfect balance of the age distribution of cases and controls, a consequence of the matching.

The analysis of these data is aimed at studying the risk associated with the use of oestrogens as well as with a history of gall bladder disease, and how these risks may be modified by the other factors shown in Table 5.1. When illustrating methods which involve matching a single control to a single case, the first of the four selected controls is used. A listing of the complete set of data is presented in Appendix III.

Table 5.1 Characteristics of cases and controls in Los Angeles study of endometrial cancer

Variable	Level	Cases	Controls	RR[a]
Age (years)	55–59	1	4	
	60–64	12	43	
	65–69	15	60	
	70–74	21	77	
	75–79	6	37	
	80+	8	31	
Mean		70.7	70.8	
S.D.		6.4	6.2	
Gall-bladder disease	Yes	17	24	3.5
	No	46	228	1.0
Hypertension	Yes	26	82	1.5
	No	37	170	1.0
Obesity	Yes	41	126	1.6
	No	16	81	1.0
	Unk	6	45	0.7
Other drugs	Yes	56	176	3.5
(non-oestrogen)	No	7	76	1.0
Oestrogens (any)	Yes	56	127	7.9
	No	7	125	1.0
Conjugated	None	12	143	1.0
oestrogen: amount	0.1–0.299	16	45	4.2
(mg/day)	0.3–0.625	15	41	4.4
	0.626+	16	19	10.0
	Unk	4	4	11.9
Conjugated	None	12	143	1.0
oestrogen: duration	1–11	6	26	2.8
(months)	12–47	12	32	4.5
	48–95	10	17	7.0
	96+	17	23	8.8
	Unk	6	11	6.5

[a] Relative risks calculated from unmatched data; RR = 1.0 identifies baseline category

5.2 Matched pairs: dichotomous exposure

The simplest example of matched data occurs when there is $1:1$ pair matching of cases with controls and a single binary exposure. This is a special case of the situation considered in § 4.4, wherein each stratum consists of one case-control pair. The possible outcomes are represented by four 2×2 tables:

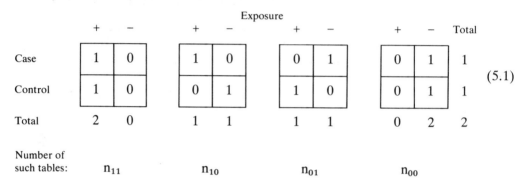

$$(5.1)$$

Number of such tables:	n_{11}	n_{10}	n_{01}	n_{00}

The most suitable statistical model for making inferences about the odds ratio with matched or very finely stratified data is to determine the conditional probability of the number of exposed cases in each stratum, assuming that the marginal totals of that stratum are fixed (§ 4.2). For tables in which there are zero marginal totals, i.e., for the extreme tables in which either both or neither the case or control are exposed to the risk factor, this conditional distribution assigns a probability of one to the observed outcome and hence contributes no information about the odds ratio. The statistical analysis uses just the *discordant* pairs, in which only the case or only the control is exposed. Denoting by $p_1 = 1\text{-}q_1$ and $p_0 = 1\text{-}q_0$ the exposure probabilities for case and control, respectively, the probability of observing a case-control pair with the case only exposed is $p_1 q_0$ while that of observing a pair where only the control is exposed is $q_1 p_0$. Hence the conditional probability of observing a pair of the former variety, given that it is discordant, is

$$\pi = \frac{p_1 q_0}{p_1 q_0 + q_1 p_0} = \frac{\psi}{\psi + 1}, \qquad (5.2)$$

a function of the odds ratio ψ. This is a special case of the general formula (4.2) in which $a = n_1 = n_0 = m_1 = m_0 = 1$. It follows that the conditional probability of observing n_{10} pairs with the case exposed and control not, conditional on there being $n_{10} + n_{01}$ discordant pairs total, is given by the binomial formula with probability parameter π

$$\operatorname{pr}(n_{10} | n_{10} + n_{01}; p_0, p_1) = \binom{n_{10} + n_{01}}{n_{10}} \pi^{n_{10}} (1 - \pi)^{n_{01}}. \qquad (5.3)$$

While we will derive all statistical procedures for making inferences about ψ directly from this distribution, many can also be viewed as specializations of the general methods developed in § 4.4 for stratified samples.

Test of the null hypothesis

When $\psi = 1$, i.e., there is no association, the probabilities of the two different kinds of discordance are equal. Hence for small samples, say either n_{10} or n_{01} smaller than ten, the null hypothesis $H_0: \psi = 1$ may be tested by calculating the exact tail probabilities of the binomial distribution with probability $\pi = \frac{1}{2}$. Otherwise we use the continuity corrected version of the chi-square statistic based on the standardized value of n_{10}:

$$\chi^2 = \frac{\{|n_{10}-E(n_{10})|-\frac{1}{2}\}^2}{\text{Var}(n_{10})} = \frac{\{|n_{10} - \frac{n_{10}+n_{01}}{2}|-\frac{1}{2}\}^2}{\frac{1}{4}(n_{10}+n_{01})}, \tag{5.4}$$

which is a special case of (4.23). Known as McNemar's (1947) test for the equality of proportions in matched samples, it is often expressed

$$\chi^2 = (|n_{10}-n_{01}|-1)^2/(n_{10}+n_{01}). \tag{5.5}$$

Estimating the odds ratio

Since the maximum likelihood estimate (MLE) of the binomial parameter π is simply the observed proportion of discordant pairs in which the case is exposed, it follows that the MLE of ψ is

$$\hat{\psi} = \frac{n_{10}}{n_{01}}, \tag{5.6}$$

i.e., the ratio of the two types of discordant pairs. This is essentially the only instance when the conditional MLE (4.25) discussed for stratified data can readily be calculated. It is interesting that $\hat{\psi}$ is also the Mantel-Haenszel (M-H) estimate (4.26) applied to matched pair data.

Confidence limits

Exact $100(1-\alpha)\%$ confidence intervals for the binomial parameter π in (5.2) may be determined from the charts of Pearson and Hartley (1966). Alternatively, they may be computed from the tail probabilities of the binomial distribution, using the formulae

$$\pi_L = \frac{n_{10}}{n_{10}+(n_{01}+1)F_{\alpha/2}(2n_{01}+2,2n_{10})}.$$

and

$$\pi_U = \frac{(n_{10}+1)F_{\alpha/2}(2n_{10}+2,2n_{01})}{n_{01}+(n_{10}+1)F_{\alpha/2}(2n_{10}+2,2n_{01})}. \tag{5.7}$$

Here $F_{\alpha/2}(\nu_1,\nu_2)$ denotes the upper $100(\alpha/2)$ percentile of the F distribution with ν_1 and ν_2 degrees of freedom, in terms of which the cumulative binomial distribution may be expressed (Pearson & Hartley, 1966).

Approximate confidence limits for π are based on the normal approximation to the binomial tail probabilities. These are computed from the quadratic equations

$$\frac{n_{10} - \pi_L(n_{10} + n_{01}) - \tfrac{1}{2}}{\sqrt{(n_{10} + n_{01})\pi_L(1 - \pi_L)}} = Z_{\alpha/2}$$

and   (5.8)

$$\frac{n_{10} - \pi_U(n_{10} + n_{01}) + \tfrac{1}{2}}{\sqrt{(n_{10} + n_{01})\pi_U(1 - \pi_U)}} = -Z_{\alpha/2}$$

where $Z_{\alpha/2}$ is the upper $100\alpha/2$ percentage point of the normal distribution.

Once limits for π are found, whether from (5.7) or (5.8), they are converted into limits for ψ by using the inverse transformation

$$\psi = \frac{\pi}{1 - \pi}.$$ (5.9)

Alternatively, substituting for π_L and π_U in (5.8), one can write the equations somewhat more simply as

$$\frac{n_{10} - \psi_L n_{01} - \tfrac{1}{2}(1 + \psi_L)}{\sqrt{(n_{10} + n_{01})\psi_L}} = Z_{\alpha/2}$$

                                                                                                      (5.10)

$$\frac{n_{10} - \psi_U n_{01} + \tfrac{1}{2}(1 + \psi_U)}{\sqrt{(n_{10} + n_{01})\psi_U}} = -Z_{\alpha/2}$$

and solve directly for ψ_L and ψ_U.

Adjustment for confounding variables

One problem which occurs frequently in practice is that of adjusting for the confounding effects of a variable on which cases and controls have not been matched. In a study of the effects of a particular occupational exposure on lung cancer, for example, cases and controls may be matched on age and calendar year of diagnosis but not on smoking history. It would have been standard procedure in the past to adjust for the smoking effects by restricting the analysis to those case-control sets which were homogeneous for smoking according to some prescribed definition. Depending upon the stringency of the criteria for "same smoking history", this procedure could well result in the loss of a major portion of the data from analysis and is therefore wasteful. A much more satisfactory technique for control of confounding in a matched analysis is to model the effects of the confounding variables in a multivariate equation which also includes the exposures of interest (see § 7.2).

Testing for heterogeneity of the relative risk

It is important to note that the modifying effect of a variable is not altered by its use for case-control matching. Interaction effects can be estimated just as well from matched as from unmatched data. For example, if both the incidence of the disease and the prevalence of a confounding variable vary throughout the region of study, one might well choose controls matched for place of residence. It would be appropriate and prudent to investigate if the relative risk associated with the exposure of interest was the same throughout the region. Partitioning the matched case-control pairs into subgroups on the basis of the variable of interest, in this case place of residence, enables separate relative risk estimates to be calculated for each subgroup and compared.

This approach could also be used to study the interaction effects of variables besides those used for matching. But, it then entails the same loss of information noted to occur when controlling for the confounding effects of such variables, since the analysis must be restricted to matched sets which are homogeneous for the additional variable(s).

With 1:1 pair matching the easiest way to test for the homogeneity of the odds ratios ψ in several subgroups is in terms of the associated probabilities π defined by (5.2). With H separate subgroups, one simply arranges the frequencies of discordant pairs in a $2 \times H$ table

	Subgroup			
	1	2	...	H
n_{10}				
n_{01}				

and carries out the appropriate test for independence or trend (see § 4.5). More advanced and flexible techniques for modelling interaction effects are presented in Chapter 7.

Example: We begin the illustrative analysis of the Los Angeles endometrial cancer study by confining attention to the first of the four controls and considering exposure as "ever having taken any oestrogen". This yields the following distribution of the 63 case-control pairs:

		Control	
		Exposed	Non-exposed
Case	Exposed	27	29
	Non-exposed	3	4

Hence the ML estimate of the relative risk is $29/3 = 9.67$ and the statistic (5.4) for testing the null hypothesis is

$$\chi^2 = \frac{\{|29-3|-1\}^2}{32} = 19.53,$$

corresponding to a significance level of $p = 0.000005$.

Ninety-five percent confidence limits based on the exact binomial distribution (5.7) are.

$$\pi_L = \frac{29}{29 + 4(2.42)} = 0.75 \text{ corresponding to } \psi'_L = 3.0$$

and

$$\pi_U = \frac{30(4.96)}{3 + 30(4.96)} = 0.97 \text{ corresponding to } \psi'_U = 49.6$$

where $2.42 = F_{.025}(8,58)$ and $4.96 = F_{.025}(60,6)$. Limits based on the normal approximation are found as solutions to the equations (5.10)

$$29-3\psi'_L-{}^{1}/_{2}(1+\psi'_L) = 1.96\sqrt{32\psi'_L}$$

and

$$29-3\psi'_U+{}^{1}/_{2}(1+\psi'_U) = -1.96\sqrt{32\psi'_U}\ ,$$

the solutions being $\psi'_L = 2.8$ and $\psi'_U = 39.7$, respectively.

Similar calculations may be made for the effect of a history of gall-bladder disease on endometrial cancer incidence. Here the overall matched pair data are

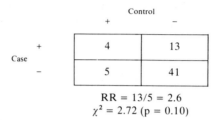

$$RR = 13/5 = 2.6$$
$$\chi^2 = 2.72\ (p = 0.10)$$

Dividing the pairs according to the age of the case (and hence also the control) we find

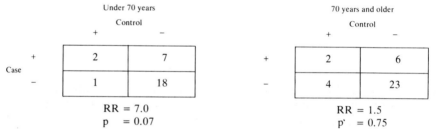

where the two p-values were obtained from the tail probabilities of the binomial distribution with $\pi = {}^{1}/_{2}$ in view of the small numbers. To test for the homogeneity of the two relative risks in the different age groups we form the 2×2 table

	Age		
	<70	≥70	
n_{10}	7	6	13
n_{01}	1	4	5
	8	10	18

for which the usual (corrected) chi-square is $\chi^2 = 0.59$, $p = 0.44$. Thus there is no evidence for a modifying effect of age on the relative risk for gall-bladder disease.

If we try to evaluate hypertensive disease as a confounding or modifying factor in a similar fashion, we find there is a severe loss of data because of the restriction to case-control pairs which are homogeneous for hypertension:

Hypertensive positive
Control

Case	+	−
+	1	1
−	0	6

Hypertensive negative
Control

	+	−
+	2	6
−	1	15

Only 32 of the original 63 pairs are available to estimate the relative risk associated with gall bladder disease while controlling for hypertension, and the number of discordant pairs actually used in the estimation is reduced from 18 to 8. As a measure of relative risk adjusted for hypertension we thus calculate

$$RR = 7/1 = 7.0$$

and for an adjusted test of the null hypothesis

$$\chi^2 = \frac{\{|7-1|-1\}^2}{8} = 3.13.$$

There is clearly almost no information left about how hypertension may modify the effect of a history of gall-bladder disease on cancer risk. Since only one discordant pair remains among those for which case and control are both positive for hypertension, the only possible estimates of relative risk in this category are RR = 0 and RR = ∞. In Chapter 7 we will see how the modelling approach, which assumes a certain structure for the joint effects of the two risk factors in each matched set, allows us to use more of the data to obtain adjusted estimates and tests for interaction between the two factors.

5.3 1:M matching: dichotomous exposures

One-to-one pair matching provides the most cost-effective design when cases and controls are equally "scarce". However when control subjects are more readily obtained than cases, which is often the case with rare forms of cancer, it may make sense to select two, three or even more controls matched to each case. According to the results of Ury (1975) (see also Breslow and Patton, 1979), the theoretical efficiency of a 1:M case-control ratio for estimating a relative risk of about one, relative to having complete information on the control population ($M = \infty$), is $M/(M+1)$. Thus one control per case is 50% efficient, while four per case is 80% efficient. It is clear that increasing the number of controls beyond about 5–10 brings rapidly diminishing returns, unless one is attempting to estimate accurately an extreme relative risk.

Just as for one-to-one pair matching, we can consider each case and the corresponding controls as constituting an individual stratum. With M matched controls per case, there are $2(M+1)$ possible outcomes depending upon whether or not the case is exposed and upon the number of exposed controls. Each outcome corresponds to a 2×2 table.

		Exposure +	−		+	Exposure −		+	−	Total
Case	+	1	0		1	0		1	0	1
Control	−	M	0	...	1	M−1		0	M	M
Total		M+1	0		2	M−1		1	M	M+1

(5.11)

		+	Exposure −		+	−		+	−	Total
Case	+	0	1		0	1		0	1	1
Control	−	M	0		M−1	1	...	0	M	M
Total		M	1		M−1	2		0	M+1	M+1

The first and last tables have no alternative configuration, given the marginals, and hence contain no information with regard to ψ. The 2M remaining tables may be paired into sets of two, each having the same marginal total of exposed. For example, assuming $M \geqq 3$, the table with both the case and two controls positive is paired with the table with three controls positive and the case negative. More generally, we pair together the two tables

1	0	1
m–1	M–m+1	M
m	M–m+1	M+1

and

0	1	1
m	M–m	M
m	M–m+1	M+1

(5.12)

for $m = 1, 2, ..., M$. If, as usual, p_1 denotes the probability that the case is exposed and p_0 the probability that a control is exposed, the probabilities of the two alternative outcomes in (5.12) may be written

$$\binom{M}{m-1} p_1 p_0^{m-1}(1-p_0)^{M-m+1} \text{ and } \binom{M}{m}(1-p_1)p_0^m(1-p_0)^{M-m},$$

respectively. Therefore the conditional probability of the outcome shown on the left, given the marginal totals, is

$$\text{pr(case exposed} \mid \text{m exposed among case} + \text{controls)} = \frac{m\psi}{m\psi + M-m+1}. \quad (5.13)$$

This illustrates once again the fact that consideration of the conditional distribution given the marginals eliminates the nuisance parameters and leaves the probabilities expressed solely in terms of the odds ratio ψ.

The full results of such a matched study may be summarized in the table:

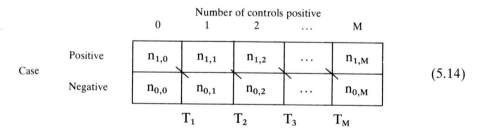

		0	1	2	...	M	
	Positive	$n_{1,0}$	$n_{1,1}$	$n_{1,2}$	...	$n_{1,M}$	
Case							(5.14)
	Negative	$n_{0,0}$	$n_{0,1}$	$n_{0,2}$	...	$n_{0,M}$	
		T_1	T_2	T_3		T_M	

where the entry $n_{1,2}$, for example, is the number of matched sets in which the case and exactly two of the controls are exposed. The diagonal lines in (5.14) indicate the pairing of frequencies according to (5.12), i.e., $n_{1,m-1}$ with $n_{0,m}$, while the totals $T_m = n_{1,m-1} + n_{0,m}$ are the number of matched sets with exactly m subjects exposed. The conditional probability of the entire set of data may be written as a product of binomial distributions with probabilities (5.13) and is proportional to

$$\prod_{m=1}^{M} \left(\frac{m\psi}{m\psi+M-m+1}\right)^{n_{1,m-1}} \left(\frac{M-m+1}{m\psi+M-m+1}\right)^{n_{0,m}} \quad (5.15)$$

Conditional means and variances of the basic frequencies are

$$E(n_{1,m-1}|T_m;\psi) = \frac{T_m m\psi}{m\psi+M-m+1},$$

and $\qquad\qquad\qquad\qquad\qquad\qquad\qquad\qquad\qquad\qquad\qquad$ (5.16)

$$Var(n_{1,m-1}|T_m;\psi) = \frac{T_m m\psi(M-m+1)}{(m\psi+M-m+1)^2},$$

respectively.

Estimation

The conditional MLE i.e., the value $\hat{\psi}$ which maximizes (5.15), is obtained as the solution of the equation

$$\sum_{m=1}^{M} n_{1,m-1} = \sum_{m=1}^{M} \frac{T_m m\psi}{m\psi+M-m+1} \quad (5.17)$$

equating the total observed and expected numbers of exposed cases (see 4.25)[1]. While its solution in general requires iterative numerical calculations, a closed form expression for the case $M = 2$ is available (Miettinen, 1970). A more simply computed estimate is given by the robust formula (4.26) of Mantel and Haenszel, which in this case reduces to

$$\hat{\psi}_{mh} = \frac{\sum_{m=1}^{M} (M-m+1)n_{1,m-1}}{\sum_{m=1}^{M} mn_{0,m}} \quad . \quad (5.18)$$

Test of null hypothesis

As usual this is obtained by comparing the total number of exposed cases with its expectation under the null hypothesis. When $\psi = 1$ the means and variances (5.16) reduce to $T_m m/(M+1)$ and $T_m m(M-m+1)/(M+1)^2$, respectively. Hence the continuity corrected test statistic may be written

$$\chi^2 = \frac{\left\{\left|\sum_{m=1}^{M} (n_{1,m-1} - \frac{T_m m}{M+1})\right| - {}^1/_2\right\}^2}{\frac{1}{(M+1)^2} \sum_{m=1}^{M} T_m m(M-m+1)}$$

---

[1] Note that the number $n_{1,M}$ of sets with the case and all the controls exposed contributes equally to both observed and expected values and is hence ignored.

$$= \frac{\left\{\left|\sum_{m=1}^{M}(M-m+1)n_{1,m-1} - \sum_{m=1}^{M} mn_{0,m}\right| - \frac{1}{2}(M+1)\right\}^2}{\sum_{m=1}^{M} T_m m(M-m+1)} . \tag{5.19}$$

This is a special case of the summary chi-square formula (4.23), which has been derived both by Miettinen (1970) and Pike and Morrow (1970).

Confidence limits

Approximate confidence limits for ψ analogous to those of (4.27) are obtained from the chi-square statistic for testing hypotheses of the form $H:\psi=\psi_0$. This is similar to (5.19) but with means and variances valid for arbitrary ψ. The equations for upper and lower $100(1-\alpha)\%$ limits may thus be written

$$\frac{\sum_{m=1}^{M}\{n_{1,m-1}-E(n_{1,m-1}|T_m;\psi_L)\}-\frac{1}{2}}{\sqrt{\sum_{m=1}^{M} Var(n_{1,m-1}|T_m;\psi_L)}} = Z_{\alpha/2}$$

and   (5.20)

$$\frac{\sum_{m=1}^{M}\{n_{1,m-1}-E(n_{1,m-1}|T_m;\psi_U)\}+\frac{1}{2}}{\sqrt{\sum_{m=1}^{M} Var(n_{1,m-1}|T_m;\psi_U)}} = -Z_{\alpha/2}$$

where E and Var are as defined in (5.16). Numerical methods are required to solve these equations.

Somewhat easier to calculate are the limits for $\log\psi$ proposed by Miettinen (1970) and based on the large sample properties of the conditional probability (5.15). According to the general theory outlined in the following chapter (§ 6.4), the approximate variance of $\log\hat{\psi}$ is

$$Var(\log\hat{\psi}) = \left[\sum_{m=1}^{M}\frac{T_m m\psi(M-m+1)}{(m\psi+M-m+1)^2}\right]^{-1} . \tag{5.21}$$

Substituting either the MLE or M-H estimate of ψ in (5.21) to yield an estimated variance, approximate confidence limits are thus

$$\log\psi_L, \log\psi_U = \log\hat{\psi} \pm Z_{\alpha/2}\sqrt{Var(\log\hat{\psi})}$$

i.e.,   (5.22)

$$\psi_L,\psi_U = \hat{\psi}\exp\{\pm Z_{\alpha/2}\sqrt{Var(\log\hat{\psi})}\} .$$

Alternatively, the test-based procedure (4.20) may be used to approximate the variance, and thus the confidence limits, using only the point estimate and chi-square test statistic. This is subject to the usual problem of underestimating the variance when ψ departs markedly from unity.

Homogeneity of the relative risk

Suppose that the matched sets have been divided into H subgroups, and that separate estimates of the odds ratio are obtained for each one. In order not to lose too much data from analysis, due to non-homogeneity of cases and controls, such subgroups are most usefully formed on the basis of variables already used for matching. The approach we shall continue to use for evaluating the statistical significance of the heterogeneity of the different estimates is to compare the observed number of exposed cases within each subgroup to that expected under the hypothesis that the same relative risk applies to all of them. Thus the statistic is a special case of that suggested in (4.32), with each matched set forming a stratum, except that the exact conditional means and variances (5.16) are used in place of the asymptotic ones.

More formally let us denote by $n_{1,m,h}$ the number of matched sets with the case and m out of M controls exposed in the hth group, by $n_{0,m,h}$ the number of matched sets where the case is unexposed, and set $T_{m,h} = n_{1,m-1,h} + n_{0,m,h}$. Then the statistic for heterogeneity may be written

$$\sum_{h=1}^{H} \left[\frac{\left\{ \sum_{m=1}^{M} n_{1,m-1,h} - E(n_{1,m-1,h} | T_{m,h};\hat{\psi}) \right\}^2}{\sum_{m=1}^{M} \text{Var}(n_{1,m-1,h} | T_{m,h};\hat{\psi})} \right] \qquad (5.23)$$

where $\hat{\psi}$ is an overall estimate of the odds ratio (MLE or M-H) based on the combined data from all H subgroups. This statistic should be referred to tables of chi-square on H-1 degrees of freedom.

If the subgroups correspond to levels $x_1, \ldots, x_H$ of some quantitative variable, a single degree of freedom chi-square test for a trend in the odds ratios is obtained as

$$\frac{\left[\sum_{h=1}^{H} x_h \left\{ \sum_{m=1}^{M} n_{1,m-1,h} - E(n_{1,m-1,h} | T_{m,h};\hat{\psi}) \right\} \right]^2}{\sum_{h=1}^{H} x_h^2 \text{Var}_h - \left[\left(\sum_{h=1}^{H} x_h \text{Var}_h \right)^2 \Big/ \sum_{h=1}^{H} \text{Var}_h \right]}, \qquad (5.24)$$

where the $\text{Var}_h = \sum_{m=1}^{M} \text{Var}(n_{1,m-1,h} | T_{m,h};\hat{\psi})$ are the variances for each subgroup shown in the denominator of (5.23). Note the similarity in form between this statistic and its analog (4.31) for stratified data. When the x's are equally spaced Δ units apart, then a continuity correction of $\Delta/2$ should be applied to the numerator before squaring.

Example continued: To illustrate these methods we repeat the analyses carried out at the end of the last section, but this time we use all four controls for each case rather than just a single one. Considering as the exposure variable whether or not the subject ever used oestrogen, the basic data (5.14) are

		Number of controls exposed					
		0	1	2	3	4	Total
Case	Exposed	3	17	16	15	5	56
	Unexposed	0	4	1	1	1	7
		7	18	17	16		

The total number of exposed cases in the paired sets is $3+17+16+15 = 51$. According to (5.17), we find the MLE by equating this figure to its expected value,

$$51 = \frac{7\psi}{\psi+4} + \frac{36\psi}{2\psi+3} + \frac{51\psi}{3\psi+2} + \frac{64\psi}{4\psi+1}.$$

The solution $\hat{\psi} = 7.95$, obtained by numerical means, is almost identical to that calculated from the unmatched data (Table 5.1). It may be compared with the M-H estimate, determined from (5.18) as

$$\hat{\psi}_{mh} = \frac{4\times 3 + 3\times 17 + 2\times 16 + 1\times 15}{1\times 4 + 2\times 1 + 3\times 1 + 4\times 1} = 8.46.$$

The chi-square statistic (5.19) for testing H_0 is

$$\frac{\left\{|(4\times 3 + 3\times 17 + 2\times 16 + 1\times 15) - (1\times 4 + 2\times 1 + 3\times 1 + 4\times 1)| - \frac{5}{2}\right\}^2}{7\times 1\times 4 + 18\times 2\times 3 + 17\times 3\times 2 + 16\times 4\times 1}$$

$$= \frac{\left(|110-13| - \frac{5}{2}\right)^2}{302} = 29.57,$$

which is of course highly significant ($p < 0.000001$).

To obtain approximate 95% confidence limits for ψ we solve the equations (5.20)

$$\frac{51 - \left[\frac{7\psi_L}{\psi_L+4} + \frac{36\psi_L}{2\psi_L+3} + \frac{51\psi_L}{3\psi_L+2} + \frac{64\psi_L}{4\psi_L+1}\right] - {}^1/_2}{\sqrt{\frac{28\psi_L}{(\psi_L+4)^2} + \frac{108\psi_L}{(2\psi_L+3)^2} + \frac{102\psi_L}{(3\psi_L+2)^2} + \frac{64\psi_L}{(4\psi_L+1)^2}}} = 1.96$$

and

$$\frac{51 - \left[\frac{7\psi_U}{\psi_U+4} + \frac{36\psi_U}{2\psi_U+3} + \frac{51\psi_U}{3\psi_U+2} + \frac{64\psi_U}{4\psi_U+1}\right] + {}^1/_2}{\sqrt{\frac{28\psi_U}{(\psi_U+4)^2} + \frac{108\psi_U}{(2\psi_U+3)^2} + \frac{102\psi_U}{(3\psi_U+2)^2} + \frac{64\psi_U}{(4\psi_U+1)^2}}} = -1.96,$$

this requiring numerical methods, and obtain $\psi_L = 3.3$ and $\psi_U = 19.9$. It is considerably easier to calculate the variance of $\log \hat{\psi}$ using (5.20),

$$\mathrm{Var}(\log \hat{\psi}) = \left[\frac{28\hat{\psi}}{(\hat{\psi}+4)^2} + \frac{108\hat{\psi}}{(2\hat{\psi}+3)^2} + \frac{102\hat{\psi}}{(3\hat{\psi}+2)^2} + \frac{64\hat{\psi}}{(4\hat{\psi}+1)^2}\right]^{-1} = 0.177,$$

where we have inserted the MLE $\hat{\psi} = 7.95$. Consequently approximate 95% limits on $\log \psi$ are $\log(7.95) \pm 1.96\sqrt{0.177}$, or 1.249–2.899, corresponding to limits on ψ of 3.5–18.1. Finally, the test-based procedure centred about the MLE gives

$$\psi_L, \psi_U = 7.95^{(1 \pm 1.96/\sqrt{31.16})}$$

Table 5.2 Test of heterogeneity of relative risk estimates from several groups of 1:M matched sets: Los Angeles endometrial cancer study

Data legend (column 1):

+	n_{10}	n_{11}	n_{12}	n_{13}	n_{14}
−	n_{00}	n_{01}	n_{02}	n_{03}	n_{04}
		T_1	T_2	T_3	T_4

Age group (years)	(2) Relative risk estimates $\hat{\psi}$	(3) $\hat{\psi}_{mh}$	(4) m	(5) Expectations ($\hat{\psi}$ = 7.95) $E(n_{1,m-1} \mid T_m; \hat{\psi})$	(6) Total	(7) Variances ($\hat{\psi}$ = 7.95) $Var(n_{1,m-1} \mid T_m; \hat{\psi})$	(8) Total
55–64	4.18	4.00	1	0.666		0.223	
			2	2.524	9.790	0.400	0.997
			3	3.691		0.285	
			4	2.909		0.089	
65–74	9.76	10.67	1	1.331		0.445	
			2	9.255	30.430	1.468	2.993
			3	10.149		0.785	
			4	9.695		0.295	
75+	9.12	13.50	1	2.662		0.891	
			2	3.365	10.781	0.534	1.657
			3	1.845		0.143	
			4	2.909		0.089	

Data (column 1):

55–64:

+	0	3	4	2
−	0	1	0	1
		1	3	4	3

65–74:

+	1	10	10	2
−	0	1	1	0
	2	11	11	10

75+:

+	2	4	3	1
−	0	2	0	0
	2	4	2	3

or limits of 3.8–16.4, which are somewhat narrower than the others as is typical of this approximate method, where the uncorrected χ^2 of 31.16 has been used, rather than the corrected value of 29.57.

Table 5.2 illustrates the procedures for evaluating the statistical significance of differences in the relative risk obtained from three different age strata. The data shown in column (1) sum to the pooled data from all three strata just analysed. We begin by calculating the means and variances of the frequencies $n_{1,m-1}$ in each stratum, under the hypothesis that the relative risk is constant across strata. Inserting the MLE $\hat{\psi} = 7.95$ in (5.16), for example, we have

$$E(n_{11} \mid T_2; \hat{\psi}) = \frac{3 \times 2 \times 7.95}{2 \times 7.95 + 3} = 2.524$$

$$\mathrm{Var}(n_{11} \mid T_2; \hat{\psi}) = \frac{3 \times 2 \times 3 \times 7.95}{(2 \times 7.95 + 3)^2} = 0.400,$$

and so on for the remaining entries in columns (5) and (7). The subtotals shown in columns (6) and (8) are the means and variances of the number of exposed cases in each stratum, excluding of course the contributions n_{1M} from matched sets in which the case and *all* controls are exposed. These quantities are inserted in (5.23) to obtain the test statistic, with two degrees of freedom

$$\chi^2 = \frac{(9-9.790)^2}{0.997} + \frac{(31-30.430)^2}{2.993} + \frac{(11-10.781)^2}{1.657} = 0.76.$$

Hence, there is no evidence (p = 0.68) of heterogeneity, the variations between the stratum-specific relative risk estimates shown in columns (2) and (3) being attributable to the small numbers in each table.

For the sake of completeness we compute also the single degree of freedom chi-square (5.24) for a trend in relative risk with age, although we know already that its value cannot exceed the 0.76 just obtained for the overall comparison. Assigning "doses" of $x_1 = 0$, $x_2 = 1$ and $x_3 = 2$ to the three age strata, we have

$$\chi^2 = \frac{\{(31-30.430) + 2(11-10.781) - \frac{1}{2}\}^2}{2.993 + 4 \times 1.657 - (2.993 + 2 \times 1.657)^2/(0.997 + 2.993 + 1.657)} = 0.09,$$

where a continuity correction of $\frac{1}{2}$ is applied to the numerator in view of the fact that the x's are spaced one unit apart.

5.4 Dichotomous exposure: variable number of controls

Although the study design stipulates that a fixed number of controls be matched to each case, in practice it may not always be possible to locate the full complement of controls. Even for sets in which all controls are available, some may lack information regarding certain of the risk factors. If the original design calls for 1:4 matching, for example, one may end up with most of the matched sets having data on 1 case and 4 controls, while a lesser number have 3, 2 or 1 controls. Of course, sets in which data are available only for the case, or only for the controls, provide no information about the relative risk in a matched analysis and hence need not be considered.

One approach to the analysis of matched sets containing a variable number of controls is simply to discard all those which do not contain the full number specified by design. Clearly this is a waste of important information and would be considered only if the number of sets to be discarded represented a small fraction of the total. A slight information loss might then be tolerated in order not to increase the computational burden.

Fortunately, the extra computation required is not that great. All of the tests and estimates considered in the previous section may be broken down into component parts consisting of sums or linear combinations of the observed frequencies (5.14), their means and their variances. The corresponding statistic may be generalized for use with a variable number of controls simply by computing each component part separately for the matched sets having a specified case-control ratio, and then reassembling the parts.

Arranging the data as in Table 5.3, let $n_{i,m,M}$ denote the number of matched sets containing M controls of which m are exposed and the case is (i = 1) or is not (i = 0) exposed. Let $T_{m,M} = n_{1,m-1,M} + n_{0,m,M}$ denote the number of such sets having a total of m exposed. The M-H estimate of relative risk may then be written

$$\hat{\psi}_{mh} = \frac{\sum_{M} \sum_{m=1}^{M} (M-m+1)n_{1,m-1,M}/(M+1)}{\sum_{M} \sum_{m=1}^{M} mn_{0,m,M}/(M+1)} \tag{5.25}$$

where $\sum_{M}$ denotes summation over the data in the sub-tables formed for each case-control ratio. The MLE is found as before by equating the observed and expected numbers of exposed cases, as in (5.17), except that there will be a separate contribution to the left and right hand sides of the equation for each value of M:

$$\sum_{M} \sum_{m=1}^{M} n_{1,m-1,M} = \sum_{M} \sum_{m=1}^{M} \frac{T_{m,M}m\psi}{(m\psi+M-m+1)} \tag{5.26}$$

Similarly, the statistic (5.19) for testing the null hypothesis may be written in terms of separate contributions to the observed and expected values, as well as the variance, from each sub-table:

$$\chi^2 = \frac{\left[\left| \sum_{M} \sum_{m=1}^{M} (n_{1,m-1,M} - \frac{m}{M+1} T_{m,M}) \right| - \frac{1}{2} \right]^2}{\sum_{M} \sum_{m=1}^{M} T_{m,M}m(M-m+1)/(M+1)^2} \tag{5.27}$$

Corresponding adjustments are made to the equations (5.20) and (5.21) used to find confidence intervals, as well as to the statistics (5.23) and (5.24) used to test the heterogeneity of the odds ratio in different strata.

Kodlin and McCarthy (1978) note that the M-H estimate (5.25) and summary chi-square (5.27) may each be represented in terms of weighted sums of the basic data appearing in Table 5.3. Appropriate coefficients for weighting each entry are shown in Table 5.4, of which the five parts correspond, respectively, to the numerator and denominator of the M-H estimate, the observed and expected numbers of exposed cases (excluding sets where the case and all controls are exposed), and the variance of the number of exposed cases. For example, using Part A of the table the numerator of the M-H statistic would be calculated as

$$\frac{1}{2}\,n_{1,0,1}$$

$$+\,\frac{2}{3}\,n_{1,0,2}+\frac{1}{3}\,n_{1,1,2}$$

$$+\,\frac{3}{4}\,n_{1,0,3}+\frac{2}{4}\,n_{1,1,3}+\frac{1}{4}\,n_{1,2,3}$$

$$\vdots$$

$$+\,\frac{M}{M+1}\,n_{1,0,M}+\frac{M-1}{M+1}\,n_{1,1,M}+\frac{M-2}{M+1}\,n_{1,2,M}+\ldots+\frac{1}{M+1}\,n_{1,M-1,M}.$$

Table 5.3   Data layout for a matched study involving variable number of controls

Case : control ratio	Exposure of case	Number of controls exposed				
		0	1	2	...	M
1:1	+	$n_{1,0,1}$	$n_{1,1,1}$			
	−	$n_{0,0,1}$	$n_{0,1,1}$			
1:2	+	$n_{1,0,2}$	$n_{1,1,2}$	$n_{1,2,2}$		
	−	$n_{0,0,2}$	$n_{0,1,2}$	$n_{0,2,2}$		
⋮	⋮			⋮		
1:M	+	$n_{1,0,M}$	$n_{1,1,M}$	$n_{1,2,M}$	...	$n_{1,M,M}$
	−	$n_{0,0,M}$	$n_{0,1,M}$	$n_{0,2,M}$		$n_{0,M,M}$

Example continued: To illustrate the procedure to be followed with variable numbers of controls per case we selected another risk variable, dose of *conjugated* oestrogen, for which several subjects had missing values (Table 5.1). Four matched sets in which the case had a missing value were excluded from this analysis. The 59 remaining sets could be divided into two categories, 55 having 4 controls and 4 having 3 controls. Thus, defining "exposed" to be anything above a zero dose of conjugated oestrogen, the results were summarized:

Case: control ratio	Exposure for case	Number of controls exposed					Total
		0	1	2	3	4	
1:3	+	1	3	0	0		4
	−	0	0	0	0		0
		1	3	0			
1:4	+	4	17	11	9	2	43
	−	1	6	3	1	1	12
		10	20	12	10		

Table 5.4 Coefficients used for weighted sums in calculation of the M–H estimate and summary chi-square from matched sets with variable numbers of controls[a]

Case : control ratio	Case exposure	Number of controls exposed					
		0	1	2	3	...	M

A. Numerator of M–H estimate

1:1	+	$1/2$	0				
1:2	+	$2/3$	$1/3$	0			
1:3	+	$3/4$	$2/4$	$1/4$	0		
.				.			
1:M	+	$\frac{M}{M+1}$	$\frac{M-1}{M+1}$	$\frac{M-2}{M+1}$	$\frac{M-3}{M+1}$	...	0

B. Denominator of M–H estimate

1:1	–	0	$1/2$				
1:2	–	0	$1/3$	$2/3$			
1:3	–	0	$1/4$	$2/4$	$3/4$		
.				.			
1:M	–	0	$\frac{1}{M+1}$	$\frac{2}{M+1}$	$\frac{3}{M+1}$	...	$\frac{M}{M+1}$

Case : control ratio	Case exposure	Number of controls exposed					
		0	1	2	3	...	M

C. Observed number of exposed cases

1:1	+	0	1				
1:2	+	0	1	1			
1:3	+	0	1	1	1		
.	.			.			
.	.			.			
.	.			.			
1:M	+	0	1	1	1	...	1

D. Expected number of exposed cases (H_0)

1:1	+	$^1/_2$	0				
	−	0	$^1/_2$				
1:2	+	$^1/_3$	$^2/_3$	0			
	−	0	$^1/_3$	$^2/_3$			
1:3	+	$^1/_4$	$^2/_4$	$^3/_4$	0		
	−	0	$^1/_4$	$^2/_4$	$^3/_4$		
.	.			.			
.	.			.			
.	.			.			
1:M	+	$\dfrac{1}{M+1}$	$\dfrac{2}{M+1}$	$\dfrac{3}{M+1}$	$\dfrac{4}{M+1}$	...	0
	−	0	$\dfrac{1}{M+1}$	$\dfrac{2}{M+1}$	$\dfrac{4}{M+1}$		$\dfrac{M}{M+1}$

Case : control ratio	Case exposure	Number of controls exposed					
		0	1	2	3	...	M

E. Variance of numbers of exposed cases (H_0)

1:1 +

$1/4$	0
0	$1/4$

1:2 +

$2/9$	$2/9$	0
0	$2/9$	$2/9$

1:3 +

$3/16$	$4/16$	$3/16$	0
0	$3/16$	$4/16$	$3/16$

. . .

1:M + −

$\dfrac{M}{(M+1)^2}$	$\dfrac{2(M-1)}{(M+1)^2}$	$\dfrac{3(M-2)}{(M+1)^2}$	$\dfrac{4(M-3)}{(M+1)^2}$	...	0
0	$\dfrac{M}{(M+1)^2}$	$\dfrac{2(M-1)}{(M+1)^2}$	$\dfrac{3(M-2)}{(M+1)^2}$		$\dfrac{M}{(M+1)^2}$

ª When parts of the data are not shown, the corresponding coefficients are zero.

Accordingly, the M-H estimate, calculated from (5.25), is

$$\hat{\psi}_{mh} = \frac{\dfrac{3 \times 1}{4} + \dfrac{2 \times 3}{4} + \dfrac{4 \times 4}{5} + \dfrac{3 \times 17}{5} + \dfrac{2 \times 11}{5} + \dfrac{1 \times 9}{5}}{\dfrac{1 \times 6}{5} + \dfrac{2 \times 3}{5} + \dfrac{3 \times 1}{5} + \dfrac{4 \times 1}{5}} = \frac{21.85}{3.80} = 5.75,$$

while the equation (5.26) to be solved for the MLE is

$$45 = 1 + 3 + 4 + 17 + 11 + 9$$

$$= \frac{\psi}{\psi + 3} + \frac{3 \times 2\psi}{2\psi + 2} + \frac{10 \times \psi}{\psi + 4} + \frac{20 \times 2\psi}{2\psi + 3} + \frac{12 \times 3\psi}{3\psi + 2} + \frac{10 \times 4\psi}{4\psi + 1} \quad ,$$

yielding $\hat{\psi} = 5.53$. To test the null hypothesis we first find the mean value

$$\sum_M \sum_{m=1}^{M} \frac{mT_{m,M}}{M+1} = \frac{1 \times 1}{4} + \frac{2 \times 3}{4} + \frac{1 \times 10}{5} + \frac{2 \times 20}{5} + \frac{3 \times 12}{5} + \frac{4 \times 10}{5} = 26.95$$

and the variance

$$\sum_{M} \sum_{m=1}^{M} \frac{m(M-m+1)T_{m,M}}{(M+1)^2} = \frac{1 \times 3 \times 1}{16} + \frac{2 \times 2 \times 3}{16} + \frac{1 \times 4 \times 10}{25} + \frac{2 \times 3 \times 20}{25} + \frac{3 \times 2 \times 12}{25} + \frac{4 \times 1 \times 10}{25}$$

$$= 11.82,$$

from which the test statistic (5.27) is

$$\chi^2 = \frac{(45-26.95-^1/_2)^2}{11.82} = 26.06.$$

Ninety-five percent confidence limits for log ψ based on (5.21) are found by calculating the variance with separate contributions for $M = 3$ and $M = 4$:

$$\mathrm{Var} = \left[1 \frac{\psi \times 3}{(\psi+3)^2} + 3 \frac{2\psi \times 2}{(2\psi+2)^2} + 10 \frac{\psi \times 4}{(\psi+4)^2} + 20 \frac{2\psi \times 3}{(2\psi+3)^2} + 12 \frac{3\psi \times 2}{(3\psi+2)^2} + 10 \frac{4\psi \times 1}{(4\psi+1)^2} \right]^{-1} = 0.125,$$

where we have inserted the MLE for ψ. Consequently the confidence limits are

$$\psi_L, \psi_U = 5.53 \times \exp(\pm 1.96\sqrt{0.125})$$
$$= (2.76, 11.1).$$

5.5 Multiple exposure levels: single control

Restriction of a risk variable to two levels may waste important information about the effects of the full range of exposures actually experienced (§ 4.5). More detailed results are obtained if the case and control in each matched pair are classified instead into one of several exposure categories. The data are usefully summarized as in Table 5.5, where the entry n_{kh} denotes the number of pairs in which the case is exposed at level k and the control at level h of K possible levels. The marginal totals $n_{k.}$ and $n_{.k}$ represent, respectively, the total number of cases and total number of controls which are exposed at level k. This situation has been studied in some detail by Pike, Casagrande and Smith (1975).

Table 5.5   Representation of data from a matched pair study with K exposure categories

Exposure level for case	Exposure level for control				
	1	2	...	K	Total
1	n_{11}	n_{12}	...	n_{1K}	$n_{1.}$
2	n_{21}	n_{22}	...	n_{2K}	$n_{2.}$
.	.	.		.	.
.	.	.		.	.
.	.	.		.	.
K	n_{K1}	n_{K2}	...	n_{KK}	$n_{K.}$
Total	$n_{.1}$	$n_{.2}$		$n_{.K}$	$n_{..}$

Following the general principles of conditional inference outlined in § 4.2 and § 4.3, we approach the analysis of such data by considering the probability of the outcome in each matched pair conditional on the combined set of exposures for case and control. Pairs in which both members are exposed to the same level are uninformative about the relative risk since for them the conditional probability of the observed outcome is unity. Hence the statistical analysis does not utilize the diagonal entries n_{kk} in Table 5.5. The off-diagonal entries in the table may be grouped into sets of two representing all pairs having a particular combination of different exposures. Thus, for $k \neq h$, $N_{kh} = n_{kh} + n_{hk}$ represents the number of matched pairs in which the exposures are at levels k and h, without specifying which is associated with the case and which with the control.. If ψ_{kh} denotes the relative risk of disease for level k *versus* that for level h, then the conditional distribution of n_{kh} given N_{kh} is binominal (cf. 5.3):

$$\text{pr}(n_{kh} \mid N_{kh}) = \binom{N_{kh}}{n_{kh}} \left(\frac{\psi_{kh}}{1 + \psi_{kh}}\right)^{n_{kh}} \left(\frac{1}{1 + \psi_{kh}}\right)^{n_{hk}} . \qquad (5.28)$$

The (conditional) distribution of the entire set of data consists of the product of $K(K-1)/2$ such binomials, one for each of the entries n_{kh} above the diagonal $(k < h)$ in Table 5.5.

Estimation of relative risk

As noted in § 4.5 for the combination of multiple exposure level data across several strata, the summary estimates of relative risk for different pairs of exposure levels may not display the consistency expected of them. The same phenomenon occurs with matched pairs. Here the odds ratio relating levels k and h of exposure may be calculated from the pairs showing exposure to these two levels only (cf. 5.6) as the ratio

$$\hat{\psi}_{kh} = \frac{n_{kh}}{n_{hk}} .$$

According to their interpretation as ratios of incidence rates for level k *versus* level h, assumed to be constant across the matching factors, the estimated odds ratios ought to satisfy, within the bounds of sampling error, the consistency relationship

$$\psi_{kh} = \frac{\psi_k}{\psi_h} , \qquad (5.29)$$

where $\psi_k = \psi_{k1}$ and $\psi_h = \psi_{h1}$ denote the odds ratios for levels k and h relative to level 1 (baseline). To the extent that the individual estimates $\hat{\psi}_{kh}$ do not satisfy this condition, at least within the limits of random variation, the assumption of constant relative risks across the factors used for matching is called into question.

In order to ensure that the estimated relative risks do display such consistency it is necessary to *build the relationship into a model* for the observed data. The model will contain K−1 parameters $\psi_2, \ldots, \psi_K$ whose ratios are assumed to represent the relative risks for each pair of levels as in (5.29). It is an example of the general conditional model for matched data which will be discussed at greater length in Chapter 7. MLEs for the parameters in the model are found from the usual set of formulae equating observed and expected values of the numbers of cases exposed to each level. There are K–1 equations in K–1 unknowns, namely[1]

$$\sum_{h:h \neq k} n_{kh} = \sum_{h:h \neq k} N_{kh} \frac{\psi_k}{\psi_k + \psi_h} \tag{5.30}$$

for $k = 2, ..., K$. Solution requires numerical methods. Variances for the estimates are also available, but discussion of their derivation and computation is perhaps best left until presentation of the general model (§ 7.3). Approximate confidence limits for the parameters ψ_k may be based on these variances.

Test of the null hypothesis

A test of the hypothesis $H_0 : \psi_2 = \psi_3 = ... = \psi_K = 1$ that there is no effect of exposure on risk is obtained by comparing the observed numbers of cases exposed at each level to that expected, standardizing by the corresponding variance-covariance matrix. Since all the probabilities $\psi_k/(\psi_k + \psi_h)$ in (5.30) are equal to $1/2$ under H_0, the means, variances and covariances of the marginal totals shown in Table 5.5 are readily calculated to be

$$E(n_{k.}) = 1/2 (n_{k.} + n_{.k})$$
$$\text{Var}(n_{k.}) = 1/4 (n_{k.} + n_{.k}) - 1/2 n_{kk} \tag{5.31}$$
and
$$\text{Cov}(n_{k.}, n_{h.}) = -1/4 N_{kh}, \text{ for } h \neq k.,$$

respectively. Only the first K–1 of these are used to form the test statistic, defined by

$$(O-E)^T V^{-1} (O-E) \tag{5.32}$$

where O and E denote the K–1 dimensional vectors of observed and expected values of the $n_{k.}$, while V is the corresponding $(K-1) \times (K-1)$ dimensional covariance matrix. This has a nominal χ^2_{K-1} distribution under the null hypothesis. First proposed by Stuart (1955), it is a special case of the general summary chi-square (4.41) used for testing homogeneity with stratified data (Mantel & Byar, 1978).

If dose levels $x_1, ..., x_K$ are assigned to the K exposure levels, a test for a linear trend in the (log) relative risks ψ_k with increasing dose may be based on the statistic[2]

$$\frac{\left\{ \sum_{k<h}\sum (n_{kh} - n_{hk})(x_k - x_h) \right\}^2}{\sum_{k<h}\sum N_{kh}(x_k - x_h)^2} . \tag{5.33}$$

To make a continuity correction the absolute value of the numerator term inside the brackets is reduced by half of the difference between adjacent doses, provided these

---

[1] Here $\sum_{h:h \neq k}$ means summation over the indices h which are not equal to a fixed k, i.e., $\sum_{h:h \neq 3} n_{3h} = n_{31} + n_{32} + n_{34} + ...$

[2] Here and below $\sum_{k<h}\sum$ denotes summation over all K(K–1)/2 *pairs* of indices (k, h) with k<h.

are equally spaced. This statistic, a special case of (4.43), should be referred to tables of chi-square with one degree of freedom.

Testing for consistency of the odds ratio

In order to test for consistency in the estimated odds ratios, which as explained earlier (§ 4.5) is a consequence of our usual assumptions about the constancy of the relative risk, we compare the frequencies observed in Table 5.5 with those expected under the hypothesis (5.29) using the usual chi-square formula. More specifically, the test statistic is defined by

$$\sum_{k<h}\sum \left\{ n_{kh} - N_{kh} \frac{\hat{\psi}_k}{\hat{\psi}_k + \hat{\psi}_h} \right\}^2 \times \frac{(\hat{\psi}_k + \hat{\psi}_h)^2}{N_{kh}\hat{\psi}_k\hat{\psi}_h}$$

$$= \sum_{k<h}\sum \frac{(n_{kh}\hat{\psi}_h - n_{hk}\hat{\psi}_k)^2}{N_{kh}\hat{\psi}_k\hat{\psi}_h}, \qquad (5.34)$$

where the $\hat{\psi}_k$ are the ML estimates obtained from (5.30).

This statistic should be referred to tables of chi-square with $K(K-1)/2 - (K-1)$ = $(K-1)(K-2)/2$ degrees of freedom. A significant result would lead one to reject the hypothesis of consistency and to search for matching variables which modified the relative risks. However, this test is not likely to be as sensitive to such interactions as the more direct methods based on the modelling approach.

Example continued: We have already remarked that for 4 of 63 cases from the Los Angeles endometrial cancer study the dose level of conjugated oestrogen was unknown. However, this variable was known for the first matched control in all sets. Using four levels of exposure, (1) none, (2) 0.1–0.299 mg, (3) 0.3–0.625 mg and (4) 0.626+ mg, the data for the 59 matched pairs are presented in Table 5.6.

To estimate the relative risk parameters ψ_2, ψ_3, ψ_4, for levels 2, 3 and 4 *versus* level 1, assuming consistency, we set up the equations (5.30):

Table 5.6 Average doses of conjugated oestrogen used by cases and matched controls: Los Angeles endometrial cancer study

Average dose for case (mg)	Average dose for control (mg)				
	0	0.1–0.299	0.3–0.625	0.626+	Total
0	6	2	3	1	12
0.1–0.299	9	4	2	1	16
0.3–0.625	9	2	3	1	15
0.626+	12	1	2	1	16
Total	36	9	10	4	59

$$9 + 2 + 1 = 11 \frac{\psi_2}{1 + \psi_2} + 4 \frac{\psi_2}{\psi_2 + \psi_3} + 2 \frac{\psi_2}{\psi_2 + \psi_4}$$

$$9 + 2 + 1 = 12 \frac{\psi_3}{1 + \psi_3} + 4 \frac{\psi_3}{\psi_2 + \psi_3} + 3 \frac{\psi_3}{\psi_3 + \psi_4}$$

$$12 + 1 + 2 = 13 \frac{\psi_4}{1 + \psi_4} + 2 \frac{\psi_4}{\psi_2 + \psi_4} + 3 \frac{\psi_4}{\psi_3 + \psi_4} .$$

Their solution, obtained by numerical methods, is $\hat{\psi}_2 = 4.59$, $\hat{\psi}_3 = 3.55$ and $\hat{\psi}_4 = 8.33$. These values may be inserted in (5.34) to test the assumption of consistency, yielding

$$\frac{(2 \times 4.59 - 9 \times 1)^2}{11 \times 1 \times 4.59} + \frac{(3 \times 3.55 - 9 \times 1)^2}{12 \times 1 \times 3.55} + \frac{(1 \times 8.33 - 12 \times 1)^2}{13 \times 1 \times 8.33}$$

$$+ \frac{(2 \times 3.55 - 2 \times 4.59)^2}{4 \times 4.59 \times 3.55} + \frac{(1 \times 8.33 - 1 \times 4.59)^2}{2 \times 4.59 \times 8.33} + \frac{(1 \times 8.33 - 2 \times 3.55)^2}{3 \times 3.55 \times 8.33} = 0.46,$$

which when referred to tables of chi-square with $(4-1)(4-2)/2 = 3$ degrees of freedom gives p = 0.93. In other words, the observed data satisfy the consistency hypothesis extremely well.

In order to carry out the global test of the null hypothesis we calculate the means

$$E(n_{1.}) = \frac{1}{2}(36 + 12) = 24$$
$$E(n_{2.}) = \frac{1}{2}(9 + 16) = 12.5$$
$$E(n_{3.}) = \frac{1}{2}(10 + 15) = 12.5,$$

variances

$$Var(n_{1.}) = \frac{1}{4}(36 + 12) - \frac{1}{2}6 = 9$$
$$Var(n_{2.}) = \frac{1}{4}(9 + 16) - \frac{1}{2}4 = 4.25$$
$$Var(n_{3.}) = \frac{1}{4}(10 + 15) - \frac{1}{2}3 = 4.75$$

and covariances

$$Cov(n_{1.}, n_{2.}) = -\frac{1}{4}(2 + 9) = -2.75$$
$$Cov(n_{1.}, n_{3.}) = -\frac{1}{4}(3 + 9) = -3$$
$$Cov(n_{2.}, n_{3.}) = -\frac{1}{4}(2 + 2) = -1$$

according to (5.31). The test statistic (5.32) is then

$$(36 - 24, 9 - 12.5, 10 - 12.5) \begin{bmatrix} 9 & -2.75 & -3 \\ -2.75 & 4.25 & -1 \\ -3 & -1 & 4.75 \end{bmatrix}^{-1} \begin{pmatrix} 36 - 24 \\ 9 - 12.5 \\ 10 - 12.5 \end{pmatrix}$$

$$= (12, -3.5, -2.5) \begin{bmatrix} 0.234 & 0.196 & 0.189 \\ 0.196 & 0.412 & 0.210 \\ 0.189 & 0.210 & 0.374 \end{bmatrix} \begin{pmatrix} 12 \\ -3.5 \\ -2.5 \end{pmatrix}$$

$$= 16.96,$$

which is highly significant (p = 0.001) as shown by reference to tables of chi-square with three degrees of freedom. Assigning dose levels of $x_1 = 1$, $x_2 = 2$, $x_3 = 3$ and $x_4 = 4$ to the four exposure levels, we next calculate the test for trend using (5.33). This is

$$\frac{[(2-9)(1-2) + (3-9)(1-3) + (1-12)(1-4) + (2-2)(2-3) + (1-1)(2-4) + (1-2)(3-4) - \frac{1}{2}]^2}{11(1-2)^2 + 12(1-3)^2 + 13(1-4)^2 + 4(2-3)^2 + 2(2-4)^2 + 3(3-4)^2} = 14.43,$$

an even more significant result (p = 0.0001) which indicates that most of the variation in risk among the four exposure levels is accounted for by the linear increase. The contribution of $16.96 - 14.43 = 2.53$

from the remaining two degrees of freedom is not statistically significant. Note that we have used the continuity correction of $^1/_2$ in the numerator of this statistic, as is appropriate since the assigned x's are spaced one unit apart.

5.6 More complex situations

One lesson learned from the preceding sections is that the types of matched data which can be analysed easily using elementary methods are extremely limited. While the calculations are reasonably tractable in the case of a single dichotomous risk variable, with both single or multiple controls, estimation of a consistent set of relative risks for polytomous exposures requires solution of a system of non-linear equations even for matched pairs. More complicated still are the situations involving multiple controls together with a single exposure variable at multiple levels, or multiple exposure variables with any combination of controls. The control of confounding, or evaluation of effect modification, by variables not used for matching may require that we discard from analysis much of the relevant data.

Certain of the limitations imposed by the elementary methods can be overcome using multivariate analysis. Just as we noted earlier for stratified samples, multivariate analysis of matched data is carried out in the context of an explicit mathematical model relating each individual's exposures to his risk for disease. Such modelling is especially valuable in dealing with quantitative variables as it permits their effect on risk to be summarized by a few parameters. Chapter 6 introduces for this purpose the linear logistic regression model, showing that its structure is well suited for determining the multiplicative effects of one or more risk factors on disease rates. Chapter 7 extends the model for use with matched or finely stratified samples. Since all the tests and estimates considered in this chapter occur as special cases of those derived from the general model, the general-purpose computer programmes (Appendix IV) which are available to fit the multivariate model can be used (and in fact were used) to solve the equations for maximum likelihood estimation which occur in those particular problems considered above.

REFERENCES

Breslow, N. & Patton, J. (1979) *Case-control analysis of cohort studies.* In Breslow, N. & Whittemore, A., eds, *Energy and Health,* Philadelphia. Society for Industrial and Applied Mathematics, pp. 226–242

Kodlin, D. & McCarthy, N. (1978) Reserpine and breast cancer. *Cancer, 41,* 761–768

Mack, T.M., Pike, M.C., Henderson, B.E., Pfeffer, R.I., Gerkins, V.R., Arthur, B.S. & Brown, S.E. (1976) Estrogens and endometrial cancer in a retirement community. *New Engl. J. Med., 294,* 1262–1267

McNemar, Q. (1947) Note on the sampling error of the difference between correlated proportions or percentages. *Psychometrika, 12,* 153–157

Mantel, N. & Byar, D. (1978) Marginal homogeneity, symmetry and independence. *Commun. Stat. Theory Meth., A7 (10),* 956–976

Miettinen, O.S. (1970) Estimation of relative risk from individually matched series. *Biometrics, 26,* 75–86

Pearson E.S. & Hartley, H.O. (1966) *Biometrika Tables for Statisticians,* Vol. I (3rd Edition), Cambridge, Cambridge University Press

Pike, M.C., Casagrande, J. & Smith, P.G. (1975) Statistical analysis of individually matched case-control studies in epidemiology: factor under study a discrete variable taking multiple values. *Br. J. prev. soc. Med., 29,* 196–201

Pike, M.C. & Morrow, R.H. (1970) Statistical analysis of patient-control studies in epidemiology. Factor under investigation an all-or-none variable. *Br. J. prev. soc. Med., 24,* 42–44

Stuart, A. (1955) A test for homogeneity of the marginal distributions in a two way classification. *Biometrika, 42,* 412–416

Ury, H.K. (1975) Efficiency of case-control studies with multiple controls per case: continuous or dichotomous data. *Biometrics, 31,* 643–649

LIST OF SYMBOLS – CHAPTER 5 (in order of appearance)

n_{11}	number of matched pairs with both case and control exposed
n_{10}	number of matched pairs with case exposed and control not
n_{01}	number of matched pairs with control exposed and case not
n_{00}	number of matched pairs with neither case nor control exposed
p_1	probability of exposure for case
$q_1 = 1 - p_1$	probability of non-exposure for case
p_0	probability of exposure for control
$q_0 = 1 - p_0$	probability of non-exposure for control
ψ	odds ratio
π	probability that in a discordant matched pair it is the case who is exposed rather than the control
$E(\ )$	expectation of a quantity ( )
$\text{Var}(\ )$	variance of a quantity ( )
$\binom{n_1 + n_2}{n_1}$	binomial coefficient; number of ways of drawing samples of n_1 objects from a total of $n_1 + n_2$
$|x|$	absolute value of a number x
π_L	lower confidence limit for π
π_U	upper confidence limit for π
ψ_L	lower confidence limit for ψ
ψ_U	upper confidence limit for ψ
$Z_{\alpha/2}$	upper $100\alpha/2$ percentile of the standard normal distribution
$\text{pr}(\ )$	probability of an event ( )
$\text{pr}(\ |\ )$	probability of one event conditional on another
M	number of controls in each matched set
$n_{1,m}$	number of matched sets with case exposed and m controls exposed
$n_{0,m}$	number of matched sets with case not exposed and m controls exposed
T_m	number of matched sets with m exposed among case + controls (additional subscripts are added to distinguish various groups)

$E(\;\mid\;)$	expectation of a quantity conditional on the values of another
$Var(\;\mid\;)$	variance of a quantity conditional on the values of another
h	subscript indicating the hth of H groups of matched sets; e.g., $n_{1,m,h}$ is the number of matched sets with the case and m controls exposed in the hth group
M	subscript indicating the number of controls in matched set data having a variable number of controls per case; e.g., $n_{1,m,M}$ is the number of sets in which the case and m of M controls are exposed
χ_ν^2	a statistic whose (asymptotic) distribution under the null hypothesis is that of chi-square on ν degrees of freedom (when ν is not specified it is meant to be 1)
K	number of levels of a polytomous risk factor
n_{kh}	number of matched pairs where the case is exposed at level k of a polytomous variable and the control at level h
$N_{kh} = n_{kh} + n_{hk}$	number of matched pairs in which one member is at level k and the other at level h ($k \neq h$)
$n_{k.}$	sum of n_{kh} over h; number of matched pairs where the case is exposed at level k
$n_{.k}$	sum of n_{hk} over h; number of matched pairs where the control is exposed at level k
ψ_{kh}	odds ratio expressing relative risk for exposure to level k *versus* level h of a polytomous variable
ψ_k	odds ratio expressing relative risk of disease for a person exposed to level k of a polytomous factor, using level 1 as baseline ($\psi_1 = 1$)
$\hat{}$	denotes an estimate, e.g., $\hat{\psi}_k$ is an estimate of the odds ratio ψ_k
O	K–1 dimensional vector of numbers of matched pairs in which the case is exposed to one of the first K–1 levels of a polytomous factor; $\mathbf{O} = (n_{1.}, n_{2.}, ..., n_{K-1.})$
E	K–1 vector of expectations $\mathbf{E} = E(\mathbf{O}) = [E(n_{1.}), E(n_{2.}), ..., E(n_{K-1,.})]$
V	K–1 × K–1 variance-covariance matrix of which the (k,h) element is $Cov(n_{k.}, n_{h.}) = -\frac{1}{4}N_{kh}$ for $k \neq h$ or $Var(n_{k.}) = \frac{1}{4}(n_{k.} + n_{.k}) - \frac{1}{2}n_{kk}$ for k=h (see equation 5.3)

6. UNCONDITIONAL LOGISTIC REGRESSION FOR LARGE STRATA

6.1   Introduction to the logistic model

6.2   General definition of the logistic model

6.3   Adaptation of the logistic model to case-control studies

6.4   Likelihood inference: an outline

6.5   Combining results from 2×2 tables

6.6   Qualitative analysis of grouped data from Ille-et-Vilaine

6.7   Quantitative analysis of grouped data

6.8   Regression adjustment for confounders

6.9   Analysis of continuous data

6.10 Interpretation of regression coefficients

6.11 Transforming continuous risk variables

6.12 Studies of interaction in a series of 2×2 tables

CHAPTER 6

UNCONDITIONAL LOGISTIC REGRESSION
FOR LARGE STRATA

The elementary techniques described above for stratified analysis of case-control studies, and in particular the Mantel-Haenszel combined relative risk estimate and test statistic, have served epidemiologists well for over two decades. Most of the calculations are simple enough for an investigator to carry out himself, although this often means devoting considerable time to routine chores. Some of the boredom may be alleviated through the use of modern programmable calculators, for which the methods are ideally suited. By working closely with his data, examining them in tabular form, calculating relative risks separately for each stratum, and so on, the researcher can spot trends or inconsistencies he might not otherwise have noticed. Errors in the data may be discovered in this way, and new hypotheses generated.

Nevertheless there are certain limitations inherent in the elementary techniques that must be recognized. If many potentially confounding factors must be controlled simultaneously, a stratified analysis will ultimately break down. Individual strata simply become so large in number and small in size that many of them contain only cases or only controls. This means that substantial amounts of data are effectively lost from the analysis. There are similar limits on the number of categories into which continuous risk factors can be broken down for calculation of separate estimates of relative risk. It is desirable to leave them as continuous variables for purposes of interpolation and extrapolation. The inconsistencies arising from the selection of different levels of a variable to serve as baseline have already been noted, and while often relatively minor, these can be irritating. Limitations are likewise imposed on the extent to which one can analyse the joint effects of several risk factors. Perhaps even more important are the deficiencies in the elementary methods for evaluating interactions among risk and nuisance variables. The usual tests are notoriously lacking in statistical power against patterns of interaction which one might well expect to observe in practice. Other than calculating a separate estimate for each stratum, no provision is made for incorporating such interactions into the estimates of relative risk.

Access to high-speed computing machinery and appropriate statistical software removes these limitations and opens up new possibilities for the statistical analysis of case-control data. By entering a few simple commands into a computer terminal, the investigator can carry out a range of exploratory analyses which could take days or weeks to perform by hand, even with a programmable calculator. He has a great deal of flexibility in choosing how variables are treated in the analysis, how they are categorized, or how they are transformed. The possibilities for multivariate analysis are virtually limitless. Such methods should, of course, be used in conjunction with tabular presentation of the basic data. Liberal use of charts and graphs to represent the results of the analyses is also recommended.

The basic tool which allows the scope of case-control study analysis to be thus broadened is the linear logistic regression model. Here we introduce the logistic model as a method for multivariate analysis of prospective or cohort studies, which reflects the historical fact that the model was specifically designed for, and first used with, such investigations. Its equal suitability for use in case-control investigations follows as a logical consequence. We replicate the stratified analyses of Chapter 4 using the modelling approach, and then extend these analyses by the inclusion of additional variables so as to illustrate the full power and potential of the method.

Unfortunately the level of statistical sophistication demanded from the reader for full appreciation of the modelling approach is more advanced than it has been in the past. While we have attempted to make the discussion as intelligible as possible for the non-specialist, familiarity with certain aspects of statistical theory, especially linear models and likelihood inference, will undoubtedly facilitate complete understanding.

6.1 Introduction to the logistic model

Whether using the follow-up or case-control approach to study design, cancer epidemiologists typically collect data on a number of variables which may influence disease risk. Each combination of different levels of these variables defines a category for which an estimate of the probability of disease development is to be made. For example, we way want to determine the risk of lung cancer for a man aged 55 years who has worked 30 years as a telephone linesman and smoked 20 cigarettes per day since his late teens.

If a large enough population were available for study, and if we had unlimited time and money, an obvious approach to this problem would be to collect sufficient numbers of subjects in each category in order to make a precise estimate of risk for each category separately. Of course in the case-control situation these risk estimates would not be absolute, but instead would be relative to that for a designated baseline category. With such a vast amount of data there would be no need to borrow information from neighbouring categories, i.e., those having identical levels for some of the risk variables and similar levels for the remainder, in order to get stable estimates of risk.

Epidemiological studies of cancer, however, rarely even come close to this ideal. Often the greatest limitation is simply the number of cases available for study within a reasonable time period. While this number may be perfectly adequate for assessing the relative risks associated with a few discrete levels of a single risk factor, it is usually insufficient to provide separate estimates for the large number of categories generated by combining even a few more or less continuous factors. Thus we are faced with the problem of having to make *smoothed* estimates which do utilize information from surrounding categories in order to estimate the risks in each one.

Such smoothing is carried out in terms of a *model*, which relates disease risk to the various combinations of factor levels which define each risk category *via* a *mathematical formula*. The model gives us a simplified, quantitative description of the main features of the relationship between the several risk factors and the probability of disease development. It enables us to *predict* the risk even for categories in which scant information is available. Important features for the model to have are that it provide meaningful results, describe the observed data well and, within these constraints, be as simple as possible. In view of the discussion in Chapter 2, therefore, the *parameters* of any proposed model should be readily interpretable in terms of relative risk. The model should also allow relative risks corresponding to two or more distinct factors to be represented as the product of individual relative risks, at least as a first approximation.

A model which satisfies these requirements, indeed which has in part been developed specifically to meet them, is the *linear logistic model*. It derives its name from the fact that the *logit* transform of the disease probability in each risk category is expressed as a linear function of *regression* variables whose values correspond to the levels of exposure to the risk factors. In symbols, if P denotes the disease risk, the logit transform y is defined by

$$y = \text{logit } P = \log\left(\frac{P}{1-P}\right), \tag{6.1}$$

or, conversely, expressing P in terms of y,

$$P = \frac{\exp(y)}{1 + \exp(y)}. \tag{6.2}$$

Since $P/(1-P)$ denotes the disease odds, another name for logit is *log odds*. Cox (1970) develops the theory of logistic regression in some detail.

The simplest example of logistic regression is provided by the ubiquitous 2×2 table considered in § 2.8 and § 4.2. Suppose that there is but a single factor and two risk categories, exposed and unexposed, and let P_1 and P_0 denote the associated disease probabilities. According to the discussion in § 2.8 the key parameter, which is both estimable from case-control studies and interpretable as a relative risk, is the odds ratio

$$\psi = \frac{P_1 Q_0}{P_0 Q_1}.$$

Its logarithm, i.e., the log relative risk, may be expressed

$$\beta = \log \psi = \text{logit } P_1 - \text{logit } P_0$$

as the *difference* between two logits. Let us define a single binary regression variable x by $x = 1$ for exposed and $x = 0$ for unexposed. If we write $P(x)$ for the disease probability associated with an exposure x, and $r(x) = P(x)Q_0/P_0Q(x)$ for the relative risk (odds ratio relative to $x = 0$), we have

$$\log r(x) = \beta x$$

or

$$\text{logit } P(x) = \alpha + \beta x, \tag{6.3}$$

where $\alpha = \text{logit } P_0$. There is a perfect correspondence between the two parameters α and β in the model and the two disease risks such that

$$P_1 = \frac{\exp(\alpha + \beta)}{1 + \exp(\alpha + \beta)}$$

and

$$P_0 = \frac{\exp(\alpha)}{1 + \exp(\alpha)}.$$

The formulation (6.3) focuses on the key parameter, β, and suggests how to extend the model for more complex problems.

A more interesting situation arises when there are two risk factors A and B, each at an exposed (+) and unexposed (−) level (§ 2.6). The combined levels of exposure yield four risk categories with associated disease probabilities P_{ij}:

	Factor B	
Factor A	+	−
+	P_{11}	P_{10}
−	P_{01}	P_{00}

$$(6.4)$$

Taking P_{00} as the baseline disease risk, there are three relative risks to be estimated, corresponding to the three odds ratios

$$\psi_{10} = \frac{P_{10}Q_{00}}{P_{00}Q_{10}} \approx r_A$$

$$\psi_{01} = \frac{P_{01}Q_{00}}{P_{00}Q_{01}} \approx r_B$$

and

$$\psi_{11} = \frac{P_{11}Q_{00}}{P_{00}Q_{11}} \approx r_{AB}.$$

Here r_A, r_B and r_{AB} are relative risks for single and joint exposures, relative to no exposure, as defined in § 2.6.

We are particularly interested in testing the multiplicative hypothesis $r_{AB} = r_A r_B$ under which the relative risk for exposure to A is independent of the levels of B or, equivalently, the relative risk for B is independent of exposure to A. Expressed in terms of the odds ratios this becomes

$$\psi_{11} = \psi_{10}\psi_{01}. \qquad (6.5)$$

If the hypothesis appears to fit the observed data, we should be able to summarize the risks for the three exposure categories relative to the baseline category in two numbers, *viz* the estimated relative risks for factors A and B individually. Otherwise a separate estimate for each of the three exposure categories will be required. We considered in § 4.4 some *ad hoc* tests for the multiplicative hypothesis and suggested that the Mantel-

Haenszel formula be used to estimate the individual relative risks if the hypothesis were accepted.

Estimates and tests of the multiplicative hypothesis are simply obtained in terms of a logistic regression model for the disease probabilities (6.4). Define the binary regression variable $x_1 = 1$ or 0 according to whether a person is exposed to Factor A or not, and similarly let x_2 indicate the levels of exposure to Factor B. Variables such as x_1 and x_2, which take on 0–1 values only, are sometimes called *dummy* or *indicator* variables since they serve to identify different levels of exposure rather than expressing it in quantitative terms. Note that the product x_1x_2 equals 1 only for the double exposure category. Let us define $P(x_1,x_2)$ as the disease probability, and $r(x_1,x_2)$ as the relative risk (odds ratio) relative to the unexposed category $x_1 = x_2 = 0$. Then we can *re-express* the relative risks, or equivalently the probabilities, using the model

$$\log r(x_1,x_2) = \beta_1 x_1 + \beta_2 x_2 + \gamma x_1 x_2$$

i.e.,

$$\text{logit } P(x_1,x_2) = \alpha + \beta_1 x_1 + \beta_2 x_2 + \gamma x_1 x_2. \tag{6.6}$$

Since there are four parameters α, β_1, β_2 and γ to describe the four probabilities P_{ij}, we say that the model is completely *saturated*. It imposes *no constraints* whatsoever on the relationships between the four probabilities or the corresponding odds ratios. Thus we may solve equation (6.6) explicitly for the four parameters, obtaining

$$\alpha = \text{logit } P_{00}$$

as the logit transform of the baseline disease probability,

$$\beta_1 = \log \psi_{10}$$

and

$$\beta_2 = \log \psi_{01}$$

as the log relative risks for individual exposures, and

$$\gamma = \log \left(\frac{\psi_{11}}{\psi_{10}\psi_{01}} \right) \tag{6.7}$$

$$= \text{logit } P_{11} - \text{logit } P_{10} - \text{logit } P_{01} + \text{logit } P_{00}$$

as the *interaction* parameter. It is clear from (6.7) that $\exp(\gamma)$ represents the multiplicative factor by which the relative risk for the double exposure category differs from the product of relative risks for the individual exposures. If $\gamma > 0$, a *positive interaction*, the risk accompanying the combined exposure is greater than predicted by the individual effects; if $\gamma < 0$, a *negative interaction*, the combined risk is less. Testing the multiplicative hypothesis (6.5) is equivalent to testing that the interaction parameter γ in the logistic model is equal to 0.

If the hypothesis $\gamma = 0$ is accepted by our test criterion, we would consider fitting to the data the reduced three parameter model

$$\text{logit } P(x_1,x_2) = \alpha + \beta_1 x_1 + \beta_2 x_2, \tag{6.8}$$

which re-expresses the multiplicative hypothesis in logit terms. This model does impose constraints on the four disease probabilities P_{ij}. For example, since

$$\beta_1 = \log \psi_{10} = \log \frac{\psi_{11}}{\psi_{01}}$$

now represents the log relative risk for A *whether or not* exposure to B occurs, it would be estimated by combining information from the 2×2 tables

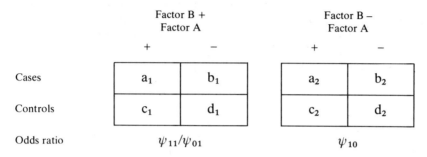

Likewise the estimate of

$$\beta_2 = \log \psi_{01} = \log \frac{\psi_{11}}{\psi_{10}}$$

would combine information from both the tables

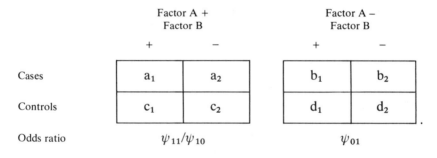

The difference between the interpretation of β_1 in (6.6) and the same parameter in (6.8) illustrates that *the meaning of the regression coefficients in a model depends on what other variables are included.* In the saturated model β_1 represents the log relative risk for A at level 0 of B only, whereas in (6.8) it represents the log relative risk for A at both levels of B. Testing the hypothesis $\beta_1 = 0$ in (6.8) is equivalent to testing the hypothesis that Factor A has no effect on risk, against the alternative hypothesis that there is an effect, but one which does not depend on B. It makes little sense to test $\beta_1 = 0$ in (6.6), or more generally to test for main effects being zero in the presence of interactions involving the same factors. Models which contain interaction terms without the corresponding main effects correspond to hypotheses of no *practical* interest (Nelder, 1977).

The regression approach is easily generalized to incorporate the effects of more than two risk factors, or risk factors at more than two levels. Suppose that Factor B occurred at three levels, say 0 = low, 1 = medium and 2 = high. There would then be six disease probabilities

	Factor B		
Factor A	High	Medium	Low
Exposed	P_{12}	P_{11}	P_{10}
Unexposed	P_{02}	P_{01}	P_{00}

and five odds ratios

$$\psi_{ij} = \frac{P_{ij} Q_{00}}{P_{00} Q_{ij}},$$

where all risks are expressed relative to P_{00} as baseline. In order to identify the three levels of Factor B, two indicator variables x_2 and x_3 are required in place of the single x_2 used earlier. These are coded as follows:

	Factor B		
	High	Medium	Low
$x_2 =$	0	1	0
$x_3 =$	1	0	0

More generally, for a factor with K levels, K–1 indicator variables will be needed to describe its effects. With x_1 defining exposure to A as before, the saturated model with six parameters is written

$$\text{logit } P_{ij} = \alpha + \beta_1 x_1 + \beta_2 x_2 + \beta_3 x_3 + \gamma_{12} x_1 x_2 + \gamma_{13} x_1 x_3,$$

where the values of the x's are determined from the factor levels i and j. Now the multiplicative hypothesis

$$\psi_{ij} = \psi_{i0} \psi_{0j}$$

corresponds to setting both interaction parameters γ_{12} and γ_{13} to zero, in which case the coefficients β_2 and β_3 represent the log relative risks for levels 1 and 2 of Factor B as compared with level 0.

If instead there are three factors A, B and C each at two levels, the disease probabilities may be denoted

	Factor C + Factor B		Factor C − Factor B	
	+	−	+	−
Factor A				
+	P_{111}	P_{101}	P_{110}	P_{100}
−	P_{011}	P_{001}	P_{010}	P_{000}

Here there are seven odds ratios $\psi_{ijk} = \dfrac{P_{ijk} Q_{000}}{P_{000} Q_{ijk}}$ to be estimated. The fully saturated model may be written

$$\text{logit } P_{ijk} = \alpha + \beta_1 x_1 + \beta_2 x_2 + \beta_3 x_3 + \gamma_{12} x_1 x_2 + \gamma_{13} x_1 x_3 + \gamma_{23} x_2 x_3 + \delta_{123} x_1 x_2 x_3, \quad (6.9)$$

where x_1, x_2 and x_3 are indicator variables which identify exposures to factors A, B and C, respectively. The last parameter δ_{123} denotes the *second order interaction* involving all three variables. It has several equivalent representations in terms of the odds ratios or disease probabilities. One of these, for example, is

$$\delta_{123} = \log \frac{\psi_{111}}{\psi_{101}\psi_{011}} - \log \frac{\psi_{110}}{\psi_{100}\psi_{010}}$$

$$= \text{logit } P_{111} - \text{logit } P_{101} - \text{logit } P_{011} + \text{logit } P_{001}$$

$$- \{\text{logit } P_{110} - \text{logit } P_{100} - \text{logit } P_{010} + \text{logit } P_{000}\},$$

viz the difference between the AB interaction at level 1 of Factor C and that same interaction at level 0 of Factor C. Other representations would be the difference between the AC interactions at the two levels of B, or the difference between the BC interactions at the two levels of A.

The advantage of expressing the disease probabilities in an equation such as (6.9) is that the higher order interactions generally turn out to be negligible. This permits the relative risks for all the cells in the complete cross-classification to be estimated using a smaller number of parameters which represent the main multiplicative effects of the important risk factors plus occasional lower order interactions. By reducing the number of independent parameters which must be estimated from the data, we achieve the smoothing which was noted earlier to be one of the primary goals of the analysis. If high-order interactions are found to be present, this alerts us to the fact that risk depends in a complicated way on the constellation of risk factors, and may not easily be summarized in a few measures.

Example: As an example of the interpretation of a three-factor regression model, suppose that in (6.9) the three main effects are present along with the two-factor AC interaction. Assume further that the values of the parameters are given by

$$\exp(\beta_1) = \psi_{100} = 2$$

$$\exp(\beta_2) = \psi_{010} = 3$$

$$\exp(\beta_3) = \psi_{001} = 4$$

and

$$\exp(\gamma_{13}) = \frac{\psi_{101}}{\psi_{100}\psi_{001}} = 2.$$

Then we can reconstruct the seven odds ratios for the three-dimensional cross-classification as the entries in the tables

	Factor C + Factor B		Factor C – Factor B	
Factor A	+	−	+	−
+	48	16	6	2
−	12	4	3	1

The relative risk of A is twice as great for those exposed to C as for those not so exposed, and vice versa. Otherwise the risks combine in a perfectly multiplicative fashion.

Further details concerning the fitting and interpretation of logistic and log linear models of the type introduced in this section are given in the elementary text by Fienberg (1977). More comprehensive accounts are given by Bishop, Fienberg and Holland (1975), Haberman (1974) and Cox (1970). Vitaliano (1978) conducts an analysis of a case-control study of skin cancer as related to sunlight exposure, using a logistic regression model with four factors, one at four levels and the remainder at two.

6.2 General definition of the logistic model

So far the logistic model has been used solely as a means of relating disease probabilities to one or more categorical risk factors whose levels are represented by indicator variables. More generally the model relates a dichotomous outcome variable y which, in our context, denotes whether ($y = 1$) or not ($y = 0$) the individual develops the disease during the study period, to a series of K regression variables $\underset{\sim}{x} = (x_1, \ldots, x_K)$ via the equation

$$\mathrm{pr}(y = 1 \,|\, \mathbf{x}) = \frac{\exp(\alpha + \Sigma \beta_k x_k)}{1 + \exp(\alpha + \Sigma \beta_k x_k)} \tag{6.10}$$

or, equivalently,

$$\mathrm{logit}\ \mathrm{pr}(y = 1 \,|\, \mathbf{x}) = \alpha + \sum_{k=1}^{K} \beta_k x_k.$$

This formulation implies that the relative risk for individuals having two different sets $\underset{\sim}{x}^*$ and x of risk variables is

$$\mathrm{RR} = \frac{P(\mathbf{x}^*)\,\{1 - P(\mathbf{x})\}}{P(\mathbf{x})\,\{1 - P(\mathbf{x}^*)\}} = \exp\Big\{\sum_{k=1}^{K} \beta_k (x_k^* - x_k)\Big\}. \tag{6.11}$$

Thus α represents the log odds of disease risk for a person with a standard $(\mathbf{x} = \mathbf{0})$ set of regression variables, while $\exp(\beta_k)$ is the fraction by which this risk is increased (or decreased) for every unit change in x_k. A large number of possible relationships may be represented in this form by including among the x's indicator variables and continuous measurements, transformations of such measurements, and cross-product or interaction variables.

As we saw in the last chapter, one important means of controlling the effects of nuisance or confounding variables is by stratification of the study population on the basis of combinations of levels of these variables. When conducting similar analyses in the context of logistic regression, it is convenient to generalize the model further so as to isolate the stratum effects, which are often of little intrinsic interest, from the effects of the risk factors under study. With $P_i(\mathbf{x})$ denoting the disease probability in stratum i for an individual with risk variables $\mathbf{x}$, we may write

$$\text{logit } P_i(\mathbf{x}) = \alpha_i + \sum_{k=1}^{K} \beta_k x_k. \tag{6.12}$$

If none of the regression variables are interaction terms involving the factors used for stratification, a consequence of (6.12) is that the relative risks associated with the risk factors under study are constant over strata. By including such interaction terms among the x's, one may model changes in the relative risk which accompany changes in the stratification variables. The fact that the parameters of the logistic model are so easily interpretable in terms of relative risk is, as we have said, one of the main reasons for using the model.

The earliest applications of this model were in prospective studies of coronary heart disease in which $\mathbf{x}$ represented such risk factors as age, blood pressure, serum cholesterol and cigarette consumption (Cornfield, 1962; Truett, Cornfield & Kannel, 1967). In these investigations the authors used linear discriminant analysis to estimate the parameters, an approach which is strictly valid only if the x's have multivariate normal distributions among both diseased and non-diseased (see § 6.3). The generality of the method was enhanced considerably by the introduction of maximum likelihood estimation procedures (Walker & Duncan, 1967; Day & Kerridge, 1967; Cox, 1970). These are now available in several computer packages, including the General Linear Interactive Modelling system (GLIM) distributed by the Royal Statistical Society (Baker & Nelder, 1978).

We noted in § 2.8 that for a long study it is appropriate to partition the time axis into several intervals and use these as one of the criteria for forming strata. In the present context this means that the quantity $P_i(\mathbf{x})$ refers more specifically to the *conditional* probability of developing disease during the time interval specified by the ith stratum, given that the subject was disease-free at its start. For follow-up or cohort studies, if we are to use conventional computer programmes for logistic regression with conditional probabilities, separate data records must be read into the computer for *each stratum* in which an individual appears. Thomson (1977) discusses in some detail the problems of estimation in this situation.

A limiting form of the logistic model for conditional probabilities, obtained by allowing the time intervals used for stratification to become infinitesimally small, is known as the *proportional hazards* model (Cox, 1972). Here the ratio of incidence rates for individuals with exposures x^* and x is given exactly by the right-hand side of equation (6.11). This approach has the conceptual advantage of eliminating the odds ratio approximation altogether, and thus obviates the rare disease assumption. The model has a history of successful use in the statistical analysis of survival studies, and it is becoming increasingly clear that many of the analytic techniques developed for use in that field can also be applied in epidemiology (Breslow, 1975, 1978). Prentice and Breslow (1978) present a detailed mathematical treatment of the role of the proportional hazards model in the analysis of case-control study data. Methodological techniques stemming from the model are identical to those presented in Chapter 7 on matched data.

6.3 Adaptation of the logistic model to case-control studies[1]

According to the logistic model as just defined, the exposures x are regarded as fixed quantities while the response variable y is random. This fits precisely the cohort study situation because it is not known in advance whether or not, or when, a given individual will develop the disease. With the case-control approach, on the other hand, subjects are selected on the basis of their disease status. It is their history of risk factor exposures, as determined by retrospective interview or other means, which should properly be regarded as the random outcome. Thus an important question, addressed in this section, is: how can the logistic model for disease probabilities, which has such a simple and desirable interpretation *vis-à-vis* relative risk, be adapted for use with a sample of cases and controls?

If there is but a single binary risk factor with study subjects classified simply as exposed *versus* unexposed, the answer to this is perfectly clear. Recall first of all our demonstration in § 2.8 that the odds ratio ψ of disease probabilities for exposed *versus* unexposed is identical to the odds ratio of exposure probabilities for diseased *versus* disease-free. When drawing inferences about ψ on the basis of data in 2×2 tables (4.1), it makes absolutely no difference whether the marginal totals m_1 and m_0 corresponding to the two exposure categories are fixed, as in a cohort study, or whether the margins n_1 and n_0 of diseased and disease-free are fixed, as in a case-control study. The estimates, tests and confidence intervals for ψ derived in § 4.1 and § 4.2 in no way depend on how the data in the tables are obtained. Hence we have already demonstrated for 2×2 tables that *inferences about relative risk are made by applying to case-control data precisely the same set of calculations as would be applied to cohort data from the same population.*

This identity of inferential procedures, whether sampling is carried out according to a cohort or case-control design, is in fact a fundamental property of the general logistic model. We illustrate this feature with a simple calculation involving conditional probabilities (Mantel, 1973; Seigel & Greenhouse, 1973) which lends a good deal of plausibility to the deeper mathematical results discussed afterwards. It suffices to consider the model (6.10) for disease probabilities in a single population, as results for the

---

[1] This section, which is particularly abstract, deals with the logical basis for the application of logistic regression to case-control data. Readers interested only in practical applications can go directly to § 6.5.

stratified situation are quite analogous. Suppose the indicator variable z denotes whether (z = 1) or not (z = 0) someone is sampled, and let us define

$$\pi_1 = \text{pr}(z = 1 \mid y = 1)$$

to be the probability that a diseased person is included in the study as a case and

$$\pi_0 = \text{pr}(z = 1 \mid y = 0)$$

to be the probability of including a disease-free person in the study as a control. Typically π_1 is near unity, i.e., most potential cases are sampled for the study, while π_0 has a lower order of magnitude.

Consider now the conditional probability that a person is diseased, given that he has risk variables **x** *and that he was sampled for the case-control study.* Using Bayes' Theorem (Armitage, 1975) we compute $\text{pr}(y = 1 \mid z = 1, \mathbf{x})$

$$= \frac{\text{pr}(z = 1 \mid y = 1, \mathbf{x}) \, \text{pr}(y = 1 \mid \mathbf{x})}{\text{pr}(z = 1 \mid y = 0, \mathbf{x}) \, \text{pr}(y = 0 \mid \mathbf{x}) + \text{pr}(z = 1 \mid y = 1, \mathbf{x}) \, \text{pr}(y = 1 \mid \mathbf{x})}$$

$$= \frac{\pi_1 \exp(\alpha + \Sigma \beta_k x_k)}{\pi_0 + \pi_1 \exp(\alpha + \Sigma \beta_k x_k)}$$

$$= \frac{\exp(\alpha^* + \Sigma \beta_k x_k)}{1 + \exp(\alpha^* + \Sigma \beta_k x_k)}$$

where $\alpha^* = \alpha + \log(\pi_1 / \pi_0)$. In other words, the disease probabilities for those in the sample continue to be given by the logistic model with precisely the same βs, albeit a different value for α. This observation alone would suffice to justify the application of (6.10) to case-control data provided we could also assume that the probabilities of inclusion in the study were independent for different individuals. However, unless a separate decision was made on whether or not to include each potential case or control in the sample, this will not be true. In most studies some slight dependencies are introduced because the total numbers of cases and controls are fixed in advance by design. Hence a somewhat more complicated theory is required.

One assumption made implicitly in the course of this derivation deserves further emphasis. This is that *the sampling probabilities depend only on disease status and not on the exposures.* In symbols, $\text{pr}(z = 1 \mid y, \mathbf{x}) = \text{pr}(z = 1 \mid y) = \pi_y$ for y = 1 and 0. With a stratified design and analysis these sampling fractions may vary from stratum to stratum, but again should not depend on the values of the risk variables. An illustration of the magnitude of the bias which may accompany violations of this assumption was made earlier in § 2.8.

Since case-control studies typically involve *separate samples* of fixed size from the diseased and disease-free populations, the independent probabilities are those of risk variables given disease status. If the sample contains n_1 cases and n_0 controls, the likelihood of the data is a product of n_1 terms of the form $\text{pr}(\mathbf{x} \mid y = 1)$ and n_0 of the form $\text{pr}(\mathbf{x} \mid y = 0)$. Using basic rules of conditional probability, each of these can be expressed

$$pr(\mathbf{x}|y) = \frac{pr(y|\mathbf{x})pr(\mathbf{x})}{pr(y)} \qquad (6.13)$$

as the product of the conditional probabilities of disease given exposure, specified by the logistic model, times the ratio of unconditional probabilities for exposure and disease.

How one approaches the estimation of the relative risk parameters $\boldsymbol{\beta}$ from (6.13) depends to a large extent on assumptions made about the mechanism generating the data, i.e., about the joint probability distribution for $\mathbf{x}$ and y. The key issue is whether the $\mathbf{x}$ variables themselves, without knowledge of the associated y's, contain any information about the parameters of interest. Such a condition would be expressed mathematically through dependence of the marginal distribution $pr(\mathbf{x})$ on $\boldsymbol{\beta}$ as well as on other parameters, in which case better estimates of $\boldsymbol{\beta}$ could in principle be obtained by using the entire likelihood (6.13) rather than by using only the portion of that likelihood specified by (6.10).

An example in which the $\mathbf{x}$'s do contain information on their own about the relative risk was alluded to in § 6.2. In early applications of logistic regression to cohort studies, the regression variables were assumed to have multivariate normal distributions in each disease category (Truett, Cornfield & Karrel, 1967). If such distributions are centred around expected values of μ_1 for diseased individuals and μ_0 for controls, and have a common covariance matrix Σ, then the corresponding relative risk parameters can be computed to be

$$\boldsymbol{\beta} = \Sigma^{-1}(\mu_1 - \mu_0).$$

Estimation of $\boldsymbol{\beta}$ from the full likelihood (6.13) thus entails calculation of the sample means $\bar{x}_1$ and $\bar{x}_0$ of the regression variables among cases and controls, of the pooled covariance matrix S_p^2, and substitution of these quantities in place of μ_1, μ_0 and Σ, respectively. While this procedure yields the most efficient estimates of $\boldsymbol{\beta}$ *provided the assumptions of multivariate normality hold,* severe bias can result if they do not (Halperin, Blackwelder & Verter, 1971; Efron, 1975; Press & Wilson, 1978). It is therefore not recommended for estimation of relative risks, although it may be useful in the early exploratory phases of an analysis to help determine which risk factors contribute significantly to the multivariate equation.

In most practical situations, the $\mathbf{x}$ variables are distinctly non-normal. Indeed, many if not all of them will be discrete and limited to a few possible values. It is therefore prudent to make as few assumptions as possible about their distribution. This can be accomplished by allowing $pr(\mathbf{x})$ in (6.13) to remain completely arbitrary, or else to assume that it depends on a (rather large) set of parameters which are functionally independent of $\boldsymbol{\beta}$. Then, following general principles of statistical inference, one could either try to estimate $\boldsymbol{\beta}$ and $pr(\mathbf{x})$ jointly using (6.13); or else one could try to *eliminate* the $pr(\mathbf{x})$ term by deriving an appropriate *conditional likelihood* (Cox & Hinkley, 1974).

If we decide on the first course, namely joint estimation, a rather remarkable thing happens. Providing $pr(\mathbf{x})$ is assumed to remain completely arbitrary, the joint maximum likelihood estimate $\hat{\boldsymbol{\beta}}$ turns out to be identical to that based only on the portion of the likelihood which is specified by the linear logistic model. Furthermore, the standard errors and covariances for $\hat{\beta}$ generated from partial and full likelihoods also agree. This fact was first noted by Anderson (1972) for the case in which $\mathbf{x}$ was a discrete variable, and established for the general situation by Prentice and Pyke (1979).

Another approach to the likelihood (6.13) is to eliminate the nuisance parameters through consideration of an appropriate conditional distribution. Suppose that a case-control study of $n = n_1 + n_0$ subjects yields the exposure vectors $\mathbf{x}_1, \ldots, \mathbf{x}_n$, but it is not specified which of them pertain to the cases and which to the controls. The conditional probability that the first n_1 $\mathbf{x}$'s in fact go with the cases, as observed, and the remainder with the controls may be written

$$\frac{\prod\limits_{j=1}^{n_1} \mathrm{pr}(\mathbf{x}_j | y = 1) \prod\limits_{j=n_1+1}^{n_1+n_0} \mathrm{pr}(\mathbf{x}_j | y = 0)}{\sum\limits_{\iota} \prod\limits_{j=1}^{n_1} \mathrm{pr}(\mathbf{x}_{\iota_j} | y = 1) \prod\limits_{j=n_1+1}^{n_1+n_0} \mathrm{pr}(\mathbf{x}_{\iota_j} | y = 0)} \tag{6.14}$$

where the sum in the denominator is over all the $\binom{n}{n_1}$ ways of dividing the numbers from 1 to n into one group $\{\iota_1, \ldots, \iota_{n_1}\}$ of size n_1 and its complement $\{\iota_{n_1+1}, \ldots, \iota_n\}$. Using (6.10) and (6.13) it can be calculated that (6.14) reduces to

$$\frac{\prod\limits_{j=1}^{n_1} \exp(\Sigma \beta_k x_{jk})}{\sum\limits_{\iota} \prod\limits_{j=1}^{n_1} \exp(\Sigma \beta_k x_{\iota_j k})}, \tag{6.15}$$

where x_{jk} denotes the value of the kth regression variable for the jth subject and the sum in the denominator is again over all possible choices of n_1 subjects out of n (Prentice & Breslow, 1978; Breslow et al., 1978). This likelihood depends only on the β parameters of interest. However, when n_1 and n_0 are large, the number of summands in the denominator is so great as to rule out its use in practice. Fortunately, as these quantities increase, the conditional maximum likelihood estimate and the standard errors based on (6.15) are almost certain to be numerically close to those obtained by applying the unconditional likelihood (6.10) (Efron, 1975; Farewell, 1979).

In summary, unless the marginal distribution of the risk variables in the sample is assumed to contain some information about the relative risk, methods of estimation based on the joint exposure likelihood yield essentially the same numerical results as do those based on the disease probability model. This justifies the application to case-control data of precisely the same analytic techniques used with cohort studies.

6.4 Likelihood inference: an outline[1]

We have now introduced the logistic regression model as a natural generalization of the odds ratio approach to relative risk estimation, and argued that it may be directly

---

[1] This section also treats material which is quite technical and is not required for appreciation of the applications of the methods. The reader who lacks formal mathematical or statistical training is advised to skim through it on a first reading, and then refer back to the section while working through the examples.

applied to case-control study data with disease status (case *versus* control) treated as the "dependent" or response variable. Subsequent sections of this chapter will illustrate its application to several problems of varying complexity. With one exception, the illustrative analyses may all be carried out using standard computer programmes for the fitting of linear logistic models by maximum likelihood.

Input to GLIM or other standard programmes is in the form of a *rectangular data array*, consisting of a list of values on a fixed number of variables for each subject in the study, with different subjects on different rows. The variables are typically in the order $(y, x_1, \ldots, x_K)$, where y equals 1 or 0 according to whether the subject is a case or control, while the x's represent various discrete and/or continuous regression variables to be related to y. *Output* usually consists of estimates of the regression coefficients for each variable, a variance/covariance matrix for the estimated coefficients, and one or more test statistics which measure the goodness of fit of the model to the observed data. It is not necessary to have a detailed understanding of the arithmetical operations linking the inputs to the outputs in order to be able to use the programme. Researchers in many fields have long used similar programmes for ordinary (least squares) fitting of multiple regression equations, with considerable success. Nevertheless, some appreciation of the fundamental concepts involved can help to dispel the uneasiness which accompanies what otherwise might seem a rather "black box" approach to data analysis. In this section we outline briefly the key features of likelihood inference in the hopes that it may lay the logical foundation for the interpretation of the outputs. More detailed expositions of this material can be found in the books by Cox (1970), Haberman (1974), Bishop, Fienberg and Holland (1975) and Fienberg (1977).

Statistical inference starts with an expression for the probability, or likelihood, of the observed data. This depends on a number of unknown parameters which represent quantitative features of the population from which the data are sampled. In our situation the likelihood is composed of a product of terms of the form (6.10), one for each subject. The α's and β's are the unknown parameters, interest being focused on the β's because of their ready interpretation *vis-à-vis* relative risk.

Estimates of the parameters are selected to be those values which maximize the likelihood or rather, and what is equivalent, those which maximize its logarithm. The parameters thus estimated, which are often denoted $\hat{\alpha}$ and $\hat{\beta}$, are inserted back into the individual likelihoods (6.10) to calculate the *fitted* or *predicted* probability $\hat{P}$ of being a case for each study subject. If we subtract twice the maximized log likelihood from zero, which is the absolute maximum achieved as all the 'fitted values $\hat{P}$ approach the observed y's, and sum up over all individuals in the sample, we obtain the expression

$$G = -2\Sigma\{y\log\hat{P} + (1-y)\log(1-\hat{P})\} \qquad (6.16)$$

for the *log likelihood statistic*[1]. Although G as given here does not have any well defined distribution itself, differences between G statistics for different models may be interpreted as chi-squares (see below).

Other important statistics in likelihood analysis are defined in terms of the first and second derivatives of the log likelihood function. The vector of its first partial derivatives

---

[1] The statistic (6.16) is called the *deviance* in GLIM.

is known as the efficient score, $\mathbf{S} = \mathbf{S}(\alpha,\beta)$, while the negative of the matrix of second partial derivatives is the *information matrix,* denoted $\mathbf{I} = \mathbf{I}(\alpha,\beta)$. The variance/covariance matrix of the estimated parameters is obtained from the inverted information matrix, evaluated at the maximum likelihood estimate (MLE):

$$\text{Covariance matrix for } (\hat{\alpha},\hat{\beta}) = \mathbf{I}^{-1}(\hat{\alpha},\hat{\beta}). \tag{6.17}$$

Another specification of the MLE is as the value α,β for which the efficient score is zero.

Likelihood inference typically proceeds by fitting a *nested hierarchy* of models, each one containing the last. For example, we might start with the model

(1) $\text{logit pr}(y\,|\,\mathbf{x}) = \alpha$

which specifies that the disease probabilities do not depend on the regression variables, i.e., that the log relative risk for different $\mathbf{x}$'s is zero. This would be elaborated in a second model

(2) $\text{logit pr}(y\,|\,\mathbf{x}) = \alpha + \beta_1 x_1,$

for which the log relative risk associated with risk factor x_1 is allowed to be non-zero. A further generalization is then to

(3) $\text{logit pr}(y\,|\,\mathbf{x}) = \alpha + \beta_1 x_1 + \beta_2 x_2 + \beta_3 x_3,$

in which the coefficients for two more variables, one of which might for instance be an interaction involving x_1, are also allowed to be non-zero.

At each stage we obtain the MLEs of the coefficients in the model, together with their estimated variances and covariances. We also carry out a test for the significance of the additional parameters, which is logically equivalent to testing whether the current model fits better than the last one. Three tests are available. The *likelihood ratio test* is simply the difference of the maximized log likelihood statistics (6.16) for the two models. If G_1, G_2 and G_3 denote the values of these statistics for models 1, 2 and 3, respectively, then necessarily $G_3 \leqq G_2 \leqq G_1$. Each hypothesis is less restrictive than the last and its fitted probabilities $\hat{P}$ will therefore generally be closer to the observed y's. $G_1 - G_2$ tests the hypothesis $\beta_1 = 0$, i.e., the significance of x_1 as a risk factor, while $G_2 - G_3$ evaluates the additional contributions of x_2 and x_3 after the effect of x_1 is accounted for.

The *score statistic* for testing the significance of the additional parameters is based on the efficient score evaluated at the MLE for the previous model, appropriately augmented with zeros. For example, the score test of Model 2 against Model 1 is given by

$$S_2 = \mathbf{S}(\hat{\alpha},0)^\mathrm{T}\, \mathbf{I}^{-1}(\hat{\alpha},0)\, \mathbf{S}(\hat{\alpha},0) \tag{6.18}$$

where $\mathbf{S}$ and $\mathbf{I}$ are calculated for Model 2 whereas $\hat{\alpha}$ is the MLE for Model 1. Similarly the score test of the hypothesis $\beta_2 = \beta_3 = 0$ in Model 3 is

$$S_3 = \mathbf{S}(\hat{\alpha},\hat{\beta}_1,0,0)^\mathrm{T}\, \mathbf{I}^{-1}(\hat{\alpha},\hat{\beta}_1,0,0)\, \mathbf{S}(\hat{\alpha},\hat{\beta}_1,0,0).$$

A third test for the significance of the additional parameters in a model is simply to compare their estimated values against 0, using their standard errors as a reference.

Thus to test $\beta_1 = 0$ in Model 2 we would calculate the *standardized regression coefficient*

$$Z_1 = \frac{\hat{\beta}_1}{\sqrt{\mathrm{Var}(\hat{\beta}_1)}}$$

where $\mathrm{Var}(\hat{\beta}_1)$ was the appropriate diagonal term in the inverse information matrix for Model 2. A test statistic analogous to the previous two is based on the square of this value

$$Z_1^2 = \frac{\hat{\beta}_1^2}{\mathrm{Var}(\hat{\beta}_1)} \,.$$

Similarly, the test of $\beta_2 = \beta_3 = 0$ in Model 3 is given by the statistic

$$(\hat{\beta}_2, \hat{\beta}_3) \, \Sigma_{23}^{-1} \begin{pmatrix} \hat{\beta}_2 \\ \hat{\beta}_3 \end{pmatrix},$$

where Σ_{23} is the estimated variance/covariance matrix for $(\hat{\beta}_2, \hat{\beta}_3)$ in Model 3.

In large samples all three of these statistics are known to give approximately equal numerical results under the null hypothesis, and to have distributions which are chi-square with degrees of freedom equal to the number of *additional* parameters (Rao, 1965). In other words, if Model 1 holds we should have approximately

$$G_1 - G_2 \approx S_2 \approx Z_1^2 \approx \chi_1^2. \tag{6.19}$$

Similarly, all three statistics for the hypothesis $\beta_2 = \beta_3 = 0$ in Model 3 should yield similar numerical results, and will have approximate χ_2^2 distributions, if Model 2 adequately summarizes the data. The first and third statistics are most easily calculated from the output of standard programmes such as GLIM. The score statistic, while not routinely calculated by standard programmes, is mentioned here for two reasons. First, in simple situations it is identical with the elementary test statistics presented in Chapter 4, and thus provides a link between the two approaches (Day & Byar, 1979). Second, the nominal chi-square distribution is known to approximate that of the score statistic more closely in small samples, so that its use is less likely to lead to erroneous conclusions of statistical significance (Lininger et al., 1979).

Two other statistics should be mentioned which are useful for evaluating goodness of fit with *grouped data*. These arise when there are a limited number of distinct risk categories, i.e., when the number of **x** values is sufficiently small compared with the size of the study population that quite a few individuals within each stratum have the same **x**. In this case, rather than consider each data record on its own for the analysis, it makes sense to group together those records within each stratum which have the same set of exposures. Suppose that N denotes the total number of individuals in a particular group, of whom n_1 are cases and n_0 are controls. Since the exposures are identical, the estimated probabilities $\hat{P}$ will apply equally to everyone in the group. $N\hat{P}$ may therefore be interpreted as the *expected* or fitted number of cases, while $N(1-\hat{P})$ is the expected number of controls. An appropriate version of the likelihood ratio statistic for this situation is

$$G = 2 \sum [n_1 \log(n_1/N\hat{P}) + n_0 \log\{n_0/N(1-\hat{P})\}] \tag{6.20}$$

where the sum is over all the distinct groups or risk categories. Another measure of goodness of fit of model to data is the ubiquitous chi-square statistic

$$\tilde{G} = \sum \left[\frac{(n_1 - N\hat{P})^2}{N\hat{P}} + \frac{\{n_0 - N(1-\hat{P})\}^2}{N(1-\hat{P})} \right]. \tag{6.21}$$

Unless the data are quite "thin", so that the fitted values of cases or controls for many groups are less than five, these two expressions should yield reasonably close numerical answers when the model holds.

The formulae (6.20) and (6.21) may be expressed in more familiar terms, as functions of the observed (O) and expected (E) numbers in each cell, provided we remember that the cases and controls in each group constitute *separate* cells and thus make separate contributions. The likelihood ratio statistic becomes

$$G = 2\sum O \log(O/E), \tag{6.22}$$

while the chi-square measure is

$$\tilde{G} = \sum \frac{(O-E)^2}{E}. \tag{6.23}$$

Provided the number of groups is small in relation to the total number of cases, each of the statistics G and $\tilde{G}$ have asymptotic chi-square distributions under the null hypothesis. Degrees of freedom are equal to the number of groups less the number of parameters in the logistic model. While they provide us with an overall evaluation of how well the model conforms to the data, these tests may be rather insensitive to particular types of departure from the model. Better tests are obtained by constructing a more general model, with a limited number of additional parameters which express the nature of the departure, and then testing between the two models as outlined earlier.

It should be emphasized that the methods discussed in this section, and illustrated in the remainder of the chapter, are based on *unconditional likelihoods* (6.10) and (6.12) and involve explicit estimation of the α nuisance parameters as well as of the β's. For some of the simpler problems, e.g., the combination of results from 2×2 tables, inference may be carried out also in terms of conditional likelihoods which depend only on the parameters of interest. If the number of nuisance parameters is large, and the data thin, this approach avoids some well known problems of bias (see § 7.1). It also enables exact inferences to be made (§ 4.2). Since many of the procedures in Chapter 4 and all of those in Chapters 5 and 7 are based on such conditional likelihoods, the methods discussed there would be expected to yield more accurate results for finely stratified or matched data than those presented in this chapter. However, the exact conditional procedures are too burdensome computationally for many of the problems which confront us. Thus, while we may lose some accuracy with the logistic regression approach, what we gain in return is a coherent methodology capable of handling a wide variety of problems in a uniform manner.

6.5 Combining results from 2×2 tables

As our first worked example using the logistic model, we return to the problem of combining information about the relative risk from a series of 2×2 tables. In this case there is a single exposure variable x, coded $x = 1$ for exposed and $x = 0$ for unexposed. The model (6.12) for the probabilities $P_i(x)$ of disease in the ith of I strata becomes

$$\text{logit } P_i(x) = \alpha_i + \beta x,$$

which expresses the idea that the relative risks in each stratum are given by the constant $\psi = \exp(\beta)$.

Simultaneous estimation of the α_i and β parameters as outlined in the last section leads to the estimate $\hat{\psi} = \exp(\hat{\beta})$ identified in § 4.4 as the unconditional or asymptotic maximum likelihood estimate (MLE). This has the property that the sum of the fitted values of exposed cases over all I strata is equal to the sum of the observed values. More precisely, suppose the data are laid out as in (4.21). Denote the fitted values by

$$\hat{a}_i = m_{1i}\hat{P}_{1i} = \frac{m_{1i}\exp(\hat{\alpha}_i+\hat{\beta})}{1+\exp(\hat{\alpha}_i+\hat{\beta})}$$

$$\hat{b}_i = m_{0i}\hat{P}_{0i} \quad \frac{m_{0i}\exp(\hat{\alpha}_i)}{1+\exp(\hat{\alpha}_i)}$$

(6.24)

and for the remaining cells by subtraction, $\hat{c}_i = m_{1i} - \hat{a}_i$, $\hat{d}_i = m_{0i} - \hat{b}_i$. Agreement of the observed and marginal totals means $\Sigma\hat{a}_i = \Sigma a_i$, $\Sigma\hat{b}_i = \Sigma b_i$, and so on. Since the squared deviations of observed and fitted values for the four cells in each stratum agree, i.e., $(a_i-\hat{a}_i)^2 = (b_i-\hat{b}_i)^2 = (c_i-\hat{c}_i)^2 = (d_i-\hat{d}_i)^2$, it follows that the chi-square statistic (6.23) for testing goodness of fit of the model may be written

$$\tilde{G} = \sum_{i=1}^{I} (a_i - \hat{a}_i)^2 \left\{ \frac{1}{\hat{a}_i} + \frac{1}{\hat{b}_i} + \frac{1}{\hat{c}_i} + \frac{1}{\hat{d}_i} \right\} = \sum_{i=1}^{I}(a_i - \hat{a}_i)^2/\text{Var}(a_i),$$

where we have used the variance formula (4.13). This chi-square agrees precisely with the goodness of fit statistic (4.30) derived earlier, except that we now use MLE for the parameters.

Example: To illustrate these calculations we reanalyse the grouped data from the Ille-et-Vilaine study of oesophageal cancer summarized in Table 4.1. Here the six strata are defined as ten-year age groups from 25–34 through 75+ years, while average alcohol consumption is treated as a binary risk factor with 0–79 g/day (up to one litre of wine) representing "unexposed" and anything over this amount "exposed". The data would be rearranged for computer entry as shown in Table 6.1, where 12 risk categories or groups are defined by the six strata and two levels of exposure. Within each of these the total N of cases + controls is regarded as the denominator of an observed disease proportion, while the number of cases is the numerator. The numerical results should be compared closely with those already obtained in § 4.4.

Table 6.1 Data from Table 4.5 reorganized for entry into a computer programme for linear logistic regression

Age stratum	Exposure (x=1 for 80+ g/day)	Cases	Total (cases + controls)
1	1	1	10
1	0	0	106
2	1	4	30
2	0	5	169
3	1	25	54
3	0	21	159
4	1	42	69
4	0	34	173
5	1	19	37
5	0	36	124
6	1	5	5
6	0	8	39

Results of fitting several versions of the model to these data are summarized in Table 6.2. In the first version, with six parameters, the disease probabilities may vary with each age group but not with exposure ($\beta = 0$). Considering the huge goodness of fit statistics, this assumption is clearly not tenable (p<0.00001). When a single relative risk parameter (β) is introduced the fit improves considerably. However, the chi-square ($\tilde{G} = 9.32$, p = 0.15) and log likelihood (G = 11.04, p = 0.05) statistics give somewhat different answers as to whether the differences in relative risk between strata are significantly different. Both are sufficiently large to alert us to the possibility of systematic variations in the relative risk for different age groups, which should be investigated further.

Inferences about the relative risk are made in terms of the estimate $\hat{\beta} = 1.670$ and its *standard error* 0.190[1]. We compute $\hat{\psi} = \exp(1.670) = 5.31$ as the point estimate of relative risk. Ninety-five percent confidence limits for β are given by $\beta_L = 1.670 - 1.96 \times 0.190 = 1.30$ and $\beta_U = 1.670 + 1.96 \times 0.190 = 2.04$. These correspond to bounds of $\psi_L = \exp(\beta_L) = 3.66$ and $\psi_U = \exp(\beta_U) = 7.71$ on the relative risk, which compare well with those derived in § 4.4 using two other methods.

The third model shown in Table 6.2 was fitted to see whether there was a *systematic trend in relative risk with age*. This took the form

$$\text{logit } P_i(x) = \alpha_i + \beta x + \gamma x(i-3.5),$$

where now β represents the log relative risk for a "typical" age (i = 3.5), while γ represents the linear trend in this depending on the age group indicator i. The lack of a significant improvement in the goodness of fit statistics, and the small value of $\hat{\gamma}$ as compared with its standard error, tell us that there is little evidence for such a trend.

More information about the sources of departure from model assumptions can be obtained from an examination of the *residuals*, the differences between the observed and fitted numbers of disease cases in each category (Table 6.3). As an illustration of their calculation, the fitted values for the 35–44 age category are found from (6.24) and the estimated coefficients in Table 6.2 to be

$$\hat{a}_2 = \frac{30 \times \exp(-3.512 + 1.670)}{1 + \exp(-3.512 + 1.670)} = 4.10$$

and

$$\hat{b}_2 = \frac{169 \times \exp(-3.512)}{1 + \exp(-3.512)} = 4.90.$$

---

[1] The standard error of an estimate is the square root of its estimated variance.

Table 6.2 Results of fitting several versions of the linear logistic model (6.3) to the data in Table 6.1

Model	No. of parameters	DF	Goodness-of-fit statistics		Regression coefficients Age strata (years)						Log relative risk and interactions	
			Log likelihood G	Chi-square G	25–34 $\hat{a}_1$	35–44 $\hat{a}_2$	45–54 $\hat{a}_3$	55–64 $\hat{a}_4$	65–74 $\hat{a}_5$	75+ $\hat{a}_6$	Alcohol $\hat{\beta}\pm$S.E.	Alcohol × age $\hat{\gamma}\pm$S.E.
1	6	6	90.56	101.80	−4.746	−3.050	−1.289	−0.781	−0.656	−0.869	—	—
2	7	5	11.04	9.32	−5.054	−3.512	−1.855	−1.341	−1.087	−1.092	1.670 ± 0.190	—
3	8	4	10.61	8.48	−5.182	−3.617	−1.900	−1.334	−1.049	−1.055	1.714 ± 0.201	0.125 ± 0.189

Table 6.3 Residuals from fitting model 2 of Table 6.2 to data in Table 6.1

Age stratum (years)	Exposure	Numbers of cases Observed	Expected	Variance	Standardized residual
25–34	1	1	0.33	0.32	1.19
	0	0	0.67	0.67	−0.82
35–44	1	4	4.10	3.54	−0.06
	0	5	4.90	4.75	0.05
45–54	1	25	24.50	13.4	0.14
	0	21	21.50	18.6	−0.12
55–64	1	42	40.13	16.8	0.46
	0	34	35.87	28.4	−0.35
65–74	1	19	23.74	8.51	−1.63
	0	36	31.26	23.4	0.98
75+	1	5	3.20	1.15	1.68
	0	8	9.80	7.34	−0.66
Total		200	200.00		

We easily verify that the sum of the fitted numbers of exposed cases over the six strata, $0.33 + 4.10 + 24.50 + 40.13 + 23.74 + 3.20$, equals the sum of the observed number, namely 96. This confirms the property of the maximum likelihood estimate mentioned earlier.

Variances for the O–E residuals are calculated as $N\hat{P}\hat{Q}$, where N is the denominator (total of cases and controls), $\hat{P}$ is the estimated disease probability and $\hat{Q} = 1 - \hat{P}$. Dividing each residual by its standard error gives us the *standardized residuals,* which when squared and summed produce the $\tilde{G}$ goodness of fit statistic. The greatest contribution to this comes from the last two age groups. For the 65–74 year-olds the deficit of 19 exposed cases compared with 23.74 expected indicates a relative risk smaller than that of the other groups; while for the 75+ group the excess of 5 observed to 3.20 expected implies a larger than average relative risk. The contribution from the youngest age group can be largely discounted because only one case appears. Since there does not seem to be any obvious pattern to the residuals, we feel comfortable in attributing the observed departures from the fitted model to chance phenomena.

6.6 Qualitative analysis of grouped data from Ille-et-Vilaine

In § 4.6 we applied classic Mantel-Haenszel methodology to study the joint effects of two risk factors, alcohol and tobacco, on the relative risk of oesophageal cancer in Ille-et-Vilaine. Both factors were partitioned into four levels, yielding 16 risk categories in all. Our first approach was to compute separate estimates of the age-adjusted relative risk for each such category, assigning the value 1.0 to the low alcohol, low tobacco cell. Later we estimated relative risks for each alcohol level, simultaneously adjusting for age and tobacco, and each tobacco level, simultaneously adjusting for alcohol and age. This was a cumbersome procedure which required that we construct and summarize several different series of 24 2×2 tables. The relative risks obtained for each alcohol and tobacco level were multiplied together to estimate the joint effect of these two variables. However, there was no very satisfactory way of testing the validity of the multiplicative hypothesis, and the relative risks obtained in this fashion lacked the desirable property of consistency.

In this section we demonstrate that a comprehensive and integrated analysis, which parallels the Mantel–Haenszel approach, may be carried out quite simply using the logistic model with stratification (6.12). The starting point is the grouping of the 200 cases and 775 controls into $4 \times 4 \times 6 = 96$ cells, each of which represents a combination of the categories of alcohol, tobacco and age. According to the principles outlined in § 6.3, the observations in each cell are treated in the statistical analysis as independent binomial observations, with cases representing the numerator and cases + controls the denominator. Appendix I lists the 96 binomial observations so formed. In fact, since 8 of the cells were devoid of cases and controls there are effectively only 88 observations and it is this figure that one uses to determine degrees of freedom.

As only the qualitative or categorical aspects of the data are to be considered here, the regression variables x appearing in the model are indicator variables which take the value 1 or 0 according to whether the cell (observation) in question corresponds to a given level or combination of levels of the various study factors. Even the parameter α_i in (6.12) can be regarded as the coefficient of an indicator variable which takes the value 1 for the ith stratum and 0 otherwise. Sophisticated programmes such as GLIM will automatically construct such indicators for all factors specified by the user as being categorical.

Table 6.4 shows explicitly the values of the regression variables so constructed. Since they depend only on alcohol and tobacco it suffices to show their values for the first age group only. The first three variables define the main effects of each alcohol category on risk, while the next three define the main effects of tobacco. Thus, $x_2 = 1$ for the third alcohol group and 0 otherwise, while $x_6 = 1$ for the fourth tobacco group and 0 otherwise. Cells having 0 values for all six of these variables correspond to the lowest consumption levels of both factors and are assigned a baseline relative risk of unity.

Variables x_7 to x_{15} define the totality of qualitative interactions between alcohol and tobacco. They are obtained by multiplying together the dummy variables representing the main effects:

$$x_7 = x_1 \times x_4; \; x_8 = x_1 \times x_5; \ldots; \; x_{15} = x_3 \times x_6.$$

Inclusion of all six main effect and all nine interaction variables in the equation imposes no constraints on how the relative risks vary over the 16 alcohol/tobacco cells. The 15 parameters in the model yield 15 estimated relative risks, with the value 1.0 being assigned to the baseline category. Thus the log relative risk for the third alcohol and fourth tobacco group is estimated as $\hat{\beta}_2 + \hat{\beta}_6 + \hat{\beta}_{12}$, i.e., as a contribution from the alcohol level plus one from the tobacco level plus the interaction. One obvious drawback to this method of parameterizing the interactions is that it does not lead to the ready identification of quantitative patterns which may be of particular interest. Alternative parameterizations are considered in the next section.

Table 6.5 summarizes the results of fitting several regression models using qualitative regression variables. By subtracting the goodness-of-fit (G) measures for Models 2 and 3 from that for Model 1 we obtain χ_3^2 statistics of 141.0 and 36.6, respectively, for testing the significance of alcohol and tobacco, *ignoring* the effects of the other variable. Both factors have an enormous influence on risk. Subtracting the G's for Model 4 from those for Models 2 and 3 yields χ_3^2 statistics of 128.0 and 23.6. These determine the significance of alcohol and tobacco while *adjusting* for the effects of the other variable. The adjusted chi-squares are a little smaller than the unadjusted ones, reflecting the slight correlation between alcohol and tobacco consumption. However, their magnitude

Table 6.4 Values of qualitative risk variables for the first 16 of 96 grouped data records: Ille-et-Vilaine study of oesophageal cancer

Obser-vation	Levels of age	alc	tob	Alcohol main x_1	x_2	x_3	Tobacco main x_4	x_5	x_6	Alcohol × tobacco interaction x_7	x_8	x_9	x_{10}	x_{11}	x_{12}	x_{13}	x_{14}	x_{15}
1	1	1	1	0	0	0	0	0	0	0	0	0	0	0	0	0	0	0
2	1	1	2	0	0	0	1	0	0	0	0	0	0	0	0	0	0	0
3	1	1	3	0	0	0	0	1	0	0	0	0	0	0	0	0	0	0
4	1	1	4	0	0	0	0	0	1	0	0	0	0	0	0	0	0	0
5	1	2	1	1	0	0	0	0	0	0	0	0	0	0	0	0	0	0
6	1	2	2	1	0	0	1	0	0	1	0	0	0	0	0	0	0	0
7	1	2	3	1	0	0	0	1	0	0	1	0	0	0	0	0	0	0
8	1	2	4	1	0	0	0	0	1	0	0	1	0	0	0	0	0	0
9	1	3	1	0	1	0	0	0	0	0	0	0	0	0	0	0	0	0
10	1	3	2	0	1	0	1	0	0	0	0	0	1	0	0	0	0	0
11	1	3	3	0	1	0	0	1	0	0	0	0	0	1	0	0	0	0
12	1	3	4	0	1	0	0	0	1	0	0	0	0	0	1	0	0	0
13	1	4	1	0	0	1	0	0	0	0	0	0	0	0	0	0	0	0
14	1	4	2	0	0	1	1	0	0	0	0	0	0	0	0	1	0	0
15	1	4	3	0	0	1	0	1	0	0	0	0	0	0	0	0	1	0
16	1	4	4	0	0	1	0	0	1	0	0	0	0	0	0	0	0	1

Table 6.5 Summary of goodness of fit of several logistic regression models: grouped data from the Ille-et-Vilaine study of oesophageal cancer

Model	Regression variables included[a]	No. of parameters	DF	Goodness of fit G	Hypothesis tested and/or interpretation
1	Age	6	82	246.9	No effect of alcohol or tobacco
2	Age Alcohol (1–3)	9	79	105.9	Effect of alcohol only, adjusted for age
3	Age Tobacco (4–6)	9	79	210.3	Effect of tobacco only, adjusted for age
4	Age Alcohol (1–3) Tobacco (4–6)	12	76	82.3	Main effects for alcohol and tobacco (multiplicative hypothesis), adjusted for age

[a] Numbers in parentheses correspond to variable numbers shown in Table 6.4

indicates that both variables have strong *independent* effects which are not explained by the contribution of the other.

The estimated regression coefficients for Model 2, when exponentiated, yield estimates of the risk for each alcohol level relative to baseline (0–39 g/day) which are adjusted for age but not for tobacco. Thus, $\exp(\hat{\beta}_1) = \exp(1.43) = 4.2$ is the relative risk for the 40–79 g/day group, while for the higher levels of consumption the figures are $\exp(\hat{\beta}_2) = 7.4$ and $\exp(\hat{\beta}_3) = 39.7$. These may be contrasted with the correspond-

Fig. 6.1 Log relative risk of oesophageal cancer according to four levels of alcohol consumption

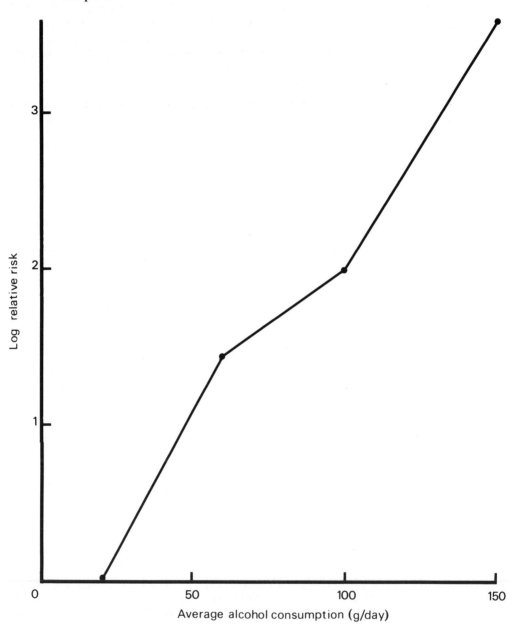

ing figures of 4.3, 8.0 and 28.6 obtained by the Mantel-Haenszel (M-H) method (Table 4.4). There is reasonably good agreement except for the highest exposure category, where there were few cases and controls in some strata. For this category the *conditional* maximum likelihood estimate (§ 4.4) was 34.9, midway between the M-H estimate and unconditional MLE. The latter estimate is probably a bit exaggerated here because of the thin data (§ 7.1).

One disadvantage of the elementary methods was that the relative risks obtained upon varying the choice of baseline category were not consistent. For example, the direct M-H estimate of the risk for the fourth alcohol level relative to the second is 8.7 rather than 28.6/4.3 = 6.7. Use of the logistic modelling approach avoids such

Fig. 6.2 Log relative risk of oesophageal cancer according to four levels of tobacco consumption

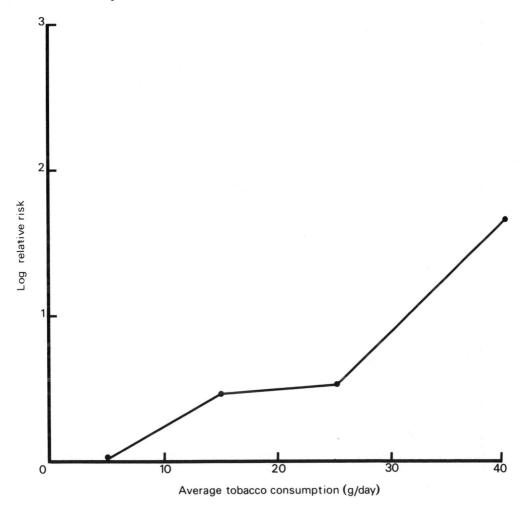

Average tobacco consumption (g/day)

discrepancies. Estimates of the log relative risks between any two categories are always obtained as the differences in the regression coefficients for those categories (with the proviso that the coefficient for the baseline category is 0), and such differences are not affected by the choice of the baseline category. Thus $\exp(\hat{\beta}_3 - \hat{\beta}_1) = 9.4$ represents the risk of level four relative to level two regardless of how the indicator variables representing the alcohol effects are coded.

Model 4 is the first reasonably satisfactory one in the sense that the goodness of fit chi-square is not significantly higher than its degrees of freedom ($\chi^2_{76} = 82.34$, p = 0.48). The fitted regression coefficients are: for alcohol $\hat{\beta}_1 = 1.44$, $\hat{\beta}_2 = 1.98$ and $\hat{\beta}_3 = 3.60$; and for tobacco $\hat{\beta}_4 = 0.44$, $\hat{\beta}_5 = 0.51$ and $\hat{\beta}_6 = 1.64$ (6.11). These show a reasonably smooth linear increase with increasing levels of consumption (Figures 6.1 and 6.2). Taking exponentials, we find estimates of relative risk for each alcohol and tobacco category relative to baseline which, according to the model, combine multiplicatively to yield the results for joint exposures to the two factors shown in Table 6.6. In view of the rather weak correlation between alcohol and tobacco consumption ($\varrho = 0.15$, see Table 4.22), it is not surprising that the alcohol relative risks obtained after adjustment for age and tobacco are only slightly smaller than those obtained after adjustment for age alone. Further evidence for the goodness of fit of the multiplicative model is presented in Table 6.7. Its entries, obtained by summing observed and fitted values over the six age categories, show consistently good agreement throughout the range of both risk factors. The greatest discrepancy is in the baseline category, with nine cases of disease against 13.7 expected. While not statistically significant, the slight lack of fit

Table 6.6 Age-adjusted relative risks for each alcohol/tobacco category according to multiplicative model: Ille-et-Vilaine oesophageal cancer study

Alcohol (g/day)	Tobacco (g/day)			
	0–9	10–19	20–29	30+
0–39	1.0	1.6	1.7	5.2
40–79	4.2	6.6	7.0	21.8
80–119	7.2	11.3	12.1	37.3
120+	36.6	56.8	61.0	188.7

Table 6.7 Observed and expected (age-adjusted) numbers of cases for each alcohol/ tobacco category according to multiplicative model: Ille-et-Vilaine oesophageal cancer study

Alcohol (g/day)	Tobacco (g/day)							
	0–9		10–19		20–29		30+	
	O	E	O	E	O	E	O	E
0–39	9	13.7	10	7.1	5	3.4	5	4.8
40–79	34	30.0	17	18.9	15	16.0	9	9.1
80–118	19	17.8	19	19.9	6	6.7	7	6.6
120+	16	15.5	12	12.1	7	6.9	10	10.5

for this category indicates that the relative risk for the other levels of exposure might possibly be even greater than that suggested by the model.

One drawback to the choice of grouping intervals used in this analysis is that in neither case does the lowest level correspond to zero consumption. To some extent the choice was dictated by necessity in that no diseased individuals abstained completely from both alcohol and tobacco, and even among controls there were very few who did not consume some alcohol. However there were a substantial number of non-smokers in the population. Thus a similar analysis was carried out using five levels of consumption for each variable: 0–24, 25–49, 50–74, 75–99 and 100+ g/day for alcohol and 0, 1–4, 5–14, 15–29 and 30+ g/day for tobacco. Results shown in Tables 6.8 and 6.9 and in Figures 6.3 and 6.4 confirm the multiplicative relationship and the linear effect of alcohol on the log relative risk. The trend with tobacco, on the other hand, is considerably changed in appearance. Even a small amount appears to increase the risk substantially and there are contra-indications to the linearity of the relationship. Figures 6.3 and 6.4 also show for comparison relative risks estimated from the *quantitative* regression models discussed in the next two sections.

It would be tempting to try to subdivide the alcohol and tobacco variables further, say into ten levels each. However even with five levels per variable there are already $5 \times 5 \times 6 = 150$ groups, and with ten levels there would be 600. The larger the number of parameters in the model, the less information there is available for estimating each one; this is reflected in increased standard errors. Further subdivision would lead one to anticipate increasingly erratic behaviour in the estimates, such as the apparent decrease in risk between the 5–14 and 15–29 g/day tobacco categories (Figure 6.4).

Table 6.8　Estimated relative risks for each alcohol/tobacco category according to the multiplicative model: Ille-et-Vilaine oesophageal cancer study

Alcohol (g/day)	Tobacco (g/day) 0	1–4	5–14	15–29	30+
0–24	1.0	4.5	7.2	5.8	19.3
25–49	1.7	7.5	11.9	9.6	31.8
50–74	4.8	21.8	34.8	27.9	92.8
75–99	6.8	30.9	49.4	39.7	131.0
100+	17.5	79.0	126.5	101.5	337.0

Table 6.9　Observed and expected (age-adjusted) numbers of cases for each alcohol/tobacco category according to the multiplicative model: Ille-et-Vilaine oesophageal cancer study

Alcohol (g/day)	Tobacco (g/day) 0 O	E	1–4 O	E	5–14 O	E	15–29 O	E	30+ O	E
0–24	0	1.3	2	1.7	8	8.2	3	3.1	4	2.7
25–49	1	1.2	6	4.5	12	11.4	5	6.1	4	4.8
50–74	2	2.4	4	4.2	25	21.7	12	13.9	4	4.8
75–99	4	1.9	3	3.1	15	19.3	14	13.4	8	6.3
100+	2	2.2	3	4.4	14	13.4	17	14.5	11	12.5

Fig. 6.3 Log relative risk of oesophageal cancer according to five levels of alcohol consumption

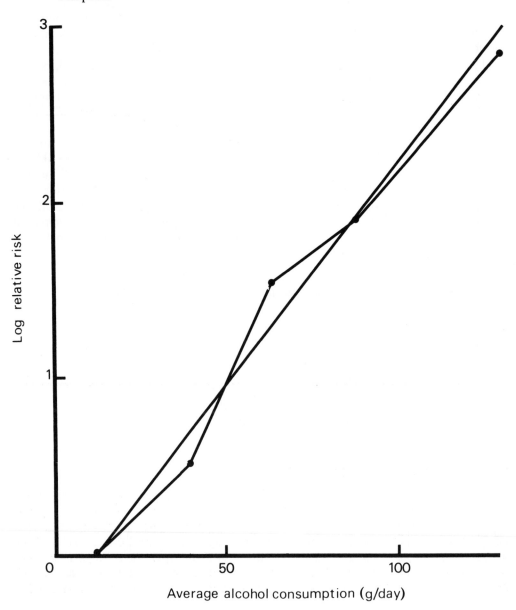

Average alcohol consumption (g/day)

Fig. 6.4 Log relative risk of oesophageal cancer according to five levels of tobacco consumption

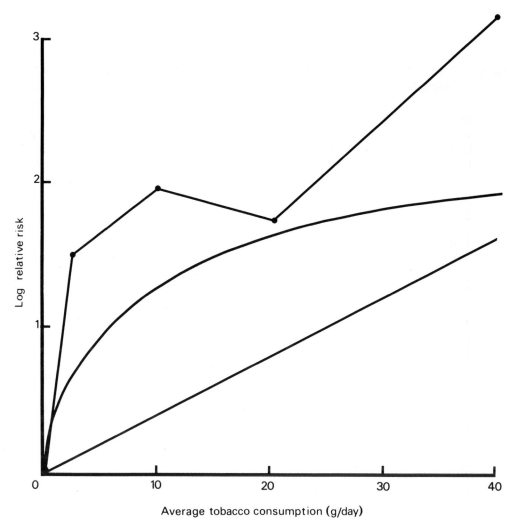

6.7 Quantitative analysis of grouped data

An important feature of the Ille-et-Vilaine data which was ignored in the preceding section is that different levels of the two risk factors have a prescribed order. It is possible to assign to each of them a quantitative value of exposure, for example the midpoint of the respective interval, or the average over the sample of the values of the underlying continuous variable within that interval. Natural values to assign to the four levels of alcohol are 20, 60, 100 and 150 g/day (Figure 6.1), which are interval midpoints except that 150 represents the approximate median of the values in the last open-ended interval above 120 g/day. Similarly, for tobacco, natural values are 5, 15, 25 and 40 g/day (Figure 6.2). Even the stratification variable is quantitative, with equally-spaced intervals centred about 30, 40, 50, 60, 70 and 80 years of age.

Quantitative aspects of the data may be accounted for in the analysis by using continuous regression variables in place of the categorical ones. There are several advantages in this approach. First, the data can often be adequately summarized by a smaller number of parameters, which facilitates interpretation. Tests for the significance of individual regression coefficients are single degree of freedom tests for trend which, as we have repeatedly emphasized, are generally more powerful than tests directed against global alternatives to the null hypothesis. This feature is especially important in exploring possible interactions, since chi-square statistics based on qualitative interaction variables tend to have rather large numbers of degrees of freedom. Quantitative interaction variables, obtained as the product of the quantitative variables representing the main effects of the corresponding factors, enable us to identify particular patterns of departure from the basic linear model.

Suppose for the moment that a single risk factor has been divided into K levels corresponding to values $x_1, ..., x_K$ of a quantitative variable. Cases and controls may be classified into one of IK cells on the basis of stratum (i) and risk factor (k). A partial selection of logistic regression models which would be appropriate to fit to the disease probabilities $P_i(x_k)$ may be outlined as follows:

Model equation logit $P_i(x_k) =$	No. of independent parameters	Goodness-of-fit statistic G	Interpretation/Description
α_i	I	G_1	Relative risk of unity in all strata: no effect of risk factor
$\alpha_i + \beta_1 x_k$	I + 1	G_2	Linear increase in log-relative risk with exposure, same slope for each stratum
$\alpha_i + \beta_1 x_k + \beta_2 x_k^2$	I + 2	G_3	Quadratic effect of exposure on log-relative risk
$\alpha_i + \beta_i x_k$	2I	G_4	Linear effect of exposure, but slope varies depending on stratum
$\alpha_i + \beta_k$	I + K − 1	G_5	Individual relative risk for each exposure level
$\alpha_i + \beta_k + \gamma_{ik}$	IK	$G_6 = 0$	No constraints at all: separate relative risks in each stratum

$\beta_k = \gamma_{ik} = 0$ by convention for k = 1 and all i.

By comparing the statistics corresponding to different models one may test several hypotheses. For example $G_1 – G_5$, a χ^2_{K-1} statistic, provides an unstructured (qualitative) test for the effects of the risk factor like those considered in the last section. *Its value would not be changed by a re-ordering of the exposure categories.* $G_1 – G_2$, which has but a single degree of freedom, yields a much more specific test for linear trend in log relative risk with increasing exposure. A global test of departures from the linear model is provided by G_2–G_5, on $K-2$ degrees of freedom, while G_2–G_3 is a χ_1^2 statistic specifically designed to test for curvature in the regression line. Finally, G_2–G_4 is a χ_{I-1}^2 statistic testing the parallelism of the regression lines in the I strata. Lack of parallelism means that the relative risks for different exposure levels vary from one stratum to another, i.e., that there are interactions between stratification variables and risk factors. Notice that the goodness-of-fit statistic for model 6 is 0. Since the number of independent parameters equals the number of observations, there is perfect agreement between model and data in this case.

A similar but somewhat more elaborate set of models was fitted to the 96 grouped data records from Ille-et-Vilaine, treating the two risk factors alternately as qualitative and quantitative variables at four levels each. The values assigned to each level are as indicated above, namely 20, 60, 100 and 150 g/day for alcohol and 5, 15, 25 and 40 g/day for tobacco. In fact these x values were not used in the regression analyses in their original form, since this would have led to computational problems, especially with the square terms. Instead, alcohol consumption was expressed in units of 100 g/day, with values 0.2, 0.6, 1.0 and 1.5, while tobacco was expressed in units of 10 g/day. It is sometimes helpful to go even further and to *standardize* all regression variables, i.e., scale and centre them so that they have approximate mean values of zero and variances of unity, before proceeding with the numerical analyses.

Table 6.10 summarizes the results. In identifying the various models we have used the following shorthand: ALCGRP and TOBGRP denote the qualitative effects of alcohol and tobacco, each representing three indicator regression variables; ALC and TOB are single variables which represent the quantitative effects. All models contain the six stratum parameters α_i which express the qualitative effects of age. Model 1 is identical with Model 4 of Table 6.5, both alcohol and tobacco consumption being treated as qualitative factors which combine multiplicatively.

Comparing Models 1 and 2 there is some slight evidence that the increase in log relative risk with alcohol may not be purely linear ($\chi_2^2 = 5.07$, p = 0.08); however, since the specific test for curvature obtained by comparing Models 2 and 3 is not at all significant ($\chi_1^2 = 0.11$, p = 0.95), we feel reasonably confident in attributing these deviations from a straight line relationship to chance. Linearity of the trend with tobacco, at least as based on the grouping into four levels, seems quite adequate; compare Model 4 with Models 1 and 5. Thus, Model 6, containing just one term for each of alcohol and tobacco, fits the data nearly as well as a model with four more parameters representing the non-linear effects of the two risk variables. From the regression coefficients[1] for Model 6, $\hat{\beta}_{ALC} = 2.55$ and $\hat{\beta}_{TOB} = 0.409$, we estimate that the risk of oesophageal cancer increases by a factor of $\exp(0.255) = 1.29$ for every additional 10 grams of alcohol consumed per day, and by $\exp(0.409) = 1.51$ for each additional 10 grams of tobacco.

Model 7 contains a quantitative term representing the linear × linear interaction of alcohol and tobacco. A significant value for its coefficient would have indicated a trend in the slope of the alcohol relationship with increasing consumption of tobacco, or

---

[1] Remember that for these calculations alcohol was expressed in units of 100 g/day and tobacco in 10-gram units.

Table 6.10 Results of fitting various logistic models with qualitative and quantitative regression variables to grouped data from the Ille-et-Vilaine study of oesophageal cancer

Model	Parameters fitted (in addition to stratum or age effects)	DF	Goodness of fit G	Hypothesis tested/interpretation
1	ALCGRP + TOBGRP	76	82.34	Multiplicative model with qualitative risk variables
2	TOBGRP + ALC	78	87.41	Linear effect of alcohol
3	TOBGRP + ALC + ALC^2	77	87.01	Linear + quadratic effects of alcohol
4	ALCGRP + TOB	78	84.53	Linear effects of tobacco
5	ALCGRP + TOB + TOB^2	77	83.73	Linear + quadratic effects of tobacco
6	ALC + TOB	80	89.02	Linear effects of alcohol and tobacco
7	ALC + TOB + ALC × TOB	79	88.05	Linear × linear alcohol/tobacco interaction
8	ALCGRP + TOBGRP + ALC × TOB	75	81.37	Linear × linear alcohol/tobacco interaction in qualitative model
9	ALCGRP + TOBGRP + ALC × AGE	75	80.08	Linear increase in slope of alcohol effect with age
10	ALCGRP + TOBGRP + TOB × AGE	75	82.33	Linear increase in slope of tobacco effect with age

KEY: ALCGRP = indicator variables for alcohol levels
TOBGRP = indicator variables for tobacco levels
AGE = quantitative age variable
ALC = quantitative alcohol variable
TOB = quantitative tobacco variable

equivalently a trend in the tobacco relationship with alcohol. However, there is no evidence for such a trend ($\chi_1^2 = 0.97$, p = 0.32). Model 8 illustrates that quantitative interaction terms may be used even when the model expresses the main effects qualitatively. Subtracting G_8 from G_1 leads to a nearly identical test for the quantitative alcohol × tobacco interaction ($\chi_1^2 = 0.97$, p = 0.32). Quantitative interaction variables may be quite valuable in giving some specificity to the search for interactions even if one does not want to assume a particular form for the main effects.

The last two models search for similar quantitative interactions with the stratification variable. A negative regression coefficient for the ALC × AGE term in Model 9 indicates a tendency for the alcohol relative risk to diminish with advancing age. However, it is not a significant trend ($\chi_1^2 = 2.28$, p = 0.13). There is no indication at all of a systematic change in the tobacco effect with age. Thus our previous conclusions based on the qualitative analysis of interactions are in this example further supported by the quantitative approach.

6.8 Regression adjustment for confounders

Stratification, whether in the context of M-H methodology or logistic regression, has traditionally been used to control the confounding effects of nuisance factors. Typically, we define a separate stratum for each combination of levels of the nuisance factors, assigning to each one a parameter in the model. If there are several such factors, or if they occur at very many levels, the total number of strata can become quite large. For example, with three stratifying factors at 3, 4 and 5 levels, respectively, the total number of α parameters in (6.2) is $3 \times 4 \times 5 = 60$. Since the available data usually place severe limitations on the number of strata which may be incorporated in the analysis, alternative methods for the control of confounding must be considered.

From the discussion in § 6.1 it is clear that the *practice of stratification is tantamount to saturating the effects of the nuisance factors with parameters.* Not only the main effects, but also all the first and higher order interaction terms are represented. This practice is unnecessary, however, unless we have good reason to believe that such higher order interactions are present. An obvious alternative to stratification for the control of confounding variables is to incorporate their effects directly into the model. This allows us much more flexibility in deciding which of the higher order interaction terms to retain and which to discard. The approach may be especially efficacious with continuous nuisance factors whose effects can be adequately summarized in a few quantitative regression variables.

This does not mean, however, that risk and nuisance variables are treated symmetrically in the analysis. For risk factors our goal is to identify the most important ones and quantify their influence in a precise and meaningful way. This implies that we *economize* on the number of parameters used to represent them and that we retain in the multivariate risk equation only those which have reasonably significant effects.

For nuisance factors, on the other hand, the effects on disease have presumably already been conceded, or in any event are not the specific concern of the study. They are included only to ensure that the estimates of relative risk are free from possible confounding effects, and no specific meaning is to be attached to their coefficients. *Hence, known confounding variables should be included in the equation regardless of statistical significance if such inclusion changes the estimated coefficients of the risk variables by any appreciable degree* (§ 3.4).

We illustrate the regression adjustment for confounding effects with the grouped data from Ille-et-Vilaine, specifically the age adjustment of estimates in the qualitative multiplicative model (Model 4, Table 6.5). Table 6.11 compares the previous estimates, obtained using stratification in six age groups, to estimates for which quantitative adjustments were made by introducing polynomial expressions in age group into the equation. Let i denote the age stratum, j the alcohol group, and k the tobacco group. The left-hand column presents the unadjusted estimates, based on an equation of the form

$$\text{logit } P_{ijk} = \alpha_0 + \beta_j(\text{alc}) + \beta_k(\text{tob})$$

where age does not appear at all. The next column shows the changes in the alcohol and tobacco coefficients upon introduction of a single linear term in age

$$\text{logit } P_{ijk} = \alpha_0 + \alpha_1 i + \beta_j(\text{alc}) + \beta_k(\text{tob}).$$

The third column shows the effect of adding a quadratic age term $\alpha_2 i^2$, and so on.

Comparing G's for the extreme left- and right-hand columns of Table 6.11 it is clear that age has an enormous influence on risk ($\chi_5^2 = 126.5$). Nevertheless, the differences between these two columns in the relative risk estimates for alcohol and tobacco are rather minor, which implies that the confounding effects of age are quite weak. The explanation for this phenomenon has been given in § 3.3. While age is strongly related to risk, it has only a weak correlation with the level of exposure to alcohol and tobacco (Table 4.2) and hence would not be expected to be a strong confounder.

Inclusion of a single linear term in age group results in an enormous improvement in overall fit and brings the estimated coefficients quite close to those obtained *via* stratification. Fitting both linear and quadratic terms yields results which are virtually identical to those obtained with higher degrees of adjustment. These comparisons, which are typical of our experience with quantitative nuisance factors, indicate that effective control of confounding is often obtainable by inclusion of a few polynomial terms in the regression equation, thus obviating the need for stratification. The regression method of adjustment should generally work well unless disease incidence or the exposure to other risk factors depends in a complicated, non-linear way on the nuisance variables.

Table 6.11   Estimate of log relative risk for each alcohol and tobacco category according to the degree of adjustment for age: Ille-et-Vilaine oesophageal cancer study

Risk category	Type of analysis Unadjusted	Polynomial adjustment for age group				Stratification in six age groups
		Linear	Quadratic	Cubic	Quartic	
Tobacco (g/day)						
0–9	0.0	0.0	0.0	0.0	0.0	0.0
10–19	0.39	0.46	0.44	0.43	0.43	0.44
20–29	0.43	0.55	0.51	0.50	0.50	0.51
30+	0.99	1.52	1.63	1.63	1.64	1.64
Alcohol (g/day)						
0–39	0.0	0.0	0.0	0.0	0.0	0.0
40–79	1.23	1.53	1.44	1.44	1.44	1.44
80–119	2.00	2.17	1.99	2.00	1.99	1.98
120+	3.18	3.60	3.57	3.58	3.59	3.60
Goodness-of-fit statistic G	208.8	101.9	84.6	84.0	83.8	82.3
Degrees of freedom	81	80	79	78	77	76

6.9 Analysis of continuous data

The full power of the regression approach to case-control studies is obtained when continuous risk variables are analysed in the original form in which they were recorded, rather than by grouping into intervals whose endpoints are often arbitrarily chosen. This permits the incorporation of many more variables than would be possible using grouped data, their joint effects being summarized by a relatively small number of parameters. Of course such an increase in power and flexibility is not without associated costs. Perhaps the most serious are potential errors in the estimated relative risks arising from a *mis-specification* of the model. Careful exploration of the adequacy of the postulated relationships is essential to avoid over-interpretation of the data. Transformations and interaction terms should be used where required to improve the fit.

Another cost associated with the use of continuous risk variables is monetary. Since individual data records for each subject must be processed repeatedly during the iterative fitting process, large amounts of computer time can be required to analyse a comprehensive series of models. With the Ille-et-Vilaine study, for example, only 88 data records were required for the grouped data analyses of § 6.6 and 6.7. All 975 records, one for each subject, were needed for the continuous analysis, and computer costs for fitting equivalent models were 5–10 times higher. Of course additional information is contained in the original, continuous data which is undoubtedly worth the price of extraction, especially when one considers that costs of data processing and analysis are only a small part of the total cost of any study.

In the first series of continuous models fitted to the Ille-et-Vilaine data we used quantitative variables representing alcohol and tobacco consumption as well as various transformations of these. "Alcohol" (ALC) was a true continuous variable in that it took on 163 separate values between 0 and 268 g/day (inclusive) among the 975 study subjects. 'Tobacco" (TOB), on the other hand, had been recorded as a discrete variable with nine levels. For the analyses reported here quantitative values were assigned to each such level, as they had been earlier for the grouped data analyses:

Coding of quantitative tobacco variable

Level	Interval (g/day)	Assigned value (x)
1	0	0.0
2	1–4	2.5
3	5–9	7.5
4	10–14	12.5
5	15–19	17.5
6	20–29	25.0
7	30–39	35.0
8	40–49	45.0
9	50+	60.0

As an alternative to using ALC and TOB as linear terms in the model, transformations of each of these were considered. A particularly appropriate transformation for variables which represent dose rates of continuous exposures is the log transform. Postulating a log-linear relation of the form $\log RR(x) = \alpha + \beta \log(x)$ means that risk itself is proportional to a power of dose, x^{β}, a relationship known to occur frequently from both human and animal studies (see § 6.11). Since both ALC and TOB took on 0 values it was necessary to "start" the logs by adding 1 to each before transforming it, in order to avoid infinities. Note that with either the original (ALC and TOB) or the transformed [LOG(ALC + 1) and LOG(TOB + 1)] variables, non-consumers of both tobacco and alcohol are automatically assigned relative risks of 1.0. This is because the values of all risk variables are 0 for individuals consuming no alcohol and no tobacco.

Table 6.12 presents the results. The first model, which includes linear terms for each of alcohol and tobacco, may be compared with Model 6, Table 6.10, of the grouped data analysis. Agreement between the two sets of coefficients is remarkably good: the log relative risk is estimated to increase by 0.255 (grouped) or 0.260 (continuous) for every additional 10 grams of alcohol, while for 10 grams of tobacco the corresponding figures are 0.409 and 0.405.

In contrast to the situation with grouped data, the goodness-of-fit statistics shown in the fourth column of Table 6.12 should not be interpreted as chi-squares with the indicated degrees of freedom. Because the number of cases in each "group" is 0 or 1 according to whether the record refers to a case or control, a direct comparison of observed and expected numbers is not helpful in determining the adequacy of the model. Instead the *differences* between the measures for nested models evaluate their relative goodness of fit, as explained in § 6.4.

Table 6.12 Logistic regression analysis of continuous risk variables: Ille-et-Vilaine oesophageal cancer study

Model	No. of param- eters[a]	DF	Goodness of fit G	Regression coefficients for each risk variable (standardized coefficients in parentheses)[b]						
				ALC	TOB	LOG (ALC+1)	LOG (TOB+1)	ALC^2	TOB^2	LOG^2 (TOB+1)
1	8	967	695.4	0.0260 (10.00)	0.0405 (5.13)					
2	8	967	749.5		0.0411 (5.47)	0.933 (7.02)				
3	8	967	683.2	0.0252 (9.66)			0.539 (9.33)			
4	8	967	734.8			0.890 (6.73)	0.555 (6.19)			
5	9	966	693.9	0.0257 (9.88)	0.0648 (3.05)				-0.0006 (1.24)	
6	9	966	682.8	0.0202 (2.52)			0.539 (5.77)	0.0033 (0.65)		
7	9	966	681.1	0.0251 (9.61)			0.965 (3.05)			-0.114 (1.44)

[a] Includes the six age terms α_i in addition to the alcohol and tobacco parameters shown

[b] Both ALC and TOB are expressed in units of g/day.

For Model 2 of Table 6.12, the effect of alcohol consumption is expressed on a logarithmic rather than an arithmetic scale. In view of the marked decrease in the log likelihood, the log scale is clearly not appropriate for alcohol. On the other hand, the fit is substantially improved when the effect of tobacco is expressed in this way (Model 3). Addition of square terms in ALC (Model 6) or LOG(TOB+1) (Model 7) do not result in a statistically significant improvement over the model containing these two variables alone ($G_3 - G_6 = 0.4$, p = 0.5; $G_2 - G_7 = 2.1$, p = 0.15). It is of interest to note that not even use of both linear and quadratic terms in TOB (Model 5) achieves the goodness of fit produced by expressing this variable on a log scale.

Taking ALC and LOG(TOB+1) as the basic risk variables, tests were made for interaction effects between these two factors, as well as between each of them and age. Addition of an ALC×LOG(TOB+1) interaction term to the model reduced the goodness-of-fit statistic very little, to 682.6 ($\chi_1^2 = 0.6$, p = 0.4). Likewise, no interactions of alcohol with age ($\chi_1^2 = 1.1$, p = 0.3) nor of tobacco with age ($\chi_1^2 = 0.2$, p = 0.7) were apparent. Thus the quantitative regression analysis of the continuous data confirms the lack of interaction effects noted previously in our analysis of the grouped data.

In summary, the changes in risk of oesophageal cancer associated with increased alcohol and tobacco consumption are well represented by a model in which the effects of the two factors combine multiplicatively. The proportional increase in risk accompanying additional quantities of alcohol and tobacco, expressed in units of g/day, is estimated to be

$$(TOB+1)^{0.54}\exp(0.025 \times ALC).$$

Standard errors of the regression coefficients, 0.0026 for alcohol and 0.058 for tobacco, may be used to put approximate confidence limits about the estimates. Dividing the standard errors into the coefficients themselves yields the standardized values (Table 6.12), which may be referred to tables of the normal distribution to test for the significance of individual terms in the regression equation. Clearly both alcohol and tobacco have highly significant independent effects, as has already been established using other methods.

A plot of the estimated linear increase in log relative risk with alcohol (Figure 6.3) shows excellent agreement with the results of the qualitative analyses. Similar plots for tobacco are shown in Figure 6.4. Here the situation at first appears somewhat paradoxical. The estimated relative risks from the qualitative analysis lie entirely above those based on the log transform, which in turn lie above those derived from the linear model. The explanation for this apparently bizarre phenomenon is not hard to find. It is due to the arbitrary selection of 0 as a baseline value for tobacco, which constrains all three curves to pass through the origin of the graph. Any other value for tobacco could just as well have been chosen as baseline and assigned a 0 log relative risk, in which case the curves would all be displaced so as to pass through 0 at that point. In other words *the origin of the scale of log-relative risk is completely arbitrary and it is only the shapes of the curves which have any meaning.* To compare and contrast these shapes better, Figure 6.5 shows the same three curves except that the linear curve has been displaced upwards 0.96 units and the log curve up 0.48 units. The superior fit of the model using the log term is evident from this graph.

Fig. 6.5 Log relative risk of oesophageal cancer according to five levels of tobacco consumption: not constrained to pass through origin

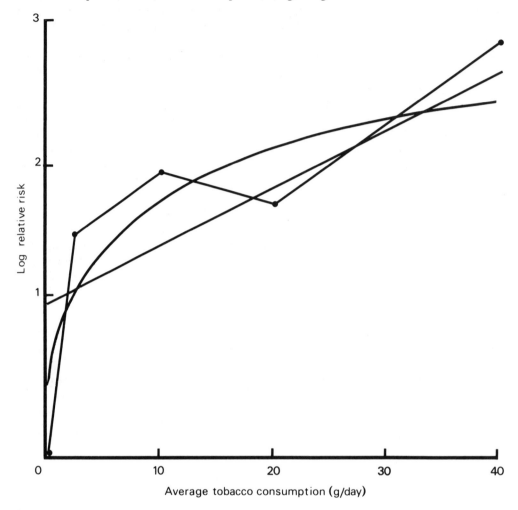

We conclude this section with an illustration of the ability of the logistic regression
model to investigate the simultaneous effects of a large number of continuous risk
variables. In order to estimate the average daily amount of alcohol consumed by each
study subject, interviewers posed separate questions regarding the pattern and frequency
of use of wine, beer, cider, aperitifs and digestives. The last two categories included
distilled beverage such as whisky (an aperitif) and brandy (a digestive). Separate
variables representing the average daily consumption of alcohol in each form were
available in the computer file. These had been obtained from the reported amounts
drunk by consideration of the usual alcoholic content: 8% by weight for wine; 3% for

beer and so on. Table 6.13 shows the distribution of each of the five beverage variables separately for cases and controls. Note that the sums of their mean values equal the means for alcohol (Table 4.1), as they should since ALC is obtained as the total of the component variables. The contributions from wine and cider are of roughly equal importance and those for beer and digestives, while lesser, are certainly not negligible. However, since so few people in this population report that they consume more than a few grams per day of aperitifs, we are already aware that it may be impossible to evaluate aperitifs as a separate risk factor.

Correlations among the five beverage variables, and of these with age and tobacco, are presented in Table 6.14 for the control population. The lack of strong correlations with age and tobacco inform us that these two variables are unlikely to confound the beverage effects to any appreciable degree. Even among the beverage variables the correlations are relatively weak, the strongest being between cider and digestives ($\varrho = 0.31$). Evidently cider drinkers tend to consume less wine, beer and aperitifs, but more digestives, than non-cider drinkers.

The rationale for using the summary alcohol variable in the statistical analysis, as done earlier, is the belief that the alcohol content of the beverages is responsible for the apparent association with oesophageal cancer and not some other characteristic such as impurities. In order to evaluate this hypothesis we fitted a series of models in which five separate beverage variables were used in place of total alcohol. The results

Table 6.13 Distribution of average daily amounts of alcohol consumption by type of beverage, for cases and controls: Ille-et-Vilaine study of oesophageal cancer

Average daily amount (g)	Beer		Cider		Type of beverage Wine		Aperitif		Digestive	
	Cases	Controls	Cases	Controls	Cases	Controls	Cases	Controls	Cases	Controls
0	141	493	76	373	28	142	105	346	76	430
1–9	21	144	12	64	30	214	90	419	55	236
10–39	18	103	49	229	63	293	5	10	58	98
40–79	11	30	39	92	52	104	0	0	10	10
80+	9	5	24	17	27	22	0	0	1	1
Mean	9.1	5.7	30.7	15.5	34.3	17.8	1.1	1.1	9.7	4.3
SD	22.7	13.7	37.4	21.6	37.1	21.2	2.6	2.0	15.1	8.9

Table 6.14 Correlations between alcoholic beverage variables, tobacco and age in control population: Ille-et-Vilaine study of oesophageal cancer

	Age	Tobacco	Beer	Cider	Wine	Aperitif	Digestive
Beer	−0.18	0.20	1.00				
Cider	0.08	−0.10	−0.16	1.00			
Wine	−0.04	0.16	0.07	−0.27	1.00		
Aperitif	−0.09	0.15	0.09	−0.11	0.21	1.00	
Digestive	0.13	0.04	−0.03	0.31	−0.02	0.06	1.00

Table 6.15 Logistic regression analysis of continuous beverage variables: Ille-et-Vilaine oesophageal cancer study

Model	No. of parameters[a]	DF	Goodness of fit G	Regression coefficients for each risk variable (standardized coefficients in parentheses)						
				LOG (TOB+1)	ALC	Beer	Cider	Wine	Aperitif	Digestive
1	8	967	683.2	0.539 (9.33)	0.0252 (9.66)					
2	12	963	674.3	0.546 (5.70)		0.0252 (4.55)	0.0281 (7.33)	0.0312 (7.80)	−0.0660 (−1.48)	0.0120 (1.30)
3	11	964	676.6	0.535 (5.61)		0.0247 (4.48)	0.0284 (7.43)	0.0301 (7.70)		0.0109 (1.27)
4	10	965	678.2	0.537 (5.64)		0.0248 (4.52)	0.0299 (8.19)	0.0304 (7.83)		
5	8	967	793.2	0.592 (6.90)	0.0156 (3.09)					
6	8	967	766.4	0.690 (7.46)			0.0178 (5.86)			
7	8	967	766.3	0.536 (6.24)				0.0194 (5.89)		
8	8	967	802.6	0.627 (7.26)					−0.0109 (0.28)	
9	8	967	786.6	0.624 (7.16)						0.0291 (3.87)

[a] Includes six age parameters in addition to those shown

are shown in Table 6.15, of which the first line is simply a repeat of Model 3, Table 6.12 Model 2 shows that beer, cider and wine each have highly significant independent effects on the risk of oesophageal cancer. It is remarkable how close all three coefficients are to the 0.0252 estimated for total alcohol, which lends support to the idea that alcohol *per se* is responsible for the effect. On the other hand, the coefficients for the two distilled beverage categories are not significantly different from zero, and that for aperitifs is even negative.

Before jumping to the conclusion that the aperitifs and digestives have a lesser effect, or even no effect in proportion to their alcohol content, we should consider the data presented in Table 6.13. Since fewer people in the population consume large amounts of aperitifs or digestives there is less information available for evaluating their role, a fact which is reflected in higher standard errors for their coefficients in comparison with the other variables. The upper 95% confidence intervals for the log relative risks are 0.0216 for aperitifs and 0.0288 for digestives, and the latter at least is quite consistent with the range of values for beer, cider and wine. To test formally the hypothesis that the coefficients for all five beverage variables are equal we have merely to compare the goodness-of-fit statistics for Models 1 and 2. Since Model 1 uses the sum of the beverage variables as a single regression variable (ALC), it constrains the coefficients to be equal and is consequently contained in Model 2. The value of the test statistic is $G_1 - G_2 = 8.9$ which, when referred to tables of χ_4^2, gives p = 0.06, a result bordering on statistical significance.

To go one step further we can *partition* the χ_4^2 value into single degree of freedom components by considering two intermediate models: 1A, in which the coefficients for beer, cider and wine only were assumed equal; and 1B, in which all coefficients were assumed equal except for aperitifs. These yield goodness-of-fit statistics of $G_{1A} = 678.9$ and $G_{1B} = 675.3$. Hence we may write $G_1 - G_2 = (G_1 - G_{1A}) + (G_{1A} - G_{1B}) + (G_{1B} - G_2)$, i.e., $8.9 = 4.3 + 3.6 + 1.0$, partitioning the χ_4^2 statistic into two χ_1^2's and one χ_2^2. The first, $G_1 - G_{1A}$, tests whether aperitifs have an effect different from the average of the remaining beverages ($p = 0.04$); the second, $G_{1A} - G_{1B}$, whether digestives differ from the remaining three ($p = 0.06$); and the last, $G_{1B} - G_2$, tests for differences among the coefficients of beer, cider and wine ($p = 0.60$). But, since the particular partitioning was suggested by the data rather than from *a priori* considerations, we are faced with *a multiple comparisons* dilemma and should discount the observed p values.

In the last analysis the situation is somewhat ambiguous. While digestives appear to have lesser effects than the other variables, and aperitifs no effect at all, we cannot rule out at conventional levels of statistical significance the possibility that all beverages contribute to the risk in proportion to their alcohol content.

6.10 Interpretation of regression coefficients

The preceding example considered a model with 12 independent parameters, each of which had a reasonably clear and straightforward interpretation. Six of the parameters, the α's attached to the six age strata, were included only to account for possible confounding effects of age. Since age effects were not of special interest, their estimates were not even presented in Table 6.15. However, the controls were obtained as a reasonably random sample of the adult male population so that differences between the α's could be interpreted in terms of log relative risks for the corresponding age groups. (From the α coefficients in Table 6.2, for example, it appears that risk does not change much with age beyond 55 years.) On the other hand, had the sample been stratified by design on the basis of age, no meaning at all could be attached to the α parameters since the effects of age on risk would then be completely confounded with the sampling fractions for different ages (§ 6.3).

While there is generally little interest in the actual values taken on by the α estimates, apart from knowing that the variables they represent have been "accounted for", this is hardly true for the β's. These we have repeatedly interpreted as indicating the change in risk associated with changes in the corresponding regression variables. It is a little disconcerting, therefore, to realize that the *estimated regression coefficients may change drastically according to what other variables are included in the model*. Such changes are to be anticipated whenever there is *collinearity* among the regression variables, meaning simply that their values tend to be correlated in the sampled data. Mosteller and Tukey (1977) provide a good discussion of this problem, which is fundamental to all regression models. Here we consider a few of the main issues, mostly by means of example.

In the Ille-et-Vilaine data there was a remarkable lack of collinearity among age and the levels of consumption of tobacco and total alcohol (Table 4.2). Consequently the estimated relative risks associated with each of these factors were little affected by which others were accounted for in the equation. For example, the (age-adjusted) relative risks for the four alcohol categories were 1.0, 4.2, 7.4 and 39.7 without inclusion of tobacco in the analysis, and 1.0, 4.2, 7.2 and 36.6 with such inclusion (Table 6.6).

A better illustration of the effects of collinearity is provided by the analyses of the contributions of individual alcoholic beverages (Table 6.15). We note first that neither the coefficients nor the standard errors of beer, cider and wine are much affected by the presence or absence of aperitif or digestive in the equation (Models 2–4), provided all three of the alcoholic beverages with significant effects are included. One would anticipate such a result if either (1) there was no correlation between the beverage variables, or (2) aperitif and digestive had no effect on risk beyond that explained by such a correlation (§ 3.4). However, when any one of beer, cider or wine is used as the *only* alcohol variable (Models 5–7), its coefficient and degree of statistical significance are noticeably reduced. This reflects the fact that cider is *negatively* correlated with both wine ($\varrho = -0.27$) and beer ($\varrho = -0.16$). Since an individual consuming a large amount of cider tends to consume less than the average amount of the other beverages, his apparent cancer risk relative to someone who drinks no cider is reduced unless the effects of these other beverage variables are accounted for by inclusion in the equation.

A different type of change occurs when digestive is used as the only alcohol variable (Model 9). Here the coefficient increases markedly from its value when all alcoholic beverage variables are included, and attains an apparently high level of statistical significance. The explanation now is the *positive* correlation of digestive with cider ($\varrho = 0.31$), such that when cider is not included in the equation, digestive serves, at least partially, as a *proxy* for its effects. After accounting for the effects of cider the coefficient for digestive falls to a non-significant level. On the other hand, since the correlations of digestive with beer and wine are essentially zero (Table 6.14), one would not expect the digestive coefficient to be much altered by the presence of these latter two variables.

Collinearity is bound to arise when both a variable and its square are included in the same equation. Compare, for example, Model 3 with Model 7 in Table 6.12. Introduction of the square term in LOG(TOB + 1) results in an almost doubling of the coefficient for the linear term, from 0.539 to 0.965. At the same time the standardized value decreases, from 9.33 to 3.05, indicating a roughly sixfold increase in the standard error. This is true in spite of the fact that the coefficient of the added variable, $LOG^2(TOB+1)$, is not statistically significant at all. Indeed, if we were to evaluate the significance of the tobacco effect only on the basis of the standardized coefficients in the quadratic model, we would be sorely misled. The significance of the trend in risk with increased tobacco consumption is well expressed by the single linear term in Model 3; and the large standard errors for LOG(TOB + 1) and $LOG^2(TOB + 1)$ in Model 7 tell us not that these variables are unimportant, but rather that there are many different sets of coefficients for them which express more or less equally well the relationship found in the data. This example illustrates that there is little point in trying to interpret individual coefficients and standard errors in a polynomial regression. A plot of the fitted relationship over the range of the regression variables conveys a much more accurate impression of what the equation means.

A similar type of artificial association can arise between one variable representing the main effects of a factor and others representing its interactions, at least if care is not taken in how these interactions are coded. For example, in order to investigate the interaction between age and alcohol we added to Model 3 of Table 6.12 a variable ALC × AGEGRP, where AGEGRP took on the values 1 to 6 of the age group. Although this improved the goodness of fit only slightly, from G = 683.2 to G = 682.1, and the interaction terms had a non-significant regression coefficient, its inclusion in the equation markedly affected the coefficient of ALC. The estimated regression equation (ignoring age effects) changed from

$$0.0252 \text{ ALC} + 0.539 \text{ LOG(TOB+1)}$$
$$(9.66) \qquad\qquad (9.33)$$

to

$$0.0348 \text{ALC} + 0.536 \text{LOG(TOB+1)} - 0.00246 \text{ALC} \times \text{AGEGRP},$$
$$(3.58) \qquad\quad (5.76) \qquad\qquad\qquad (-1.04)$$

and by comparing the standardized coefficients (shown in parentheses), we see that the standard error of ALC increased from 0.00261 to 0.00972. Again the explanation is the high degree of collinearity between ALC and ALC × AGEGRP, which can be substantially reduced by subtracting from AGEGRP its *modal* value of 4 before multiplying. This leads to an equation

$$0.0250 \text{ALC} + 0.536 \text{LOG(TOB+1)} - 0.00246 \text{ALC} \times (\text{AGEGRP-4})$$
$$(9.56) \qquad\quad (5.76) \qquad\qquad\qquad (-1.04)$$

which represents *exactly the same relationship* as the previous one. However, because the main effect and interaction variables have been coded to reduce the correlation between them, the changes in the coefficient and standard error of the main effect variable are much reduced. Routine coding of interaction or cross-product variables by subtracting mean or modal values from their component parts before multiplying is recommended to avoid the anomalies provoked by such artificial collinearity.

A less artificial example of high correlation between two regression variables occurs when both are measuring the same fundamental quantity in a somewhat imperfect way. In attempting to relate arsenic exposure to cancer risk, for example, we might determine the arsenic concentration of both fingernails and hair of cases and controls, and use each as an indicator of chronic exposure. If these two measures turned out to be highly correlated, as they would if both were good indicators of long-term exposure, it would make little sense to attempt to evaluate their separate effects on risk by including them both in the regression equation. Instead we would take an average or composite of the two values as a single measure of arsenic exposure, and use this along with variables representing other risk factors.

Of course in some problems the collinearity between regression variables will reflect a real association between the corresponding risk factors in the population. While regression analysis is the most powerful tool available for separating out the independent associations with risk, unambiguous answers are simply not possible when collinearity is high. In some cases a judgement as to which is the proper variable, or which risk factor is more likely to play a causal role, will dictate which variables to leave in the equation. If such a judgement cannot be made, one must simply admit that precise identification of the factor responsible for the effect is impossible. To quote from Mosteller and Tukey (1977): "We must be prepared for one variable to serve as a proxy for another and worry about the possible consequences, in particular, whether the proxy's coefficient siphons off some of the coefficient we would like to have on the proper variable, or whether a variable serves well only because it is a proxy. In either case, interpretation of the regression coefficient requires very considerable care." Much of the discussion in § 3.4 on whether or not one should adjust for apparent confounding variables is relevant here.

6.11 Transforming continuous risk variables

One of the more perplexing issues facing the analyst who uses quantitative regression methods is the choice of appropriate scales on which to express continuous risk variables. He must decide between original measurements, as recorded by machine or interviewer, and such transforms as logs, square roots, reciprocals, or any number of other possibilities. Since the object is to achieve a near-linear relationship between the quantitative regression variable and log risk, it usually helps to make some plots of relative risks for grouped data as we did in Figures 6.1 to 6.4. If the data are sufficiently extensive, so that a regular pattern emerges, one can at least rule out some of the possible choices on the grounds of lack of fit. For example it was fairly clear from both graphical and quantitative analysis of the Ille-et-Vilaine data that the effects of alcohol were best expressed on the original linear scale, while for tobacco a log transform was required.

However epidemiological data are rarely sufficient to enable fine distinctions to be made between rather similar functional forms for the dose-response relationship on statistical grounds alone. Accurate measurements of human exposure to potential risk factors are not often available. Hence recourse is made to animal experimentation for elucidating fundamental aspects of the carcinogenic process. Such experiments allow one to control fairly strictly the amounts of carcinogen administered to homogenous subgroups of animals, and data derived from them are more amenable to precise quantitative analysis than are data from observational studies of human populations.

Example: One animal model which has been used to suggest relationships for human epithelial tumours is that of skin-painting experiments in mice. In an experiment reported by Lee and O'Neill (1971), mice were randomly assigned to four dosage groups each containing 300 animals. Starting at about three weeks of age, benzo[a]pyrene (BP) was painted on their shaved backs in the following dosages:

Group 1   6 μg BP/week
Group 2   12 μg BP/week
Group 3   24 μg BP/week
Group 4   48 μg BP/week

The animals were examined regularly, and the week of tumour occurrence was taken to be the first week that a skin tumour was observed. Age-specific incidence rates of skin tumours were estimated for each dosage group according to the methods of § 2.1. The number of animals developing a skin tumour for the first time during any one week was divided by the number still alive and free of skin tumours at the middle of that week. Since few new tumours would arise in any given week, these age-specific estimates tended to be highly unstable. Consequently, the four dosage groups were compared in terms of the age-specific *cumulative* incidence rates (§ 2.3).

Figure 6.6 shows log-log plots of cumulative incidence against week. These are well described by four parallel straight lines, with distances between the lines for successive dosages roughly equal. In fact the cumulative incidence $\Lambda(t; x)$ of skin tumours which occur by week t, among animals receiving BP at dose x, is well described by the equation

$$\log \Lambda(t;x) = -17.6 + 1.78 \log(x) + 2.95 \log(t-18),$$

i.e.,

$$\Lambda(t;x) = Cx^{1.78}(t-18)^{2.95},$$

where C is a constant. It follows that the ratios of cumulative incidence rates for successive dosage groups $\Lambda(t;2x) \div \Lambda(t;x)$ and hence the ratios of the age-specific rates $\lambda(t;2x) \div \lambda(t;x)$, are equal to $2^{1.78} = 3.41$. Thus, within the range of dosage and ages of animals considered in this experiment, the effect of BP on incidence can be described very simply: a doubling of dose will lead to an approximate 3.4-fold increase in the age-specific skin tumour incidence rates.

The same investigators have shown in later work (Peto et al., 1975) that the relevant time variable is in fact not the age of the animal, but rather the duration of exposure to BP. They also point out that, since the powers of dose x and time t in the fitted formula for cumulative incidence are roughly 2 and 3,

Fig. 6.6 Estimated cumulative incidence rates of skin tumours occurring among female albino mice given weekly paintings of benzo[*a*]pyrene at four dosages, with parallel regression lines fitted by maximum likelihood (from Lee & O'Neill, 1971)

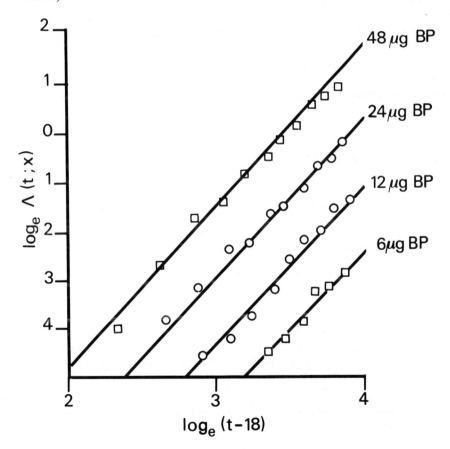

respectively, the data are consistent with a multi-stage theory for the origin of cancer wherein two of the three stages are affected by the carcinogen (Peto, 1977). Recent data for cigarette smoking and lung cancer in the British doctor study likewise suggest that incidence is proportional to the square of the dose rate (Doll & Peto, 1978).

If the linear logistic model were to be used to represent the data in the above experiment, this would take the form

$$\text{logit } P_i(x) = \alpha_i + \beta \log(x)$$

for the probability that an animal treated with x units of BP who is still at risk at age t_i develops a skin tumour within that week. The α_i parameters in turn could be modelled $\alpha_i = \alpha + \gamma \log(t_i)$ as a linear function of log age. There is no problem here with the fact that the logarithm of a zero dose is $-\infty$ and thus the estimated probability of tumour development 0, since skin tumours do not appear spontaneously on the backs of mice without treatment. For other studies, especially with humans, one could substitute a dose metameter of the form $z = \log(x + x_0)$, where x was the measured dose while x_0 represented a small *background dose* which was presumably responsible for any spontaneous cases. Although in principle it is possible to estimate x_0 from the data by maximum likelihood, this is rarely done. Special programmes would be required for such estimation since x_0 does not enter the regression equation in the same linear fashion as the other parameters. Furthermore, since different combinations of x_0 and β can give virtually identical fits to the data, the standard errors and covariances for the jointly estimated parameters tend to be large. Hence the best practice may simply be to assign x_0 some small value on the basis of *a priori* considerations. With the Ille-et-Vilaine tobacco data, we set $x_0 = 1$ and noticed that the resulting curve seemed to fit the observed data reasonably well (Figure 6.5).

6.12 Studies of interaction in a series of 2×2 tables

One of the principal advantages of using the logistic regression model is that it encourages quantitative description of how the changes in risk associated with one factor are modified by the interaction effects of other risk or nuisance variables. Since the Ille-et-Vilaine data are notably lacking in such interactions, they cannot be used to illustrate this important feature of statistical modelling. Hence in this section we analyse another set of published data, which happen to be in the form of a series of 2×2 tables, for which strong interaction effects are present.

Presence of interaction effects in a series of 2×2 tables means that the odds ratios depend systematically on the variables used for strata formation. Such dependence may have important implications for the nature of the disease process. The data we shall consider are those of Stewart and Kneale (1970) who hypothesized that the distribution of age at diagnosis for childhood cancers caused by obstetric X-rays was more concentrated or "peaked" than the age distribution of idiopathic childhood cancers. If this were so the risk ratio for irradiated *versus* non-irradiated children would also show a peak when plotted against age. The effect would presumably occur because the time of exposure for the radiogenic cases is limited to the period of gestation, while for other cancers it could vary over a broader age span.

Such variations are detected by the addition of interaction terms to the logistic model. In § 6.5 we considered a model in which the log relative risk was assumed to change linearly over the six age strata. More generally one might define several different regression variables, including transformations and cross-product terms, from factors such as age and time which are used to define strata. Let us denote by z_{il} the value of the lth variable for the ith stratum $(i = 1, ..., I; l = 1, ..., L)$. Then the interaction model may be written

$$\text{logit } P_i(x) = \alpha_i + \beta x + \sum_{l=1}^{L} \gamma_l x z_{il}, \qquad (6.25)$$

where as usual $P_i(x)$ denotes the disease probability in the ith stratum for an exposed $(x = 1)$ or unexposed $(x = 0)$ individual. A consequence of this formulation is that the log relative risk for the ith stratum is expressed

$$\log \psi = \log \frac{P_i(1)Q_i(0)}{P_i(0)Q_i(1)} = \beta + \sum_{l=1}^{L} \gamma_l z_{il}$$

as a linear function of the regression variables z, with the "constant" term β denoting the baseline log relative risk for the group having covariate values $\mathbf{z} = \mathbf{0}$. It is best to code the covariates in such a way that $\mathbf{z} = \mathbf{0}$ corresponds to some "typical" individual.

Summary data from the Oxford Childhood Cancer Survey and associated studies reported by Kneale (1971) are presented in Appendix II. Cases were ascertained as all children under ten years of age in England and Wales who died of cancer (leukaemia or solid tumours) during the period 1954–65. For each of these a neighbourhood control of the same age was selected who was alive and well at the time the case died. Only "traced" pairs, for whom both case and control mothers could be found and interviewed, were analysed. The published data ignore the exact pairing but do preserve the stratification by age and year of birth.

Exposure in this example is simply a question of whether or not the study subjects received *in utero* irradiation, as reported by the mother. The stratification variables were age at death, from 0 to 9 years, and year of birth, from 1944 to 1964. Because of the limited period of case ascertainment, not all 210 possible combinations of these factors appear. For example, among childhood cancer patients born in 1944, only those who died at age 9 are represented. A total of 120 such strata were available.

In order to estimate the overall relative risk of obstetric radiation, and to determine whether, and if so how, it varied with age and year, we fitted several versions of the model (6.25). Five different regression variables were used: $z_1 = $ year of birth, coded $z_1 = -10$ for 1944, ..., $z_1 = 10$ for 1964; $z_2 = z_1^2 - 22$; $z_3 = $ age at death, coded -9 for age 0, -7 for age 1, ..., 9 for age 9; $z_4 = z_3^2 - 33$; and $z_5 = z_1 \times z_3$. Different subsets of these were entered into the regression equation so as to detect particular kinds of trends and patterns in the relative risk.

Results of the analysis are shown in Table 6.16. Degrees of freedom (DF) for each model were obtained in the usual manner by subtracting the number of parameters, in this case the 120 α's plus additional β and γ terms, from the number of binomial observations, namely 240. The first model, which includes only the α's, assumes that the relative risk is unity in each stratum. In view of the large goodness-of-fit statistics, this supposition is clearly untenable. The second model specifies a constant relative

Table 6.16 Results of fitting several logistic regression models with interactions: Oxford study of obstetric radiation and childhood cancer[a]

Model	No. of parameters	DF	Goodness-of-fit statistics		Regression coefficients ± S.E.	Interactions with				
			G	$\tilde{G}$	Log RR ($\hat{\beta}$)	YR^b ($\hat{\gamma}_1$)	YR^2-22^c ($\hat{\gamma}_2$)	AGE^d ($\hat{\gamma}_3$)	AGE^2-33^c ($\hat{\gamma}_4$)	$YR \times AGE$ ($\hat{\gamma}_5$)
1	0	120	207.89	196.74						
2	1	119	124.29	118.75	0.5102±0.0564					
3	2	118	116.96	112.52	0.5218±0.0567	−0.0390±0.0145				
4	3	117	111.57	108.74	0.5707±0.0611	−0.0450±0.0150	0.0068±0.0030			
5	3	117	116.33	112.75	0.5297±0.0576	−0.0312±0.0176		0.0105±0.0133		
6	6	114	110.20	107.32	0.4738±0.1308	−0.0411±0.0182	0.0029±0.0057	0.0069±0.0134	0.0025±0.0028	−0.0054±0.0063

[a] From Breslow (1976); data from Kneale (1971)
[b] YR is coded as follows: 1944 = −10, 1945 = −9, ..., 1963 = 9, 1964 = 10.
[c] Constants subtracted from square of AGE and YR so that variables sum to zero over tables
[d] AGE is coded as follows: 9 years = 9, 8 years = 7, 7 years = 5, ..., 1 year = −7, 0 year = −9.

risk for obstetric radiation, estimated as $\hat{\psi} = \exp(0.5102) = 1.67$. Since the chi-square statistics for it are close to their mean values (DF), they might be taken as evidence of a good fit. However the introduction of a linear interaction term in year of birth (Model 3) results in a significant improvement ($G_2 - G_3 = 124.29 - 116.96 = 7.3$, $p = 0.007$). Hence there is reasonably strong evidence for a decrease in relative risk with year of birth. Additional improvement in fit occurs when a quadratic term in year is added to the model, which would indicate a degree of curvature in the regression line. However it is of lesser statistical significance ($G_3 - G_4 = 5.39$, $p = 0.02$). Figure 6.7 shows age-adjusted estimates of the log-relative risk for each year, together with linear and quadratic regression lines as fitted by Models 3 and 4. This illustrates graphically the nature of the decline in the radiation effect over time.

Absolutely no improvements in fit accompanied the addition to the model of either linear or quadratic terms in age: compare Models 3 *versus* 5 and 4 *versus* 6. The quadratic term would be expected to be particularly sensitive to a peak in relative risk as a function of age. The lack of evidence for any such peak argues against the hypothesis that the age distributions for radiogenic and idiopathic cancers are different. Improvements in radiological technology probably account for the declining effect with year of birth (Bithel & Stewart, 1975).

Fig. 6.7 Age-adjusted estimates of log relative risk (odds ratio) for obstetric radiation each with approximate 80 percent confidence limits and both linear and quadratic regression lines (from Breslow, 1976; data from Kneale, 1971)

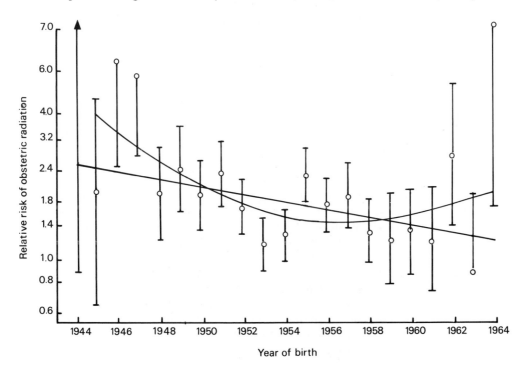

Table 6.17 Comparison of the log relative risk and its interaction with year of birth, depending on the degree of polynomial adjustment for age and year: Oxford study of obstetric radiation and childhood cancer[a]

Degree of polynomial in age and year	No. of parameters	DF	Goodness of fit $\hat{G}$	Estimates of log-relative risk and interaction $\beta \pm$ S.E.	$\hat{\gamma}_1 \pm$ S.E.
0	3	237	114.62	0.5113 ± 0.0562	-0.0343 ± 0.0136
1	5	235	113.87	0.5124 ± 0.0562	-0.0382 ± 0.0143
2	8	232	113.57	0.5124 ± 0.0562	-0.0384 ± 0.0143
3	12	228	113.55	0.5150 ± 0.0563	-0.0385 ± 0.0143
4	17	223	113.43	0.5157 ± 0.0564	-0.0385 ± 0.0143
5	23	217	113.33	0.5163 ± 0.0564	-0.0386 ± 0.0144
Stratified[b]	122	118	112.52	0.5218 ± 0.0567	-0.0390 ± 0.0145

[a] From Breslow and Powers (1978); data from Kneale (1971)
[b] From Model 3, Table 6.16

As shown in § 6.8, an alternative to a stratified analysis is simply to model the effects of the nuisance factors on disease incidence, replacing the α_i in the logistic model by quantitative terms. In order to compare the results from such an analysis with those just obtained, we considered analogs of Model 3 in which the log-relative risk was assumed to decline linearly with year of birth. Polynomials of increasing degree in age and year were used to give different degrees of adjustment for the confounding effects of these factors. Thus the models fitted were of the form

$$\text{logit } P_i(x) = \begin{cases} \alpha_0 + \beta x + \gamma_1 x z_{i1} & \text{(unadjusted)} \\ \alpha_0 + \alpha_1 z_{i1} + \alpha_3 z_{i3} + \beta x + \gamma_1 x z_{i1} & \text{(linear)} \\ \alpha_0 + \sum_1^5 \alpha_l z_{il} + \beta x + \gamma_1 x z_{i1} & \text{(quadratic)} \end{cases}$$

and so on, using third, fourth and fifth degree polynomials. The results in Table 6.17 show that increasing the degree of polynomial adjustment leads to better agreement with results of the stratified analysis (Breslow & Powers, 1978). It is somewhat surprising that there is so little improvement in the fit, and so little change in the estimated relative risks, as more terms of age and year are included. A partial explanation is, of course, that the sample was deliberately stratified to ensure that the numbers of cases and controls in each age/year stratum were equal. Thus one might not expect these two factors to contribute significantly to a model designed to discriminate cases from controls. However, as discussed in § 3.4, this identity of the marginal distributions of age and year for cases and controls is not sufficient to justify ignoring these factors in the analysis. *In general, variables used for stratification or matching in the design stage must also be accounted for in the analysis in order to obtain unbiased estimates of the relative risk.* An example which better illustrates this point is presented in § 7.6. If strata are formed at the time of analysis, rather than by design, there will be imbalances in the numbers of cases and controls within strata, and the differences between the stratified and unadjusted analyses will be more obvious than they are in Table 6.17.

REFERENCES

Anderson, J.A. (1972) Separate sample logistic discrimination. *Biometrika, 59,* 19–35

Armitage, P. (1975) *Statistical Methods in Medical Research,* Oxford, Blackwell

Baker, R.J. & Nelder, J.A. (1978) *The GLIM System. Release 3,* Oxford, Numerical Algorithms Group

Bishop, Y.M.M., Fienberg, S.E. & Holland, P.W. (1975) *Discrete Multivariate Analysis: Theory and Practice,* Cambridge, Mass., MIT Press

Bithel, J. & Stewart, A. (1975) Pre-natal irradiation and childhood malignancy: a review of British data from the Oxford Survey. *Br. J. Cancer, 31,* 271–287

Breslow, N.E. (1975) Analysis of survival data under the proportional hazards model. *Rev. Int. Stat., 43,* 45–58

Breslow, N.E. (1976) Regression analysis of the log odds ratio: a method for retrospective studies. *Biometrics, 32,* 409–416

Breslow, N.E. (1978) The proportional hazards model: applications in epidemiology. *Comm. Stat.-Theor. Meth., A7,* 315–332

Breslow, N.E., Day, N.E., Halvorsen, K.T., Prentice, R.L. & Sabai, C. (1978) Estimation of multiple relative risk functions in matched case-control studies. *Am. J. Epidemiol., 108,* 299–307

Breslow, N.E. & Powers, W. (1978) Are there two logistic regressions for retrospective studies? *Biometrics, 34,* 100–105

Cornfield, J. (1962) Joint dependence of the risk of coronary heart disease on serum cholesterol and systolic blood pressure: a discriminant function analysis. *Fed. Proc., 21,* 58–61

Cox, D.R. (1970) *The Analysis of Binary Data,* London, Methuen

Cox, D.R. (1972) Regression models and life tables (with discussion). *J. R. stat. Soc. B, 34,* 187–220

Cox, D.R. & Hinkley, D.V. (1974) *Theoretical Statistics,* London, Chapman & Hall

Day, N.E. & Byar, D.P. (1979) Testing hypotheses in case-control studies – equivalence of Mantel-Haenszel statistics and logit score tests. *Biometrics, 35,* 623–630

Day, N.E. & Kerridge, D.F. (1967) A general maximum likelihood discriminant. *Biometrics, 23,* 313–323

Doll, R. & Peto, R. (1978) Cigarette smoking and bronchial carcinoma: dose and time relationships among regular smokers and lifelong non-smokers. *J. Epidemiol. Community Health, 32,* 303–313

Efron, B. (1975) The efficiency of logistic regression compared to normal theory discriminant analysis. *J. Am. stat. Assoc., 70,* 892–898

Farewell, V.T. (1979) Some results on the estimation of logistic models based on retrospective data. *Biometrika, 66,* 27–32

Fienberg, S.E. (1977) *The Analysis of Cross-Classified Data,* Cambridge, Mass., MIT Press

Haberman, S.J. (1974) *The Analysis of Frequency Data,* Chicago, University of Chicago Press

Halperin, M., Blackwelder, W.C. & Verter, J.I. (1971) Estimation of the multivariate logistic risk function: a comparison of the discriminant function and maximum likelihood approaches. *J. chron. Dis., 24,* 125–158

Kneale, G.W. (1971) Problems arising in estimating from retrospective survey data the latent period of juvenile cancers initiated by obstetric radiography. *Biometrics, 27,* 563–590

Lee, P. & O'Neill, J. (1971) The effect of both time and dose on tumour incidence rate in benzopyrene skin painting experiments. *Br. J. Cancer, 25,* 759–770

Lininger, L., Gail, M., Green, S. & Byar, D. (1979) Comparison of four tests for equality of survival curves in the presence of stratification and censoring. *Biometrika, 63,* 419–428

Mantel, N. (1973) Synthetic retrospective studies and related topics. *Biometrics, 29,* 479–486

Mosteller, F. & Tukey, J.W. (1977) *Data Analysis and Regression: a Second Course in Statistics,* Reading, Mass., Addison & Wesley

Nelder, J.A. (1977) A reformulation of linear models. *J. R. stat. Soc. A, 140,* 48–77

Peto, R. (1977) *Epidemiology, multistage models and short-term mutagenicity tests.* In: Hiatt, H.H., Watson, J.D. & Winsten, J.A., eds. *Origins of Human Cancer,* Cold Spring Harbor, NY, Cold Spring Harbor Publications, Vol. 4, pp. 1403–1421

Peto, R., Roe, F., Lee, P., Levy, L. & Clark, J. (1975) Cancer and ageing in mice and men. *Br. J. Cancer, 32,* 411–426

Prentice, R.L. & Breslow, N.E. (1978) Retrospective studies and failure time models. *Biometrika, 65,* 153–158

Prentice, R.L. & Pyke, R. (1979) Logistic disease incidence models and case-control studies. *Biometrika, 66,* 403–411

Press, S.J. & Wilson, S. (1978) Choosing between logistic regression and discriminant analysis. *J. Am. stat. Assoc., 70,* 699–705

Rao, C.R. (1965) *Linear Statistical Inference and its Applications,* New York, Wiley

Seigel, D.G. & Greenhouse, S.W. (1973) Multiple relative risk functions in case-control studies. *Am. J. Epidemiol., 97,* 324–331

Stewart, A. & Kneale, G.W. (1970) Age-distribution of cancers caused by obstetric x-rays and their relevance to cancer latent periods. *Lancet, ii,* 4–8

Thomson, W.A., Jr (1977) On the treatment of grouped observations in life studies *Biometrics, 33,* 463–470

Truett, J., Cornfield, J. & Kannel, W. (1967) A multivariate analysis of the risk of coronary heart disease in Framingham. *J. chron. Dis., 20,* 511–524

Vitaliano, P.O. (1978) The use of logistic regression for modelling risk factors: with application to non-melanoma skin cancer. *Am. J. Epidemiol., 108,* 402–414

Walker, S.H. & Duncan, D.B. (1967) Estimation of the probability of an event as a function of several independent variables. *Biometrika, 54,* 167–179

LIST OF SYMBOLS – CHAPTER 6 (in order of appearance)

logit(p)   the logistic transform of a proportion p; $\log(\frac{p}{1-p})$

x   risk variable
ψ odds ratio
β log odds ratio

P_1	disease probability for exposed
P_0	disease probability for unexposed
$P(x)$	disease probability for exposure to an amount x
$r(x)$	relative risk of disease associated with exposure to an amount x
α	log odds for disease among unexposed
P_{ij}	disease probability associated with exposure to level i of factor A and level j of factor B
Q_{ij}	$1-P_{ij}$
ψ_{ij}	odds ratio associated with exposure to level i of factor A and level j of factor B ($\psi_{00} = 1$)
r_A	relative risk of exposure to factor A
r_B	relative risk of exposure to factor B
r_{AB}	relative risk of exposure to both factor A and factor B
β_1	log odds ratio associated with exposure to factor A
β_2	log odds ratio associated with exposure to factor B
γ	(multiplicative) interaction parameter; log of the ratio of the relative risk for combined exposure divided by the product of relative risks for individual exposures
$P(x_1,x_2)$	disease probability associated with exposure to an amount x_1 of factor A and x_2 of factor B
β_k	coefficient of variable x_k in logistic regression equation; log relative risk associated with unit increase in x_k
γ_{kl}	coefficient of cross product variable $x_k x_l$ in logistic regression equation; interaction parameter
P_{ijk}	disease probability associated with exposure to levels i of A, j of B and k of C
Q_{ijk}	$1-P_{ijk}$
ψ_{ijk}	relative risk associated with exposures to levels i of A, j of B and k of C
γ_{ijk}	coefficient of variable $x_i x_j x_k$ in logistic regression equation; second order interaction parameter
$pr(\ \mid\ )$	probability of one event given the occurrence of another
i	subscript indicating one of I strata
x	vector of risk variables associated with an individual
$P_i(x)$	disease probability associated with a vector x of risk variables in the ith stratum of the population
y	binary response variable; y = 1 for diseased, y = 0 for disease-free
π_1	sampling fraction for cases; probability that a diseased person is included in the study as a case
π_0	sampling fraction for controls; probability that a disease-free person is included in the study as a control
z	indicator sampling variable: z = 1 for inclusion in the study, z = 0 otherwise
Σ	covariance matrix for the distribution of risk variables, assumed common for cases and controls
μ_1	expected values of risk variables among cases
μ_0	expected values of risk variables among controls

$\bar{\mathbf{x}}_1$ sample mean of risk variables $\mathbf{x}$ among cases
$\bar{\mathbf{x}}_0$ sample mean of risk variables $\mathbf{x}$ among controls
$\mathbf{S}_p^2$ covariance matrix of risk variables pooled from separate samples of
                   cases and controls
$\mathbf{l}$ denotes a partition of the integers from 1 to n into two groups, one of
                   size n_1 and the other of size $n_0 = n - n_1$; e.g., if $n_1 = 2$ and $n_0 = 3$ a
                   possible partition is $l_1 = 3, l_2 = 4, l_3 = 1, l_4 = 2, l_5 = 5$ or $\mathbf{l} = (3,4,1,2,5)$
$\mathbf{x}_j$ vector of risk variables for j^{th} study subject
G   goodness-of-fit statistic based on the log likelihood
S   efficient score; vector first of first derivatives of the log likelihood function
I   information matrix; matrix of negatives of second partial derivatives of
                   the log likelihood function
Z   standardized regression coefficient (equivalent normal deviate)
$\tilde{G}$ chi-square goodness-of-fit statistic for grouped data, based on differences
                   between observed and expected values
(N.B. Subscripts on the above quantities G, $\tilde{G}$, S, I, and Z denote their values under
different models)
O   observed number of cases (or controls) in a particular cell with grouped
                   data
E   expected number of cases (or controls) in a cell, predicted by fitted model
ϱ correlation coefficient between two variables
$\varLambda(t;x)$ cumulative incidence of skin tumours by week t among animals continu-
                   ously exposed to BP at a dose rate x
$\lambda(t;x)$ age-specific incidence of skin tumours at week t among animals continu-
                   ously exposed to BP at a dose rate x
L   number of regression variables (covariates) associated with each of a
                   series of 2×2 tables
l l^{th} of L covariates associated with a series of 2×2 tables
z_{il} value of the lth covariate for the ith of a series of 2×2 tables
$\hat{\ }$ when placed over another symbol this indicates an estimate of a popula-
                   tion parameter calculated from the sampled data; or a fitted cell fre-
                   quency predicted from a model; e.g., $\hat{\beta}$ is an estimate of β

7. CONDITIONAL LOGISTIC REGRESSION FOR MATCHED SETS

7.1 Bias arising from the unconditional analysis of matched data

7.2 Multivariate analysis for matched 1:M designs: general methodology

7.3 Matched pairs with dichotomous and polytomous exposures: applications

7.4 1:M matching with single and multiple exposure variables: applications

7.5 Combining sets of 2×2 tables

7.6 Effect of ignoring the matching

CHAPTER VII

CONDITIONAL LOGISTIC REGRESSION
FOR MATCHED SETS

One of the methods for estimating the relative risk parameters β in the stratified logistic regression model was conditioning (§ 6.3). We supposed that for a given stratum composed of n_1 cases and n_0 controls we knew the unordered values $x_1, \ldots, x_n$ of the exposures for the $n = n_1 + n_0$ subjects, but did not know which values were associated with the cases and which with the controls. The conditional probability of the observed data was calculated (6.15) to be a product of terms of the form

$$\frac{\prod\limits_{j=1}^{n_1} \exp(\sum\limits_{k=1}^{K} \beta_k x_{jk})}{\sum\limits_{l} \prod\limits_{j=1}^{n_1} \exp(\sum\limits_{k=1}^{K} \beta_k x_{l_j k})}, \tag{7.1}$$

where l ranged over the $\binom{n}{n_1}$ choices of n_1 integers from among the set $\{1, 2, \ldots, n\}$.

With a single binary exposure variable x, coded $x = 1$ for exposed and $x = 0$ for unexposed, knowing the unordered x's meant knowing the total number exposed in the stratum, and thus knowing all the marginal totals in the corresponding 2×2 table. The complete data were then determined by the number of exposed cases. In these circumstances the conditional probability (7.1) is proportional to the hypergeometric distribution (4.2), used as a starting point for exact statistical inference about the odds ratio in a 2×2 table.

The conditional likelihood offers important conceptual advantages as a basis for statistical analysis of the results of a case-control study. First, it depends only on the relative risk parameters of interest and thus allows for construction of exact tests and estimates such as were described in Chapters 4 and 5 for selected problems. Second, precisely the same (conditional) likelihood is obtained whether we regard the data as arising from either (i) a prospective study of n individuals with a given set of exposures $x_1, \ldots, x_n$, the conditioning event being the observed number n_1 of cases arising in the sample; or (ii) a case-control study involving n_1 cases and n_0 controls, the conditioning event being the n observed exposure histories. The observation that these two conditional likelihoods agree, which was made in § 4.2 for the 2×2 table, confirms the fundamental point that identical methods of analysis are used whether the data have been gathered according to prospective or retrospective sampling plans.

Unfortunately, whenever the strata contain sizeable numbers of both cases and controls, the calculations required for the conditional analysis are extremely costly if not actually impossible even using large computers. Since the analysis based on the unconditional likelihood (6.12) yields essentially equivalent results, it would seem to be the method of choice in such circumstances. The conditional approach is best restricted to matched case-control designs, or to similar situations involving very fine stratification, where its use is in fact essential in order to avoid biased estimates of relative risk. We begin this chapter with an illustration of the magnitude of the bias which arises from analysing matched data with the unconditional model. Next, the conditional model is examined for several of the special problems considered in Chapters 4 and 5; many of the estimates and test statistics discussed earlier for these problems are shown to result from application of the general model. Finally, we explore the full potential of the conditional model for the multivariate analysis of matched data, largely by means of example, and discuss some of the issues which arise in its implementation.

7.1 Bias arising from the unconditional analysis of matched data

Use of the unconditional regression model (6.12) for estimation of relative risks entails explicit estimation of the α stratum parameters in addition to the β coefficients of primary interest. For matched or finely stratified data, the number of α parameters may be of the same order of magnitude as the number of observations and much greater than the number of β's. In such situations, involving a large number of nuisance parameters, it is well known that the usual techniques of likelihood inference can yield seriously biased estimates (Cox & Hinkley, 1974, p. 292). This phenomenon is perhaps best illustrated for the case of 1–1 pair matching with a single binary exposure variable x.

Returning to the general set-up of § 6.2, suppose that each of the I strata consists of a matched case-control pair and that each subject has been classified as exposed (x = 1) or unexposed (x = 0). The outcome for each pair may be represented in the form of a 2×2 table, of which there are four possible configurations, as shown in (5.1). The model to be fitted is of the form

$$\text{pr}_i(y = 1 \,|\, x) = \frac{\exp(\alpha_i + \beta x)}{1 + \exp(\alpha_i + \beta x)} \, ,$$

where $\beta = \log \psi$ is the logarithm of the relative risk, assumed constant across matched sets.

According to a well-known theory developed for logistic or log-linear models (Fienberg, 1977), unconditional maximum likelihood estimates (MLEs) for the parameters α and β are found by fitting frequencies to all cells in the $2 \times 2 \times K$ dimensional configuration such that (i) the fitted frequencies satisfy the model and (ii) their totals agree with the observed totals for each of the two dimensional marginal tables. For the n_{00} concordant pairs in which neither case nor control is exposed, and the n_{11} concordant pairs in which both are exposed, the zeros in the margin require that the fitted frequencies be exactly as observed. Such tables provide no information about the relative risk since, whatever the value of β, the nuisance parameter α_i may be chosen so that fitted and observed frequencies are identical ($\alpha_i = 0$ for tables of the first type and $\alpha_i = -\beta$ for tables of the latter to give probability $^1/_2$ of being a case or control).

The remaining $n_{10} + n_{01}$ discordant pairs have the same marginal configuration, and for these the fitted frequencies are of the form

Exposure

	+	−	
Case	μ	$1-\mu$	1
Control	$1-\mu$	μ	1
	1	1	2

where

$$\mu = \mathrm{pr}_i(y = 1 \mid x = 1) = \frac{\exp(\alpha_i + \beta)}{1 + \exp(\alpha_i + \beta)}$$

and

$$1-\mu = \mathrm{pr}_i(y = 1 \mid x = 0) = \frac{\exp(\alpha_i)}{1 + \exp(\alpha_i)},$$

which can be expressed as

$$\psi = \exp(\beta) = \left(\frac{\mu}{1-\mu}\right)^2.$$

The additional constraint satisfied by the fitted frequencies is that the total number of exposed cases, $n_{10} + n_{11}$, must equal the total of the fitted values, namely $(n_{10} + n_{01})\mu + n_{11}$. This implies $\hat{\mu} = n_{10}/(n_{10} + n_{01})$ and thus that the unconditional MLE of the relative risk is

$$\hat{\psi} = \left(\frac{\hat{\mu}}{1-\hat{\mu}}\right)^2 = \left(\frac{n_{10}}{n_{01}}\right)^2,$$

the square of the ratio of discordant pairs (Andersen, 1973, p. 69).

The estimate based on the more appropriate conditional model has already been presented in § 5.2. There we noted that the distribution of n_{10} given the total $n_{10} + n_{01}$ of discordant pairs was binomial with parameter $\pi = \psi/(1+\psi)$. It followed that the conditional MLE was the simple ratio of discordant pairs

$$\hat{\psi} = \frac{n_{10}}{n_{01}}.$$

Thus the *unconditional analysis of matched pair data results in an estimate of the odds ratio which is the square of the correct, conditional one*: a relative risk of 2 will tend to be estimated as 4 by this approach, and that of $^1/_2$ by $^1/_4$.

While the disparity between conditional and unconditional analyses is particularly dramatic for matched pairs, it persists even with other types of fine stratification. Pike, Hill and Smith (1979) have investigated by numerical means the extent of the bias in unconditional estimates obtained from a large number of strata, each having a fixed number of cases and controls. Except for matched pairs, the bias depends slightly on the proportion of the control population which is exposed, as well as on the true odds ratio. Table 7.1 presents an extension of their results. For sets having 2 cases and 2 controls each, a true odds ratio of 2 tends to be estimated in the range from 2.51 to 2.53, depending upon whether the exposure probability for controls is 0.1 or 0.3. Even with 10 cases and 10 controls per set, an asymptotic bias of approximately 4% remains for estimating a true odds ratio of $\psi = 2$, and of about 15% for estimating $\psi = 10$.

These calculations demonstrate the need for considerable caution in fitting unconditional logistic regression equations containing many strata or other nuisance parameters to limited sets of data. There are basically two choices: *one should either use individual case-control matching in the design and the conditional likelihood for analysis; or else the stratum sizes for an unconditional analysis should be kept relatively large, whether the strata are formed at the design stage or* post hoc.

7.2 Multivariate analysis for matched 1:M designs: general methodology

One design which occurs often in practice, and for which the conditional likelihood (7.1) takes a particularly simple form, is where each case is individually matched to one or several controls. The number of controls per case may either be a fixed number, M, say, or else may be allowed to vary from set to set. We considered such designs in § 5.3 and § 5.4 for estimation of the relative risk associated with a single binary exposure variable.

Suppose that the ith of I matched sets contains M_i controls in addition to the case. Denote by $x_{i0} = (x_{i01}, ..., x_{i0K})$ the K-vector of exposures for the case in this set and by $x_{ij} = (x_{ij1}, ..., x_{ijK})$ the exposure vector for the jth control ($j = 1, ..., M_i$). In other words, x_{ijk} represents the value of the kth exposure variable for the case ($j = 0$) or j^{th} control in the ith matched set. We may then write the conditional likelihood in the form (Liddell, McDonald & Thomas, 1977; Breslow et al., 1978):

$$\prod_{i=1}^{I} \frac{\exp(\sum_{k=1}^{K} \beta_k x_{i0k})}{\sum_{j=0}^{M_i} \exp(\sum_{k=1}^{K} \beta_k x_{ijk})}$$

$$= \prod_{i=1}^{I} \frac{1}{1 + \sum_{j=1}^{M_i} \exp\{\sum_{k=1}^{K} \beta_k (x_{ijk} - x_{i0k})\}}. \tag{7.2}$$

It follows from this expression that if any of the x's are matching variables, taking the same value for each member of a matched set, their contribution to the likelihood is zero and the corresponding β cannot be estimated. This is a reminder that matched designs preclude the analysis of relative risk associated with the matching variables. However by defining some x's to be interaction or cross-product terms involving both risk factors and matching variables, we may model how relative risk changes from one matched set to the next.

Table 7.1 Asymptotic mean values of unconditional maximum likelihood estimates of the odds ratio from matched sets consisting of n_1 cases and n_0 controls

True odds ratio ψ	No. of controls per set (n_0)	$p_0 = 0.1$ No. of cases per set (n_1)				$p_0 = 0.3$ No. of cases per set (n_1)				$p_0 = 0.7$ No. of cases per set (n_1)			
		1	2	4	10	1	2	4	10	1	2	4	10
1.5	1	2.25	1.81	1.64	1.55	2.25	1.83	1.65	1.56	2.25	1.86	1.67	1.57
	2	1.87	1.72	1.62	1.55	1.85	1.72	1.62	1.55	1.82	1.72	1.63	1.56
	4	1.68	1.63	1.59	1.54	1.67	1.63	1.59	1.55	1.65	1.62	1.59	1.55
	10	1.57	1.56	1.55	1.53	1.57	1.56	1.55	1.53	1.56	1.55	1.55	1.53
2	1	4.00	2.72	2.32	2.12	4.00	2.82	2.37	2.14	4.00	2.94	2.45	2.18
	2	2.97	2.51	2.27	2.11	2.90	2.53	2.29	2.13	2.76	2.52	2.32	2.15
	4	2.47	2.32	2.21	2.10	2.42	2.31	2.21	2.11	2.34	2.28	2.21	2.12
	10	2.19	2.16	2.12	2.07	2.16	2.14	2.12	2.08	2.12	2.12	2.10	2.07
5	1	25.00	10.45	6.98	5.64	25.00	12.68	8.12	6.05	25.00	14.42	9.44	6.67
	2	14.26	8.69	6.66	5.61	12.81	9.11	7.19	5.91	10.08	8.57	7.39	6.24
	4	9.30	7.40	6.31	5.55	8.20	7.22	6.46	5.74	6.83	6.58	6.27	5.84
	10	6.59	6.21	5.84	5.44	6.08	5.93	5.75	5.49	5.60	5.57	5.53	5.43
10	1	100.00	35.66	17.90	12.20	100.00	47.28	24.77	14.60	100.00	53.34	30.55	17.64
	2	50.95	24.85	16.08	12.05	42.71	26.49	18.59	13.61	27.15	21.74	18.07	14.60
	4	28.03	18.80	14.53	11.83	21.54	17.67	15.03	12.67	14.95	14.35	13.67	12.66
	10	16.16	14.28	12.81	11.44	13.34	12.87	12.34	11.60	11.46	11.42	11.34	11.18

If there is but a single matched control per case, the conditional likelihood simplifies even further to

$$\prod_{i=1}^{I} \frac{1}{1+\exp\{\sum_{k=1}^{K}\beta_k(x_{i1k}-x_{i0k})\}} . \qquad (7.3)$$

This may be recognized as the unconditional likelihood for the logistic regression model where the sampling unit is the pair and the regression variables are the *differences* in exposures for case *versus* control. The constant (α) term is assumed to be equal to 0 and each pair corresponds to a positive outcome (y = 1). This correspondence permits GLIM or other widely available computer programmes for unconditional logistic regression to be used to fit the conditional model to matched pair data (Holford, White & Kelsey, 1978).

While not yet incorporated into any of the familiar statistical packages, computer programmes are available to perform the conditional analysis for both matched (Appendix IV) and more generally stratified designs (Appendix V), using the likelihoods (7.2) and (7.1), respectively (Smith et al., 1981). These programmes calculate the following: (i) the (conditional) MLEs of the relative risk parameters; (ii) minus twice the maximized logarithm of the conditional likelihood, used as a measure of goodness of fit; (iii) the (conditional) information matrix, or negative of the matrix of second partial derivatives of the log likelihood, evaluated at the MLE; and (iv) the score statistic for testing the significance of each new set of variables added in a series of hierarchical models. These quantities are used to make inferences about the relative risk just as described in § 6.4 for the unconditional model. For example, the difference between goodness-of-fit (G) measures for a sequence of hierarchical models, in which each succeeding model represents a generalization of the preceding one, may be used to test the significance of the additional estimated parameters. This difference has an asymptotic chi-square distribution, with degrees of freedom equal to the number of additional variables incorporated in the regression equation, provided of course that the β coefficients of these variables are truly zero. Similarly, asymptotic variances and covariances of the parameter estimates in any particular model are obtained from the inverse information matrix printed out by the programme.

Now that the technology exists for conditional logistic modelling, all the types of multivariate analysis of stratified samples which were discussed in Chapter 6 can also be carried out with matched case-control data. In the next few sections we introduce these techniques by re-analysing the data already considered in Chapter 5. This will serve to indicate where the model yields results identical with the "classical" techniques, and where it goes beyond them. Later sections will extend the applications to exploit fully the potential of the model.

7.3 Matched pairs with dichotomous and polytomous exposures: applications

Our first application of the general conditional model is to analyse in this framework the matched pair data already considered at the end of § 5.2. There we used the 63 pairs consisting of the case and the first control in each matched set from the Los Angeles study of endometrial cancer (Mack et al., 1976). The analysis was directed towards obtaining an overall relative risk for oestrogens, detecting a possible interaction with age for the risk associated with gall-bladder disease, and examining the joint effects of gall-bladder disease and hypertension. Further analysis of these same matched pairs was carried out in § 5.5 to investigate the relative risks attached to different dose levels of conjugated oestrogens.

In order to carry out parallel analyses in the context of the logistic model, we defined a number of regression variables as shown in Table 7.2. The first four of these (EST, GALL, HYP, AGEGP) are dichotomous indicators for history of oestrogen use, gall-bladder disease, hypertension, and age, respectively. AGE is a continuous variable, given in years. In cases where the ages of case and control differed, although this was never by more than a year or two, AGE and AGEGP were defined as the age of the case. Hence they represent perfect matching variables which are constant within each matched set. The three binary variables, DOS1, DOS2 and DOS3, represent the four dose levels of conjugated oestrogen and thus should always appear in any equation as a group or not at all. The last variable, DOS, represents the coded dose levels of this same factor, and is used to test specifically for a trend in risk with increasing dose.

Table 7.3 shows the results of a number of regression analyses of the variables defined in Table 7.2. The statistic G for the model with no parameters, i.e., all β's assumed equal to zero, evaluates the goodness of fit to the data of the null hypothesis that none of the regression variables affects risk. Part A of the table considers the relative risk associated with a history (yes or no) of exposure to any oestrogen, as indicated by the binary variable EST. The estimated relative risk is $\hat{\psi} = \exp(\hat{\beta}) = \exp(2.269) = 9.67$, which is precisely the value found in § 5.2 as the ratio 29/3 of discordant pairs. This

Table 7.2   Definition of regression variables used in the matched pairs analysis

Variable	Code	
EST	0 1	No Yes History of any oestrogen use
GALL	0 1	No Yes History of gall-bladder disease
HYP	0 1	No Yes History of hypertension
AGEGP	0 1	Age 55–69 years Age 70–83 years
AGE	Age in years (55–83)	
DOS 1	1 0	0.1–0.299 mg/day conjugated oestrogens otherwise
DOS 2	1 0	0.3–0.625 mg/day conjugated oestrogens otherwise
DOS 3	1 0	0.626+ mg/day conjugated oestrogens otherwise
DOS	0 1 2 3	None 0.1–0.299 mg/day 0.3–0.625 mg/day } conjugated oestrogen 0.626+ mg/day

Table 7.3 Results of fitting the conditional logistic regression model to matched pairs consisting of the case and first matched control: Los Angeles study of endometrial cancer

No. of parameters	Goodness of fit (G)	Score test[a]	Regression coefficients ± standard error for each variable in equation		
0	87.34				

A. Any oestrogens

			EST		
1	62.89	21.13	2.269 ± 0.606		

B. Gall-bladder disease and age

			GALL	GALL × AGEGP	GALL × (AGE-70)
1	83.65	3.56	0.956 ± 0.526		
2	81.87	1.68	1.946 ± 1.069	-1.540 ± 1.249	
2	83.31	0.35[b]	1.052 ± 0.566		-0.066 ± 0.113

C. Hypertension/Gall-bladder disease

			GALL	HYP	GALL × HYP
1	86.53	0.81		0.325 ± 0.364	
2	82.79	3.61	0.970 ± 0.531	0.348 ± 0.364	
3	80.84	2.01	1.517 ± 0.699	0.627 ± 0.435	-1.548 ± 1.125

D. Gall-bladder disease/Hypertension

			GALL	HYP	GALL × HYP
1	83.65	3.56	0.956 ± 0.526		
2	82.79	0.86	0.970 ± 0.531	0.348 ± 0.377	
3	80.84	2.01	1.517 ± 0.699	0.627 ± 0.435	-1.548 ± 1.125

E. Dose levels of conjugated oestrogen

			DOS1	DOS2	DOS3
3	62.98	16.96	1.524 ± 0.618	1.266 ± 0.569	2.120 ± 0.693

F. Coded dose of conjugated oestrogen

			DOS	DOS × AGE	
1	65.50	14.71	0.690 ± 0.202		
2	65.50	0.00	0.693 ± 0.282	-0.001 ± 0.403	

[a] Score statistic comparing each model with the preceding model in each set, unless otherwise indicated. The first model in each set is compared with the model in which all β's are 0.
[b] After fitting one parameter model with GALL only

reflects the fact that the conditional likelihood (7.2) is identical (up to a constant of proportionality) to that used earlier as a basis of inference (5.3), so that the two analyses are entirely equivalent. Likewise, the score statistic for the test of the null hypothesis, H_0: $\psi = 1$, is identical with the *uncorrected* (for continuity) value of the χ^2 defined in (5.4), namely

$$\frac{|29-3|^2}{29+3} = 21.13.$$

This illustrates the point that many of the elementary tests are in fact score tests based on the model (Day & Byar, 1979). The corrected chi-square value is of course the more accurate and preferred one, but it has not been incorporated in the computer programme written for the general regression analysis, since it is not applicable in other situations.

Two other statistics are available for testing the null hypothesis. These are the differences in goodness-of-fit measures, 87.34–62.89 = 24.45, and the square of the standardized regression coefficient, $(2.269/0.606)^2 = 13.99$, each of which also has a nominal χ_1^2 distribution under the null hypothesis. Although the three values are somewhat disparate with these data, they all indicate a highly significant effect. The test based on the corrected score statistic is preferred when available, as this comes closest to the corresponding exact test.

Asymptotic 95% confidence limits for ψ are calculated as $\exp(2.269 \pm 1.96 \times 0.606) =$ (2.9, 31.7), the upper limit being noticeably smaller than that based on the exact conditional (binomial) distribution ($\psi_U = 49.6$) or the normal approximation to it ($\psi_U = 39.7$) which were calculated in § 5.2.

Part B of Table 7.3 presents the relative risk estimate for gall-bladder disease and its relationship to age. Just as for EST, the estimate of relative risk associated with GALL, $\exp(0.956) = 2.6 = 13/5$, and the (uncorrected) score statistic, $3.56 = (13–5)^2/18$, must agree with the values found earlier. There is better concordance between the three available tests of the null hypothesis in this (less extreme) case: 87.34–83.65 = 3.69 for the test based on G, and $(0.956/0.526)^2 = 3.30$ for that based on the standardized coefficient, are the other two values besides the score test.

For the second model in Part B the coefficient of GALL represents the log relative risk for those under 70 years of age, $\exp(1.946) = 7.0 = 7/1$, while the sum of the coefficients for GALL and GALL×AGEGP gives the log relative risk for those 70 and over, $\exp(1.946–1.540) = 1.50 = 6/4$. These are the same results as found before. Similarly, the score statistic for the additional parameter GALL×AGEGP, which tests the equality of the relative risk estimates in the two age groups, is identical to the uncorrected chi-square test for equality of the proportions 7/8 and 6/10, namely

$$\chi^2 = \frac{(7 \times 4 - 6 \times 1)^2 \times 18}{8 \times 10 \times 13 \times 5} = 1.68.$$

In § 5.2 we reported the corrected value of this chi-square as $\chi^2 = 0.59$.

The third line of Part B of the table introduces an interaction term with the continuous matching variable AGE. Here the coefficient of GALL gives the estimated relative risk for someone aged 70, $\exp(1.052) = 2.86$, while the relative risk for other ages is determined from $\exp\{1.052–0.066(AGE–70)\}$. In other words, the RR is estimated to decline by a factor $\exp(–0.066) = 0.936$ for each year of age above 70 and increase by a factor $\exp(0.066) = 1.068$ for each year below. However this tendency has no statistical significance; all three of the available tests for homogeneity give a chi-square of about 0.35 (p = 0.56). Such continuous variable modelling is of course not available with the elementary techniques.

Part C of Table 7.3 illustrates the increased analytical power which is available using regression methods. In order to estimate and test the relative risk of gall-bladder disease, while controlling for hypertension, we start with an equation containing the single variable HYP. When we add to this a second term for gall-bladder disease (line 2, part C), the model then specifies that the relative risks associated with these two variables are multiplicative, and moreover that their joint effect is multiplicative with those of the matching variables. The relative risk for GALL, adjusted for the multiplicative effects of hypertension, is estimated as $\hat{\psi} = \exp(0.970) = 2.65$, scarcely different from the unadjusted value. Likewise the null hypothesis that $\psi = 1$ is tested by $\chi^2 = 3.61$ (uncorrected), which is also rather close to the unadjusted value. By way of contrast, the adjusted estimate of RR for GALL obtained in § 5.2, where we restricted attention to the eight case-control pairs which were homogeneous for HYP and heterogeneous for GALL, gives the relatively unstable value of $\hat{\psi} = 7/1$. The difference is explained by the fact that the model uses all the case-control pairs which are discordant for at least one of GALL and HYP (see Table 7.4) to estimate the main effects of both variables. The five pairs which are discordant for both variables, not used in the elementary analysis, now contribute to the estimate of the coefficient of GALL.

In case the reader is left with the impression that something has been gained for nothing by this procedure, we hasten to point out that the elementary estimate is strictly valid under a weaker set of assumptions than that based on the model. In Chapter 5 we effectively assumed only that the relative risk of GALL was constant with respect to HYP and the matching variables. The modelling procedure supposes in addition that HYP combines multiplicatively with the matching variables; it could lead to biased estimates of the coefficient of GALL if interactions were present. Of course, in some situations, such interactions involving the matching and other confounding variables might also be modelled and added to the equation as a means of further adjustment. For example, if we suspected that not only the main effects of HYP but also the interaction between HYP and AGE were confounding the estimate of the GALL coefficient, we would fit the equation with terms for GALL, HYP and HYP × AGE. Fortunately, the higher order interactions which might necessitate such a procedure are rarely present in epidemiological studies (Miettinen, 1974).

Further insight into the assumptions which underlie the model is given by consideration of line 3 of Part C, Table 7.3. Here the addition of the interaction term GALL × HYP allows us to estimate the relative risk of each possible combination of exposures to these two risk factors, relative to those who are exposed to neither. Thus $\hat{\psi}_{10} = \exp(1.517) = 4.56$ is the estimated RR for those with gall-bladder disease only, $\hat{\psi}_{01} = \exp(0.627) = 1.87$ for those with hypertension only, and $\hat{\psi}_{11} = \exp(1.517 + 0.627 - 1.548) = 1.81$ for those having a positive history of both diseases. In summary, the relative risks are given by this bizarre-looking table:

		Gall-bladder disease	
		−	+
	−	1.00	4.56
Hypertension			
	+	1.87	1.81

However the interaction effect is not significant, as indicated by the score statistic comparing lines 2 and 3 of Table 7.3, Part C.

In effect what we have now done is to create out of GALL and HYP a joint risk variable with four exposure categories: $(-, -)$, $(-, +)$, $(+, -)$, and $(+, +)$. The estimation problem is as described in § 5.5 for matched-pair studies with a polytomous risk variable. Table 7.4 presents the distribution of the 63 matched pairs according to the joint response of case and control, following the format of Table 5.5. We readily verify that the maximum likelihood equations (5.30) for data of this type, namely

$$14 + 1 + 0 = 20 \frac{\psi_{01}}{1 + \psi_{01}} + 5 \frac{\psi_{01}}{\psi_{01} + \psi_{10}} + 1 \frac{\psi_{01}}{\psi_{01} + \psi_{11}}$$

$$6 + 4 + 0 = 7 \frac{\psi_{10}}{1 + \psi_{10}} + 5 \frac{\psi_{10}}{\psi_{01} + \psi_{10}} + 1 \frac{\psi_{10}}{\psi_{10} + \psi_{11}}$$

$$2 + 1 + 1 = 5 \frac{\psi_{11}}{1 + \psi_{11}} + 1 \frac{\psi_{11}}{\psi_{01} + \psi_{11}} + 1 \frac{\psi_{11}}{\psi_{10} + \psi_{11}} \quad ,$$

are solved by the estimates just derived using the general computer programme.

The analysis shown in Part D of Table 7.3 is identical with that in Part C except for the order of entry of the variables into the equation. If our interest is in the effects of GALL after adjustment for HYP, we would follow the sequence shown in Part D. In this example, the estimated coefficients and standard errors are not much affected by the presence of the other variable in the equation, which means that they are not confounded to any appreciable degree.

Another example of the analysis of matched-pair data with a polytomous exposure variable was presented at the end of § 5.5. There we estimated the relative risks of endometrial cancer for each of three increasing dose levels of conjugated oestrogens, using the no-dose category as baseline. In order to carry out an essentially identical analysis in the present framework, we first define the three indicator variables DOS1, DOS2 and DOS3, whose β coefficients represent the log odds ratios for each of the

Table 7.4 Histories of gall-bladder and hypertensive disease for cases and matched controls: Los Angeles study of endometrial cancer

Exposures of cases		Exposures of controls				Total
Gall bladder	Hypertension	− −	− +	+ −	+ +	
−	−	15	6	1	3	25
−	+	14	6	1	0	21
+	−	6	4	2	0	12
+	+	2	1	1	1	5
Total		37	17	5	4	63

dose levels shows in Table 7.2 relative to baseline. The conditional logistic regression model (7.3) in this case is merely a restatement of the model (5.29), in which the odds ratios corresponding to each category of exposure are assumed to be constant over the matching variables. By definition they satisfy the consistency relationship discussed earlier in § 5.5.

Part E of Table 7.3 presents the results. Regression coefficients for the three dose variables do indeed correspond to the odds ratios already estimated: $\exp(1.524) = 4.59$ for the 0.1–0.299 mg/day dose level; $\exp(1.266) = 3.55$ for 0.3–0.625 mg/day; and $\exp(2.120) = 8.33$ for over 0.625 mg/day. Likewise the score statistic for testing the null hypothesis is identical with the statistic (5.32) derived earlier, taking the value 16.96 for these data. The only important additional quantities available from the computer fit of the model are the standard errors of the parameter estimates, which enable us to put approximate confidence limits on the estimated relative risks. For example, $\exp(1.524 \pm 1.96 \times 0.618) = (1.37, 15.4)$ are the 95% limits for the 0.1–0.299 mg/day category.

In order to test for a trend in risk with increasing dose we use the single, coded dose variable DOS. Estimated relative risks for the three dose levels are then $\exp(0.690) = 1.99$, $\exp(2 \times 0.690) = 3.98$ and $\exp(3 \times 0.690) = 7.94$, respectively. Comparing the G statistics for the two dose-response models yields $65.50 - 62.98 = 2.52$, nominally a chi-square with two degrees of freedom, for testing the extent to which the linear trend adequately explains the variation in risk between dose levels. The observed departure from trend is not statistically significant ($p = 0.28$). On the other hand, the trend itself is highly significant ($p < 0.0001$) as demonstrated by the value 14.71 for the score statistic. This too is identical to the trend statistic derived earlier (5.33), except that the continuity correction is not used by the computer programme. Note that there is not the slightest hint of interaction between dose and age (line 2, part F, Table 7.3).

In summary, analyses of matched-pair data *via* the conditional logistic model yield results identical to those of the "classical" procedures presented earlier for binary and polytomous risk factors. This is hardly surprising, as the previously discussed methods were themselves based on conditional likelihoods worked out in detail for each separate problem. Nevertheless it is an important fact since it shows that the very general methodology developed here is well integrated with the techniques used in the past. Even more important, of course, are extensions to problems involving multiple and/or continuous risk variables which we next consider in the more general context of 1:M matching.

7.4 1:M matching with single and multiple exposure variables: applications

While the regression variables defined in Table 7.2 have so far in this Chapter been used exclusively with the matched-pair data, their coefficients can in fact be better estimated by taking account of the full complement of controls selected for each case. Table 7.5 presents the results of several analyses, based on the conditional likelihood (7.2), which used all the available data. Since no information was available regarding the dose and/or duration of conjugated oestrogen use by certain of the women, their data records were excluded from the analysis when fitting equations containing these variables. While a missing value for the case leads to exclusion of the entire matched

Table 7.5   Results of fitting several conditional logistic regression models to the matched sets consisting of one case and four controls: Los Angeles study of endometrial cancer

No. of parameters	Goodness of fit G	Score test	Regression coefficients ± standard error for each variable in the equation		
			A. Oestrogen use and age level (based on all 63 matched sets, 315 observations)		
			EST	EST × AGE1	EST × AGE2
0	202.79	–			
1	167.44	31.16	2.074 ± 0.421		
3	166.76	0.76	1.431 ± 0.826	0.847 ± 1.034	0.780 ± 1.154
			B. Oestrogen use and coded age level (based on all 63 matched sets, 315 observations)		
			EST	EST × AGE3	
1	167.44	31.16	2.074 ± 0.421		
2	167.05	0.39	1.664 ± 0.750	0.385 ± 0.616	
			C. Conjugated oestrogen use and age (based on 59 matched sets, 291 observations)		
			CEST	CEST × AGE1	CEST × AGE2
0	188.13				
1	159.22	27.57	1.710 ± 0.354		
3	158.28	0.89	1.583 ± 0.815	−0.081 ± 0.930	0.764 ± 1.143

set, a missing value in a control record might simply mean that the number of controls in that set was reduced by one.

In order to estimate the overall relative risk associated with a history of exposure to any oestrogen, we employed the general purpose computer programme with the single binary variable EST (Part A, Table 7.5). This yields $\hat{\psi} = \exp(2.074) = 7.95$, which is of course the same value as found in § 5.3 by solving the equation (5.17) for conditional maximum likelihood estimation. The standard error $0.421 = \sqrt{0.177}$, given by formula (5.21), has already been used to place an approximate 95% confidence interval of $\exp(2.074 \pm 1.96 \times 0.421) = (3.5, 18.1)$ about the point estimate. Likewise the score test statistic is identical to the summary chi-square defined in (5.19), but calculated without the continuity correction so as to give $(110–13)^2/302 = 31.16$ in place of the corrected value 29.57 found earlier.

Continuing the lines of the analysis shown in Table 5.2, we investigated a possible difference in the relative risk for EST in the three age groups 55–64, 65–74 and 75+ by adding to the regression equation interaction terms involving EST and age. In order to account for the breakdown of age into three groups, two binary indicator variables were defined: AGE1 = 1 for 65–74 years, and 0 otherwise; and AGE2 = 1 for 75+ years, 0 otherwise. Thus, from line 2, Part A, Table 7.5, $\exp(1.431) = 4.18$ is the estimated relative risk for women aged 55–64 years, $\exp(1.431 + 0.847) = 9.76$ for those 65–74 years, and $\exp(1.431 + 0.780) = 9.12$ for the 75+ year olds, these results agreeing with those shown in Table 5.2. While there is an apparent increase in the relative risk for the women aged 65 or more years, the score test of 0.76 shows that the differences are not statistically significant ($p = 0.68$). Note that this value agrees with that calculated earlier from the explicit formula (5.23) for the score test of interaction.

A single degree of freedom test for a trend in relative risk with increasing age is obtained by fitting a single interaction term as shown in Part B of Table 7.5. Coding AGE3 to be 0, 1 or 2 according to the subject's age group, the resulting score test for interaction is the uncorrected version of the statistic (5.24), taking the value 0.39. The corrected value calculated earlier was 0.09. Estimated relative risks for the three age categories are in this case $\exp(1.664) = 5.28$, $\exp(1.664 + 0.385) = 7.76$ and $\exp(1.664 + 2 \times 0.385) = 11.40$, respectively. However since there is no evidence that the apparent trend is real, such estimates would not normally be reported.

The flexibility of the regression approach is particularly evident when dealing with matched sets containing a variable number of controls. Part C of Table 7.5 presents

Table 7.6 Matched univariate analysis of Los Angeles study of endometrial cancer: all cases and controls used except as noted

Variable	Levels	RR	χ^{2} [a]	DF	p
Gall-bladder disease	Yes	3.69	13.83	1	0.0002
	No	1.00			
Hypertension	Yes	1.51	1.85	1	0.18
	No	1.00			
Obesity	Yes	1.76	5.70	2	0.06
	No	1.00			
	Unk	0.63			
Obesity	Yes	2.02	5.16	1	0.02
	No/Unk	1.00			
Other drugs (non-oestrogen)	Yes	3.90	10.38	1	0.001
	No	1.00			
Any oestrogens	Yes	7.96	31.16	1	<0.00001
	No	1.00			
Conjugated oestrogens[b]: dose in mg/day	None	1.00	33.22	3	<0.00001
	0.1–0.299	4.11			
	0.3–0.625	4.86			
	0.625+	10.97			
	Trend[c]	5.53	27.57	1	<0.00001
Conjugated oestrogens[d]: duration in months	None	1.00	34.93	4	<0.00001
	1–11	2.66			
	12–47	4.17			
	48–95	8.13			
	96+	10.41			
	Trend[e]	1.81	34.79	1	<0.00001

[a] Uncorrected score test
[b] Based on 59 sets, 291 observations
[c] Regression on coded dose levels: 0 = none; 1 = 0.1–0.299 mg/day; 2 = 0.3–0.625 mg/day; 3 = 0.625+ mg/day
[d] Based on 57 sets, 277 observations
[e] Regression on coded duration: 0 = none; 1 = 1–11 months; ...; 4 = 96+ months

the regression analysis of the data considered in § 5.4 on use of conjugated oestrogens. Of 59 matched sets for whom the case history of conjugated oestrogen use was known, 55 had the full complement of 4 controls while for each of the 4 others, one control was lacking information. Running the computer programme with a single binary variable CEST representing the history of use of conjugated oestrogens, we easily replicate the results already obtained: $\hat{\psi} = \exp(1.710) = 5.53$ for the estimate of relative risk and $\chi^2 = 27.57$ for the uncorrected chi-square test of the null hypothesis. It is also easy to test for constancy of the relative risk over the three age groups by addition of the interaction variables CEST×AGE1 and CEST×AGE2 to the equation. The score test for this addition, which is the generalization of (5.24) discussed in § 5.4, yields the value $\chi^2_2 = 0.89$ (p = 0.64). We did not report this result earlier because of the labour involved in the hand calculation.

Thus far in this section we have used the general methods for matched data analysis primarily in order to replicate the results already reported in Chapter 5 for particular elementary problems. The emphasis has been on demonstrating the concordance between the quantities in the computerized regression analysis, and those calculated earlier from grouped data. In the remainder of the section we carry out a full-scale multivariate analysis of the Los Angeles data much as one would do in actual practice.

As an initial step in this process, Table 7.6, which summarizes and extends the results obtained so far, presents relative risk estimates and tests of their statistical significance for each risk variable individually. Comparing the entries there with those in Table 5.1 we see that there is little to choose between the matched and unmatched analyses for this particular example (see § 7.6, however). The rather large number of "unknown" responses for obesity indicated lack of information on this item in the medical record. Grouping these with the negatives led to only a slight decrease in the goodness of fit ($\chi^2_1 = 0.75$, p = 0.39) and to a slight increase in the relative risk associated with a positive history. We therefore decided to use the dichotomy positive *versus* negative/unknown in the subsequent multivariate analyses. This meant that the final analyses used the five binary variables GALL-bladder disease, HYPertension, OBesity, NON-oestrogen drugs and any oESTrogen, none of which had missing values. There were also two polytomous variables representing DOSe and DURation of conjugated oestrogen, both of which had missing values.

Table 7.7 presents the results for a series of multivariate analyses involving the five binary risk factors and several of their two-factor interactions. Model 2 contains just the main effects of each variable. Their β coefficients have been exponentiated for presentation so as to facilitate their interpretation in terms of relative risk. In fact the estimates of RR for gall-bladder disease and oestrogen use do not change much from the univariate analysis (Table 7.6), while those for the other three variables are all somewhat smaller. The coefficient for hypertension becomes slightly negative, while those for obesity and non-oestrogen drugs are reduced to non-significant levels. The reduction for non-oestrogen drugs is particularly striking, and inspection of the original data indicates this is due to a high degree of confounding with oestrogen use: for the controls, only 16 or 21.1% of 76 who did not take non-oestrogen drugs had a history of oestrogen use, *versus* 111 or 63.1% of 176 who did take non-oestrogen drugs (Table 7.8).

Models 3–5 explore the consequences of dropping from the equation those variables which do not have significant main effects. The confounding between other drugs and

Table 7.7 Matched multivariate analysis of five binary risk factors and their interactions: Los Angeles study of endometrial cancer

Model	No. of parameters	Goodness of fit G	Score test[a]	Relative risks (exponentiated regression coefficients) for each variable in the equation. Standardized regression coefficients in parentheses									
				GALL	HYP	OB	NON	EST	GALL×EST	OB×EST	NON×EST	GALL×OB	GALL×NON
1	0	202.79											
2	5	153.74	42.75	3.63 (3.12)	0.82 (−0.55)	1.61 (1.31)	1.95 (1.31)	6.78 (4.21)					
3	4	154.04	42.63[b]	3.59 (3.10)		1.58 (1.27)	1.85 (1.23)	6.58 (4.17)					
4	3	155.64	41.74[b]	3.58 (3.10)		1.67 (1.43)		7.69 (4.62)					
5	3	155.68	41.42[b]	3.63 (3.12)			2.00 (1.39)	6.79 (4.22)					
6	2	157.74	39.92[b]	3.58 (3.10)				8.29 (4.81)					
7	3	153.46	4.66	18.07 (3.28)				14.88 (4.41)	0.128 (−2.06)				
8	4	151.58	4.39[c]	17.19 (3.23)		1.63 (1.35)		13.74 (4.27)	0.136 (−2.01)				
9	5	151.50	0.43	17.84 (3.26)		2.85 (1.13)		19.92 (3.43)	0.132 (−2.02)	0.532 (−0.65)			
10	6	151.00	0.17	14.78 (2.72)		2.46 (0.93)		18.98 (3.43)	0.127 (−2.05)	0.576 (−0.56)		1.39 (0.41)	
11	4	151.17	4.92[d]	19.45 (3.32)			2.14 (1.46)	12.28 (4.03)	0.120 (−2.12)				
12	5	148.75	2.23	22.51 (3.27)			8.63 (1.80)	54.60 (3.07)	0.103 (−2.14)		0.156 (−1.42)		
13	6	148.04	0.68	9.36 (1.55)			4.94 (1.23)	40.36 (2.94)	0.089 (−2.22)		0.225 (−1.11)		2.98 (0.81)

[a] Score test with respect to preceding model, unless otherwise noted
[b] Score test for all variables in model (with respect to Model 1)
[c] Score test versus Model 4
[d] Score test versus Model 5

Table 7.8 Joint distribution of cases and controls according to selected risk factors: Los Angeles study of endometrial cancer

A. Gall-bladder disease and oestrogens

	Gall-bladder disease negative		Gall-bladder disease positive		Totals
	Oestrogen−	Oestrogen+	Oestrogen−	Oestrogen+	
Cases	3	43	4	13	63
Controls	117	111	8	16	252
Relative risks					
Unmatched	1.0	15.1	19.5	31.7	
Matched[a]	1.0	14.9	18.1	34.5	

B. Oestrogen and non-oestrogen drug use

	Other drugs negative		Other drugs positive		Totals
	Oestrogen−	Oestrogen+	Oestrogen−	Oestrogen+	
Cases	1	6	6	50	63
Controls	60	16	65	111	252
Relative risks					
Unmatched	1.0	22.5	5.5	27.0	
Matched[b]	1.0	54.6	8.6	73.5	

[a] From Model 7, Table 7.7.
[b] From Model 12, Table 7.7 (hence adjusted for gall-bladder disease)

oestrogen is evident from the fact that the coefficient for the latter depends most noticeably on whether or not the former is present. Subtracting the goodness-of-fit statistics between Models 6 and 2 yields $\chi_3^2 = 4.00$ (p = 0.26) for testing the joint contribution of hypertension, obesity and non-oestrogen drug use to the equation.

The contrast between Models 7 and 6 shows that there is a strong and statistically significant (p = 0.03) *negative* interaction between the two variables that have substantial main effects on risk, namely gall-bladder disease and oestrogens. The basic data contributing to this negative interaction are shown in Part A of Table 7.8, together with relative risks estimated *via* the model, e.g., RR = $14.9 \times 18.1 \times 0.128 = 34.5$ for the double exposure category. The interaction effect itself is perhaps best illustrated by contrasting the RR of 14.9 for oestrogens among those who had no history of gall-bladder disease with the RR of 34.5/18.1 = 1.9 among those with such a history.

Similar negative interactions are evident in Models 10 and 12 for obesity with oestrogens, and other drugs with oestrogens, respectively. From the unmatched data, shown in Part B of Table 7.8, we see that the instability in the regression coefficients for Model 12 stems from the fact that only a single case falls in the joint "non-exposed" category. While they are statistically significant only in the case of gall-bladder disease, the data suggest that there are negative interactions of oestrogen use with the other factors which are possibly linked to endometrial cancer. Given that a woman is already at elevated risk from her history of gall-bladder disease, obesity, or non-oestrogen drug use, the further increase in risk from use of oestrogens is not nearly as important as when she is not exposed to other risk factors. This same observation, that oestrogen use interacts negatively with traditional risk factors for endometrial cancer, such as hypertension and obesity, has been made in other case-control studies (Smith et al., 1975). It suggests that the effects of oestrogen use are more likely to combine additively rather than multiplicatively with those of other factors. Another interesting feature of the relationship, which could not be investigated in the Los Angeles study, is that the excess risk is much smaller among ex-users compared with continuing users of oestrogen (Jick et al., 1979).

So far our analysis has accounted only for the fact of oestrogen use and not of dose or duration. Unfortunately, information about one or both of these items was lacking for nine cancer cases, leading to the exclusion of the corresponding matched sets from the analysis, and for one control in each of seven of the remaining 54 sets. Moreover, the drug tended to be administered at one of a few standard doses, which precluded analysis of this variable as a true continuous variable. Instead both dose and duration were treated as ordered categorical variables, and arbitrary scale values were assigned to the increasing levels for regression analysis of trends (see Tables 7.2 and 7.6).

A series of analyses which investigate the effect of dose and/or duration of conjugated oestrogen exposure on risk is presented in Table 7.9. In part A of the table we first fit the main effect for oestrogen exposure followed by a single variable DOS representing the trend in risk with coded dose level. Since women with EST = 1 but DOS = 0 use oestrogens but not the conjugated variety, the coefficient of EST determines the relative risk for women taking only non-conjugated oestrogens, $\exp(1.451)$ = 4.3. Estimated relative risks for the three dose levels of conjugated oestrogen are $\exp(1.451 + 0.402) = 6.4$, $\exp(1.451 + 2 \times 0.402) = 9.5$ and $\exp(1.451 + 3 \times 0.402)$ = 14.3, respectively. The third model is a generalization of the second in that the effects of the individual dose levels are allowed to vary independently rather than being determined by the trend. While the estimated relative risks for dose levels 1 and 2 are rather similar, there is no strong evidence for a deviation from the fitted trend ($\chi_2^2 = 2.41$, p = 0.30). As shown in Model 4, there is a significant trend with duration, even after accounting for the dose effects.

Part B of the table considers in a similar way the effect of duration of exposure. Here there is a smooth progression in risk, and the fit of the linear trend in coded duration level seems quite adequate ($\chi_3^2 = 1.11$, p = 0.78). The trend in dose continues to be significant even after adjustment for duration (Model 3, Part B).

In Part C of the table we simultaneously fit separate effects for both dose and duration. Since the sums of both DOS1 + DOS2 + DOS3 and DUR1 + DUR2 + DUR3 + DUR4 equal the variable CEST defined above, it was necessary to drop one of these indicator variables from the equation in order to avoid linear dependence among the variables and to obtain unique estimates of all coefficients; this explains the absence of DOS1 from the list of variables. Comparing Model 2 with Model 1 shows that the effects of dose and duration are reasonably multiplicative; addition of the linear interaction term results in only a slight improvement in goodness of fit($\chi_1^2 = 0.59$, p = 0.44). In Models 3–6 we consider the effects of some of the other risk factors after

Table 7.9 Multivariate analysis of effects of dose and duration of conjugated oestrogens: Los Angeles study of endometrial cancer

Regression coefficients for each variable in the equation (standardized coefficients in parentheses)

A. Effect of dose

Model	No. of parameters	Goodness of fit G	Score test[b]	EST	DOS	DOS1	DOS2	DOS3	DUR
1	1	139.86	27.22	2.088 (4.60)					
2	2	135.63	4.19	1.451 (2.59)	0.402 (2.01)				
3	4	133.20	2.41	1.856 (2.74)		0.029 (0.05)	0.023 (0.04)	1.141 (1.80)	
4	5	128.32	4.82	1.987 (2.86)		-1.101 (-1.33)	-1.116 (-1.32)	-0.013 (-0.02)	0.420 (2.15)

B. Effect of duration

Model	No. of parameters	Goodness of fit G	Score test[b]	EST	DUR	DUR1	DUR2	DUR3	DUR4	DOS
1	2	134.84	4.91[c]	1.431 (2.58)	0.309 (2.17)					
2	5	133.76	1.11	1.868 (2.73)		-0.418 (-0.58)	0.122 (0.19)	0.596 (0.88)	0.899 (1.43)	
3	6	129.52	4.22	1.946 (2.83)		-1.655 (-1.70)	-0.876 (-1.08)	-0.586 (-0.65)	-0.296 (-0.34)	0.578 (2.01)

Table 7.9 (contd)

C. Dose, duration and other variables

				EST	DOS2	DOS3	DUR1	DUR2	DUR3	DUR4	DUR×DOS	GALL	GALL×EST	NON	OB
1	7	127.63	6.25[d]	2.020 (2.90)	-0.024 (-0.05)	1.175 (2.07)	-0.961 (-1.18)	-0.131 (-0.19)	0.251 (0.33)	0.404 (0.57)					
			5.35[e]												
2	8	127.04	0.59	2.024 (2.91)	-0.835 (-1.03)	-0.416 (-0.53)	-0.395 (-0.35)	-0.555 (-0.39)	-0.464 (-0.61)	0.254 (0.19)	0.179 (0.77)				
3	8	118.91	9.54	2.083 (2.81)	-0.725 (-0.86)	-0.019 (-0.03)	0.470 (0.59)	0.283 (0.38)	-0.049 (-0.09)	1.136 (1.95)		1.498 (2.93)			
4	9	117.06	1.87	2.433 (2.99)	-0.708 (-0.85)	-0.034 (-0.05)	0.357 (0.45)	0.276 (0.37)	0.000 (0.00)	1.111 (1.92)		2.531 (2.72)	-1.519 (-1.35)		
5	9	116.42	2.33	1.951 (2.59)	-0.694 (-0.82)	-0.008 (-0.01)	0.525 (0.65)	0.220 (0.29)	-0.076 (-0.14)	1.114 (1.90)		1.521 (2.96)		0.936 (1.50)	
6	9	113.58	5.22	2.195 (2.86)	-0.908 (-1.04)	-0.140 (-0.19)	0.356 (0.43)	0.231 (0.29)	-0.228 (-0.41)	1.242 (2.06)		1.423 (2.73)			1.059 (2.24)

[a] Based on 54 matched sets, 263 observations having known values for both dose and duration of conjugated oestrogen use
[b] Score test relative to preceding model in each Part, unless otherwise indicated
[c] Relative to Model 1, Part A
[d] Relative to Model 2, Part A
[e] Relative to Model 1, Part B

more complete adjustment for oestrogen than was possible using the binary variable EST alone. The coefficients for these variables should be contrasted with those shown in Table 7.7. Gall-bladder disease continues to stand out as an important, independent risk factor with an estimated relative risk of $\exp(1.498) = 4.5$ compared with the 3.6 found earlier (Model 6, Table 7.7). The interaction of gall-bladder disease with oestrogen use is no longer statistically significant when the dose and duration variables are included in the equation. While the coefficient for non-oestrogen drugs is little changed, obesity is now estimated to carry a relative risk of $\exp(1.059) = 2.9$, which is significantly different from 1 at the $p = 0.02$ level. Part of these differences, of course, may result because slightly different data sets were used.

In conclusion, we can simply reiterate a point which is well illustrated by the preceding example: all the techniques of multivariate analysis which were once restricted to unmatched studies are now available for use with matched data as well.

7.5 Combining sets of 2×2 tables

Besides individual case-control matching, another situation in which the calculations based on the exact conditional likelihood may be quite feasible is when information is combined from a set of 2×2 tables. We noted earlier that the conditional likelihood in this case took the form of a product of non-central hypergeometric distributions (see § 4.4 for notation):

$$\prod_{i=1}^{I} \frac{\binom{n_{1i}}{a_i} \binom{n_{0i}}{m_{1i}-a_i} \psi_i^{a_i}}{\sum_u \binom{n_{1i}}{u} \binom{n_{0i}}{m_{1i}-u} \psi_i^u}. \tag{7.4}$$

As usual, the summations in the denominator range over all possible values u which are consistent with the observed marginals in the ith table, namely $\max(0, n_{1i}-m_{0i}) \leq u \leq \min(m_{1i}, n_{1i})$. Calculation of exact tail probabilities (4.6, 4.7) and confidence intervals (4.8, 4.9) based on this distribution requires that all possible sets of tables which are compatible with the given marginals are evaluated. Their number is

$$\prod_{i=1}^{I} \{\min(m_{1i},n_{1i})-\max(0,n_{1i}-m_{0i})\},$$

i.e., the *product* of the number of possible tables at each level, which can rapidly become prohibitively large (Thomas, 1975). On the other hand, evaluation of the log-likelihood function and its first and second derivatives requires calculations which increase only in proportion to the *sum*

$$\sum_{i=1}^{I} \{\min(m_{1i},n_{1i})-\max(0,n_{1i}-m_{0i})\}$$

of the number of possible tables at each level. Hence a conditional likelihood analysis, similar to those already developed in this chapter for matched designs, is often possible for problems involving sets of 2×2 tables, even where the completely exact analysis would be unfeasible. Only if the entries in some of the tables are very large will problems be encountered in the evaluation of the binomial coefficients appearing in (7.4).

Usually cases and controls will have been grouped into strata (tables) on the basis of covariables which are thought either to confound or to modify the effect of exposure on disease. Suppose that a vector z_i of such covariables is associated with the ith table. Then there are several hypotheses about the odds ratios ψ_i which are of interest:

$$H_0: \psi_i \equiv 1$$

$$H_1: \psi_i \equiv \psi = \exp(\beta)$$

$$H_2: \psi_i = \exp(\beta + \Sigma_l \gamma_l z_{il})$$

$$H_3: \text{No restrictions on } \psi_i.$$

In Chapter 4 we concentrated on the estimation of ψ under H_1, tests of the null hypothesis H_0, and tests for constancy in the relative risk (H_1) against global alternatives (H_3). We have remarked on several occasions that these latter may be insensitive to particular patterns of interaction and that a preferred strategy is to model specific variations in the relative risk associated with the covariables using H_2. In § 6.12 several such models were fitted to the Oxford Childhood Survey data using unconditional logistic regression in which a separate α parameter was estimated for each stratum. As we saw in § 7.2, however, it is possible seriously to overestimate the relative risk with this procedure if the data are thin. Hence it will often be preferable to use instead the conditional likelihood, which may be written

$$\prod_{i=1}^{1} \frac{\binom{n_{1i}}{a_i}\binom{n_{0i}}{m_{1i}-a_i} \exp\{a_i(\beta + \Sigma_l \gamma_l z_{il})\}}{\sum_u \binom{n_{1i}}{u}\binom{n_{0i}}{m_{1i}-u} \exp\{u(\beta + \Sigma_l \gamma_l z_{il})\}}. \tag{7.5}$$

A listing of a computer programme for fitting models of the form H_2 to sets of 2×2 tables using the conditional likelihood is given in Appendix VI. This programme may be used as an alternative to that of Thomas (1975) for finding the exact MLE of the relative risk in H_1, provided of course that exact tests and confidence intervals are not also desired. Zelen (1971) develops exact tests for the constancy of the odds ratio against alternatives of the form H_2 with a single covariable, and also against the global alternative H_3. We presented in (4.31) the score statistic based on (7.5) for testing H_1 against H_2 with a single covariable.

If the data in each table are truly extensive it may be burdensome to evaluate the binomial coefficients in (7.5). In this case an asymptotic procedure is available. Rather than use the exact conditional means and variances of the table entries a_i under hypothesized values for the odds ratios ψ_i, which are required by the iterative likelihood fitting procedure, one can use instead the asymptotic means and variances defined by (4.11) and (4.13). This substitution yields likelihood equations and an information matrix which are identical to those obtained by applying a two-stage maximization procedure to the *unconditional* likelihood function whereby one first solves the equations for the α coefficients in terms of β and γ (Richards, 1961). The estimates $\hat{\beta}$ and $\hat{\gamma}$ so obtained, as well as their standard errors and covariances, are thus identical to those obtained using unconditional logistic regression (Breslow, 1976). The advantage is that the unconditional model is fitted without explicit estimation of all the nuisance

. This is a serious consideration if there are many tables, since the required
f parameters may exhaust the capacity of the available computer. Nevertheless,
ter how they are calculated, the unconditional estimates may be subject to bias
uch circumstances and the conditional analysis is preferred whenever it is compu-
ationally feasible.

To illustrate the use of the conditional likelihood with a set of 2×2 tables we found
new estimates of the parameters β and γ_1, representing the log relative risk of obstetric
radiation and its linear decrease with calendar time, which we estimated earlier from the
Oxford Childhood Cancer Survey Data using unconditional logistic regression (6.12).
We recall that several estimates for these parameters were made depending on the
degree of polynomial adjustment for the stratifying variables age and calendar year.
In fact, for the last line in Table 6.17 where the confounding effects of age and year
were completely saturated, we avoided explicit estimation of separate α parameters for
each of the 120 2×2 tables by using the technique just discussed.

The parameter estimates and standard errors calculated directly from the conditional
likelihood (7.5) were

$$\hat{\beta} = 0.5165 \pm 0.0564$$

and

$$\hat{\gamma}_1 = -0.0385 \pm 0.0144 .$$

It is of considerable theoretical interest that these quantities are closer to those obtained from the unconditional fifth degree polynomial model than to those obtained
with the saturated model (see last two lines, Table 6.17). This suggests that the confounding effects of age and year are suitably accounted for by the polynomial regression, and that inclusion of additional nuisance parameters in the equation serves only
to increase bias of the type considered in § 7.1. However, because of the exceptionally
large sample (over 5 000 cases and controls) the inflation of the relative risk estimates
due to the excess of nuisance parameters was not terribly serious.

7.6 Effect of ignoring the matching

Prior to the advent of methods for the multivariate analysis of case-control studies,
in particular those based on the conditional likelihood (7.2), it was common practice
to ignore the matching in the analysis. In simple problems one often found that taking
explicit account of the matched pairs or sets did not seriously alter the estimate of
relative risk. With the Los Angeles study of endometrial cancer, for example, there
were only slight differences between the unmatched (Table 7.5) and matched (Table
7.6) estimates for each risk variable considered individually. However, the agreement
is not always as good, and there has been considerable confusion regarding the conditions under which incorporation of the matching in the analysis is necessary.

A sufficient and widely-quoted condition for the 'poolability' of data across matched
sets or strata is that the *stratification variables are either:* (i) *conditionally independent*
of disease status given the risk factors; or (ii) *conditionally independent of the risk*
factors given disease status. If either of these conditions is satisfied, both pooled and
matched analyses provide (asymptotically) unbiased estimates of the relative risk for

a dichotomous exposure (Bishop, Fienberg & Holland, 1975). [Whittemore (1978) has shown that, contrary to popular belief, both types of analyses may sometimes yield equivalent results even if conditions (i) and (ii) are both violated.] In matched studies condition (i) is more relevant since the matching variables are guaranteed to be uncorrelated with disease in the sample as a whole. Of course this does not ensure that they have the same distributions among cases and controls conditionally, within categories defined by the risk factors. Therefore an unmatched analysis may give biased results.

One result of using an unmatched analysis with data collected in a matched design, however, is that the *direction of the bias tends towards conservatism*. Relative risk estimates from the pooled data tend on average to be closer to unity than those calculated from the matched sets. This phenomenon was noted in § 3.4 when pooling data from two 2×2 tables, where the ratio of cases to controls in each table was constant. Seigel and Greenhouse (1973) show that the same thing happens if matched pairs are formed at random from among the cases and controls within each of two strata, and the data are then pooled for analysis. Armitage (1975) gives a slightly more general formulation. He supposes that there are I matched sets with exposure probabilities $p_{1i} = 1 - q_{1i}$ for the cases and $p_{0i} = 1 - q_{0i}$ for the controls, and that the odds ratio $\psi = p_{1i}q_{0i}/(p_{0i}q_{1i})$ is constant across all sets. It follows that the estimate of relative risk calculated as the cross-products ratio from the 2×2 table formed by pooling all the data tends towards the value

$$\frac{\Sigma p_{1i} \Sigma q_{0i}}{\Sigma p_{0i} \Sigma q_{1i}}$$

$$= \psi \frac{\Sigma q_{1i}\vartheta_i \Sigma q_{0i}}{\Sigma q_{0i}\vartheta_i \Sigma q_{1i}} \tag{7.6}$$

where $\vartheta_i = p_{0i}/q_{0i}$. For $\psi > 1$ the bias term multiplying ψ in (7.6) is less than one, unless the exposure probabilities p_{0i} are constant across sets (in which case there is no bias). Similarly, for $\psi < 1$, the bias term exceeds unity. Thus, failure to account for the matching in the analysis can (and often does) result in conservatively biased estimates of the relative risk.

A related question is to consider the cost, in terms of a loss of efficiency in the analysis, of using a matched analysis when in fact the matching was unnecessary to avoid bias. Suppose that the exposure probabilities p_{0i} in the above model are all equal to the constant p_0, so that both matched and unmatched analyses tend to estimate correctly the true odds ratio ψ. According to (4.18), the large sample variance of the pooled estimate of $\log \psi$ is

$$\frac{1}{I} \left\{ \frac{1}{p_1} + \frac{1}{q_1} + \frac{1}{p_0} + \frac{1}{q_0} \right\} = \frac{p_1 q_1 + p_0 q_0}{I p_1 q_1 p_0 q_0}.$$

Standard calculations show that the large sample variance of the estimate of $\log \psi$ based on the matched pairs in this situation is

$$\frac{p_1 q_0 + q_1 p_0}{I p_1 q_1 p_0 q_0}.$$

Consequently, using the ratio of variances to measure the relative precision of the two estimates, the efficiency of the matched pairs analysis when pairing at random is

$$\text{eff} = \frac{p_1 q_1 + p_0 q_0}{p_1 q_0 + p_0 q_1} \, . \tag{7.7}$$

When $\psi = 1$, i.e., $p_1 = p_0$, the matched pairs estimate is thus seen to be fully efficient. Otherwise eff < 1, reflecting the loss in information due to the random pairing. Nevertheless Figure 7.1 shows that the loss, which tends to be worse for intermediate values

Fig. 7.1 Loss in efficiency with a matched-pair design of using a matched statistical analysis, when the matching was unnecessary to avoid bias. Different curves correspond to different proportions exposed in the control population.

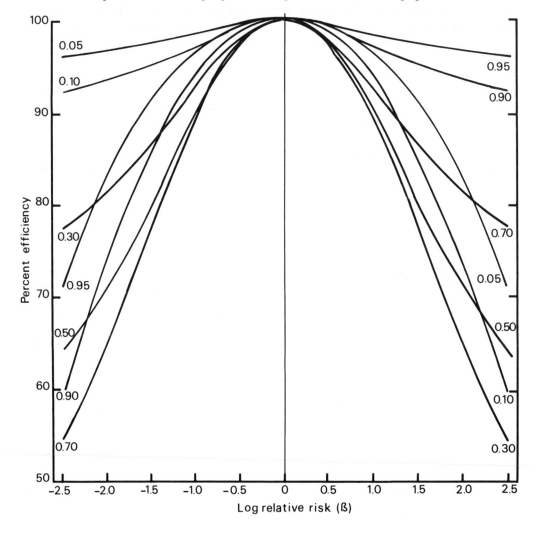

of p_0, is not terribly important unless the odds ratios being estimated are rather extreme. Pike, Hill and Smith (1979) reach similar conclusions on the basis of studies of the power of the chi-square test of the null hypothesis computed from the matched *versus* unmatched data.

While no additional theoretical studies have yet been made, it is likely that these same general conclusions regarding the bias and efficiency of matched *versus* unmatched *analyses* apply also to the estimation of multiple relative risk functions. Two numerical examples will serve to illustrate the basic points. The first contrasts the fitting of both conditional and unconditional logistic regression analyses to data from an IARC sponsored study of oesophageal cancer occurring among Singapore Chinese (de Jong et al., 1974). The analysis was based on 80 male cases and on 320 matched controls whose ages were within five years of the corresponding case. Two controls for each case were drawn from the same hospital ward as the case, while two others were selected from an orthopaedic unit. However, as there were no important differences in exposure histories between the two control groups, they were not separated in the analysis.

Table 7.10 Coefficients ($\pm$ standard errors) of variables in the multiple relative risk function, estimated using linear logistic regression analyses appropriate for both matched and unmatched samples. IARC study of oesophageal cancer among Singapore Chinese[a]

Variables in equation[b]	Matched analysis Coefficient $\pm$ S.E.	Unmatched analysis Coefficient $\pm$ S.E.
A. Interaction term excluded		
x_0 Constant		-3.2062 ± 0.3650
x_1 Dialect	1.2570 ± 0.3273	1.4145 ± 0.3301
x_2 Samsu	0.5064 ± 0.2936	0.5352 ± 0.2766
x_3 Cigarettes	0.0122 ± 0.0099	0.0121 ± 0.0095
x_4 Beverage temperature	0.7846 ± 0.1640	0.7556 ± 0.1493
Goodness-of-fit statistic (G)	197.43	336.23
B. Interaction term included		
x_0 Constant		-3.2123 ± 0.3661
x_1 Dialect	1.2559 ± 0.3280	1.4200 ± 0.3312
x_2 Samsu	0.5072 ± 0.2941	0.5303 ± 0.2774
x_3 Cigarettes	0.0123 ± 0.0099	0.0124 ± 0.0096
x_4 Beverage temperature	0.7872 ± 0.1726	0.7447 ± 0.1563
$x_5 = x_4 \times$ (age-60)	-0.0009 ± 0.0179	0.0034 ± 0.0147
Goodness-of-fit statistic (G)	197.43	336.18

[a] de Jong et al. (1974)
[b] Coding of risk variables:

$x_1 = \begin{cases} 1 \text{ Hokkien/Teochew} \\ 0 \text{ Cantonese/other} \end{cases}$ $x_3 =$ No. of cigarettes/day average

$x_2 = \begin{cases} 1 \text{ Drinkers (Samsu)} \\ 0 \text{ Abstainers} \end{cases}$ $x_4 =$ No. of beverages (0–3) drunk "burning hot"

Information was obtained regarding diet, alcohol and tobacco usage, and on various social factors including dialect group, which indicates the patient's ancestral origin within China. Only four variables are considered here: dialect group, cigarettes, samsu (a distilled liquor made from a mixture of grains) and beverage temperature (the number of beverages among tea, coffee and barley wine that the patient reported drinking at "burning hot" temperatures). The coding of these variables has been simplified from that used in the original analysis, and an interaction term between beverage temperature and age (a matching variable) was introduced to see if the log relative risk for beverage temperature changed linearly with age.

Table 7.10 presents the estimated regression coefficients and standard errors obtained by fitting the unconditional logistic model with a single stratum parameter α to the pooled data. Shown for comparison are the same quantities estimated from the conditional likelihood. With the exception of that for dialect group, the standard errors of the matched analysis are slightly larger than those for the unmatched. Small changes are evident in the regression coefficients themselves, so that this is evidently a situation in which the matching variables either have little relationship to the exposures conditional on disease status or else have little relationship to disease status conditional on exposure. As a partial confirmation of the latter interpretation, Table 7.11 shows that cases and controls have roughly equivalent average ages even within the levels of each risk factor. This analysis is incomplete, since it involves only averages and ignores possible higher order interactions of age with risk factor combinations. Nevertheless, it is consistent with the notion that the matching variables are conditionally independent of disease status given the exposures, and thus that the requirements for 'poolability' of matched data are satisfied.

Table 7.11 Average ages $\pm$ standard errors for cases and controls within levels of each risk factor: IARC study of oesophageal cancer among Singapore Chinese[a]

Risk factor	Level	Cases		Controls		Totals	
		n	Mean ± S.E.	n	Mean ± S.E.	n	Mean ± S.E.
Dialect group	Hokkien/Teochew	66	61.3 ± 1.0	160	60.6 ± 0.8	226	60.8 ± 0.6
	Cantonese/other	14	65.4 ± 2.6	160	63.0 ± 0.7	174	63.2 ± 0.6
Samsu	Drinkers	40	63.6 ± 1.2	109	62.4 ± 0.8	149	62.7 ± 0.7
	Abstainers	40	60.5 ± 1.4	211	61.5 ± 0.6	251	61.4 ± 0.6
Cigarettes	None	8	63.6 ± 5.4	55	62.8 ± 1.3	63	62.9 ± 1.3
	1–10 per day	14	65.9 ± 1.9	81	63.7 ± 1.0	95	64.0 ± 0.9
	11–20 per day	35	61.7 ± 1.0	115	62.2 ± 0.8	150	62.1 ± 0.7
	21+ per day	23	59.6 ± 1.8	69	58.2 ± 1.0	92	58.5 ± 0.9
Beverage temperature (no. "burning hot")	0	41	60.8 ± 1.4	261	61.5 ± 0.6	302	61.4 ± 0.5
	1	13	62.2 ± 2.1	31	62.8 ± 1.6	44	62.6 ± 1.3
	2	18	65.3 ± 1.9	25	63.6 ± 1.9	43	64.3 ± 1.3
	3	8	60.5 ± 2.8	3	66.3 ± 3.2	11	62.1 ± 2.3
Totals	All	80	62.0 ± 0.9	320	61.8 ± 0.5	400	61.9 ± 0.4

[a] de Jong et al. (1974)

Table 7.12 Coefficients (± standard errors) of variables in the multiple relative risk function, using a variety of analyses: Iran/IARC case-control study of oesophageal cancer in the Caspian littoral of Iran[a]

Variables in equation	Type of analysis					
	Fully matched	Stratified into				
		7 Regions, 4 Age groups	4 Regions, 4 Age groups	4 Regions	4 Age groups	Unmatched
Social class	−1.125 ± 0.254	−0.808 ± 0.212	−0.782 ± 0.206	−0.745 ± 0.201	−0.684 ± 0.180	−0.682 ± 0.179
Ownership of garden	−0.815 ± 0.250	−0.614 ± 0.222	−0.602 ± 0.219	−0.592 ± 0.218	−0.326 ± 0.191	−0.307 ± 0.190
Consumption of raw green vegetables	−0.552 ± 0.220	−0.459 ± 0.203	−0.439 ± 0.199	−0.432 ± 0.198	−0.429 ± 0.188	−0.440 ± 0.187
Consumption of cucumbers	−0.640 ± 0.217	−0.539 ± 0.196	−0.548 ± 0.192	−0.562 ± 0.192	−0.466 ± 0.182	−0.449 ± 0.181
Goodness-of-fit (G)	375.38[b]	776.54	777.60	780.80	787.04	789.56

[a] Cook-Mozaffari et al. (1979)
[b] Based on the conditional model and hence not comparable to the others

In general one must anticipate that the degree to which the matching variables are incorporated in the analysis will affect the estimates of relative risk. An example which better illustrates this phenomenon is provided by the joint Iran/IARC study of oesophageal cancer on the Caspian littoral (Cook-Mozaffari et al., 1979). In that part of the world both cancer incidence and many environmental variables show marked geographical variation. Cases and controls were therefore individually matched according to village of residence, as well as for age. Just as in the preceding example, the data were analysed using both the conditional fully matched analysis based on (7.2) and the unconditional analysis based on (6.10) in which the entire sample was considered as a single stratum. Intermediate between these two extremes, additional analyses were performed which incorporated various levels of stratification by age and by geographical area, the latter grouping the villages into regions with roughly homogeneous incidence.

Table 7.12 presents the results for males for four risk variables which appeared to be the best indicators of socioeconomic and dietary status. Substantial bias of the regression coefficients towards the origin, indicating a lesser effect on risk, is evident with the coarsely stratified and unmatched analyses. This confirms the theoretical results regarding the direction of the bias which were noted above to hold for the univariate situation. While the standard errors of the estimates increase as greater account is taken of the matching, the changes are not great and seem a small price to pay for avoiding bias.

In summary, both theoretical and numerical studies confirm that the pooling of matched or stratified samples for analysis will result in relative risk estimates which are conservatively biased in comparison with those which would be obtained using the appropriate matched analysis. In some situations, where the matching was not essential to avoid bias, the pooled and matched estimates may scarcely differ at all. Even then, however, the additional information gained from the pooled data, as reflected in the variances of the estimates, is not great. Consequently, now that appropriate and flexible methods are available for doing so, the *matching should be accounted for in the analysis whenever it has been incorporated in the design.*

While the availability of methods for multivariate analysis of matched samples certainly makes such designs more attractive, it does not follow that they should always be used. Close pair matching may result in a number of cases being lost from the study for want of an appropriate match. It may also impose severe administrative costs which could be avoided with a less restrictive design. Increasing use is being made of "population controls" obtained as an age-stratified random sample of the population from which the cases were diagnosed. Many epidemiologists believe that this is the best way to avoid the selection bias inherent in other choices of the control population. The confounding effects of other factors which are causally related to disease may be accounted for by post-hoc stratification of the sample, or by modelling them in the analysis. Such designs and analyses accomplish many of the aims intended by the use of matching, and constitute a practical alternative which may be preferred in many situations.

REFERENCES

Andersen, E.B. (1973) *Conditional Inference and Models for Measuring,* Copenhagen, Mental Hygienisk Forlag., p. 69

Armitage, P. (1975) *The use of the cross-ratio in aetiological surveys.* In: Gani, J., ed., *Perspectives in Probability and Statistics,* London, Academic Press, pp. 349–355

Bishop, Y.M.M., Fienberg, S.E. & Holland, P.W. (1975) *Discrete Multivariate Analysis: Theory and Practice,* Cambridge, Mass., MIT Press

Breslow, N.E. (1976) Regression analysis of the log odds ratio: a method for retrospective studies. *Biometrics, 32,* 409–416

Breslow, N.E., Day, N.E., Halvorsen, K.T., Prentice, R.L. & Sabai, C. (1978) Estimation of multiple relative risk functions in matched case-control studies. *Am. J. Epidemiol., 108,* 299–307

Cook-Mozaffari, P.J., Azordegan, F., Day, N.E., Ressicaud, A., Sabai, C. & Aramesh, B. (1979) Oesophageal cancer studies in the Caspian littoral of Iran: results of a case-control study. *Br. J. Cancer, 39,* 293–309

Cox, D.R. & Hinkley, D.V. (1974) *Theoretical Statistics,* London, Chapman & Hall

Day, N.E. & Byar, D. (1979) Testing hypotheses in case-control studies: equivalence of Mantel-Haenszel statistics and logit score tests. *Biometrics, 35,* 623–630

de Jong, U.W., Breslow, N.E., Goh Ewe Hong, J., Sridharan, M. & Shanmugaratnam, K. (1974) Aetiological factors in oesophageal cancer in Singapore Chinese. *Int. J. Cancer, 13,* 291–303

Fienberg, S.E. (1977) *The Analysis of Cross-Classified Categorical Data,* Cambridge, Mass., MIT Press

Holford, T.R., White, C. & Kelsey, J.L. (1978) Multivariate analysis for matched case-control studies. *Am. J. Epidemiol., 107,* 245–256

Jick, H., Watkins, R.N., Hunter, J.R., Dinan, B.J., Madsen, S., Rothman, K.J. & Walker, A.M. (1979) Replacement estrogens and endometrial cancer. *New Engl. J. Med., 300,* 218–222

Liddell, F.D.K., McDonald, J.C. & Thomas, D.C. (1977) Methods of cohort analysis: appraisal by application to asbestos mining. *J. R. stat. Soc. Ser. A, 140,* 469–491

Mack, T.M., Pike, M.C., Henderson, B.E., Pfeffer, R.I., Gerkins, V.R., Arthur, B.S. & Brown, S.E. (1976) Estrogens and endometrial cancer in a retirement community. *New Engl. J. Med., 294,* 1262–1267

Miettinen, O.S. (1974) Confounding and effect modification. *Am. J. Epidemiol., 100,* 350–353

Pike, M.C., Hill, A.P. & Smith, P.G. (1980) Bias and efficiency in logistic analyses of stratified case-control studies. *Int. J. Epidemiol., 9,* 89–95

Richards, F.S.G. (1961) A method of maximum likelihood estimation. *J. R. stat. Soc. B., 23,* 469–475

Seigel, D.G. & Greenhouse, S.W. (1973) Multiple relative risk functions in case-control studies. *Am. J. Epidemiol., 97,* 324–331

Smith, D.C., Prentice, R., Thompson, D.J. & Herrmann, W.L. (1975) Association of exogenous estrogen and endometrial carcinoma. *New Engl. J. Med., 293,* 1164–1167

Smith, P.G., Pike, M.C., Hill, A.P., Breslow, N.E. & Day, N.E. (1981) Multivariate conditional logistic analysis of stratum-matched case-control studies (submitted for publication)

Thomas, D.G. (1975) Exact and asymptotic methods for the combination of 2×2 tables. *Comput. biomed. Res., 8*, 423–446

Whittemore, A.S. (1978) Collapsibility of multidimensional contingency tables. *J. R. stat. Soc. B., 40*, 328–340

Zelen, M. (1971) The analysis of several 2×2 tables. *Biometrika, 58*, 129–137

LIST OF SYMBOLS – CHAPTER 7 (in order of appearance)

β_k	log relative risk associated with unit change in k^{th} risk variable
x_j	vector of risk variables for j^{th} study subject; $x_j = (x_{j1}, ..., x_{jk})$
n_1	number of cases
n_0	number of controls
n	total number of study subjects
l	denotes a partition of the integers from 1 to n into two groups, one of size n_1 and the other of size $n_0 = n-n_1$; e.g., if $n_1' = 2$ and $n_0 = 3$ a possible partition is $l_1 = 3, l_2 = 4, l_3 = 1, l_4 = 2, l_5 = 5$ or $l = (3,4,1,2,5)$
α_i	logit of disease probability for an individual with a standard ($x = 0$) set of risk variables in the ith stratum
$pr_i(y = 1/x)$	disease probability in the ith stratum for an individual with value x for the risk variable
ψ	odds ratio
β	log relative risk (binary exposure)
n_{00}	number of matched pairs with neither case nor control exposed
n_{01}	number of matched pairs with case unexposed and control exposed
n_{10}	number of matched pairs with case exposed and control unexposed
n_{11}	number of matched pairs with both case and control exposed
μ	in discordant matched pairs with a binary exposure variable, denotes the fitted number of exposed cases under the unconditional model
π	conditional probability that in a discordant matched pair it is the case which is exposed
M	number of controls per case (fixed)
M_i	number of controls per case in the ith matched set
I	number of matched sets
x_{ijk}	value of kth exposure variable ($k = 1, ..., K$) for case ($j = 0$) or j^{th} control ($j = 1, ..., M_i$) in the ith matched set
x_{ij}	$(x_{ij1}, ..., x_{ijK})$ exposure vector for j^{th} subject in i^{th} set
G	goodness-of-fit statistic based on the (conditional) log likelihood
a_i	number of exposed cases in i^{th} of I 2×2 tables
n_{1i}	number of cases in i^{th} table
n_{0i}	number of controls in i^{th} table
ψ_i	(expected) odds ratio associated with i^{th} of I 2×2 tables
z_{il}	value of lth covariable for i^{th} 2×2 table

$\mathbf{z}_i$	vector of covariable values for i^{th} table
γ	vector of interaction parameters in logistic model for a series of 2×2 tables
p_{1i}	exposure probability for cases in the ith stratum
q_{1i}	$1-p_{1i}$
p_{0i}	exposure probability for controls in the ith stratum
q_{0i}	$1-p_{0i}$
ϑ_i	p_{0i}/q_{0i}

APPENDIX I:

GROUPED DATA FROM THE ILLE-ET-VILAINE STUDY OF OESOPHAGEAL CANCER USED FOR ILLUSTRATION IN CHAPTERS 4 AND 6

AGE (YRS)	ALCOHOL (GM/DAY)	TOBACCO (GM/DAY)	CASES	CONTROLS
25-34	0-39	0-9	0	40
::	::	10-19	0	10
::	::	20-29	0	6
::	::	30+	0	5
::	40-79	0-9	0	27
::	::	10-19	0	7
::	::	20-29	0	4
::	::	30+	0	7
::	80-119	0-9	0	2
::	::	10-19	0	1
::	::	20-29	0	0
::	::	30+	0	2
::	120+	0-9	0	1
::	::	10-19	1	0
::	::	20-29	0	1
::	::	30+	0	2
35-44	0-39	0-9	0	60
::	::	10-19	1	13
::	::	20-29	0	7
::	::	30+	0	8
::	40-79	0-9	0	35
::	::	10-19	3	20
::	::	20-29	1	13
::	::	30+	0	8
::	80-119	0-9	0	11
::	::	10-19	0	6
::	::	20-29	0	2
::	::	30+	0	1
::	120+	0-9	2	1
::	::	10-19	0	3
::	::	20-29	2	2
::	::	30+	0	0

AGE (YRS)	ALCOHOL (GM/DAY)	TOBACCO (GM/DAY)	CASES	CONTROLS
45-54	0-39	0-9	1	45
::	::	10-19	0	18
::	::	20-29	0	10
::	::	30+	0	4
::	40-79	0-9	6	32
::	::	10-19	4	17
::	::	20-29	5	10
::	::	30+	5	2
::	80-119	0-9	3	13
::	::	10-19	6	8
::	::	20-29	1	4
::	::	30+	2	2
::	120+	0-9	4	0
::	::	10-19	3	1
::	::	20-29	2	1
::	::	30+	4	0
55-64	0-39	0-9	2	47
::	::	10-19	3	19
::	::	20-29	3	9
::	::	30+	4	2
::	40-79	0-9	9	31
::	::	10-19	6	15
::	::	20-29	4	13
::	::	30+	3	3
::	80-119	0-9	9	9
::	::	10-19	8	7
::	::	20-29	3	3
::	::	30+	4	0
::	120+	0-9	5	5
::	::	10-19	6	1
::	::	20-29	2	1
::	::	30+	5	1

AGE (YRS)	ALCOHOL (GM/DAY)	TOBACCO (GM/DAY)	CASES	CONTROLS
65-74	0-39	0-9	5	43
::	::	10-19	4	10
::	::	20-29	2	5
::	::	30+	0	2
::	40-79	0-9	17	17
::	::	10-19	3	7
::	::	20-29	5	4
::	::	30+	0	0
::	80-119	0-9	6	7
::	::	10-19	4	8
::	::	20-29	2	1
::	::	30+	1	0
::	120+	0-9	3	1
::	::	10-19	1	1
::	::	20-29	1	0
::	::	30+	1	0
75+	0-39	0-9	1	17
::	::	10-19	2	4
::	::	20-29	0	0
::	::	30+	1	2
::	40-79	0-9	2	3
::	::	10-19	1	2
::	::	20-29	0	3
::	::	30+	1	0
::	80-119	0-9	1	0
::	::	10-19	1	0
::	::	20-29	0	0
::	::	30+	0	0
::	120+	0-9	2	0
::	::	10-19	1	0
::	::	20-29	0	0
::	::	30+	0	0

APPENDIX II:

GROUPED DATA FROM THE OXFORD CHILDHOOD CANCER SURVEY USED FOR ILLUSTRATION IN CHAPTERS 6 AND 7

YEAR OF DEATH	AGE AT DEATH	X-RAYED	CASES	CONTROLS
1944	9	YES	3	0
1944	9	NO	25	28
1945	9	YES	5	2
1945	9	NO	16	19
1945	8	YES	2	2
1945	8	NO	30	30
1946	9	YES	7	1
1946	9	NO	28	34
1946	8	YES	7	2
1946	8	NO	28	33
1946	7	YES	2	0
1946	7	NO	36	38
1947	9	YES	5	1
1947	9	NO	25	29
1947	8	YES	3	1
1947	8	NO	40	42
1947	7	YES	5	1
1947	7	NO	44	48
1947	6	YES	11	2
1947	6	NO	42	51
1948	9	YES	6	4
1948	9	NO	25	27
1948	8	YES	6	4
1948	8	NO	29	31
1948	7	YES	11	2
1948	7	NO	35	44
1948	6	YES	4	1
1948	6	NO	49	52
1948	5	YES	4	7
1948	5	NO	57	54
1949	9	YES	2	4
1949	9	NO	38	36
1949	8	YES	8	3
1949	8	NO	21	26
1949	7	YES	8	5
1949	7	NO	36	39
1949	6	YES	6	3
1949	6	NO	46	49
1949	5	YES	5	2
1949	5	NO	50	53
1949	4	YES	15	4
1949	4	NO	46	57

YEAR OF DEATH	AGE AT DEATH	X-RAYED	CASES	CONTROLS
1950	9	YES	4	1
1950	9	NO	27	30
1950	8	YES	9	4
1950	8	NO	39	44
1950	7	YES	9	5
1950	7	NO	35	39
1950	6	YES	4	2
1950	6	NO	38	40
1950	5	YES	12	7
1950	5	NO	41	46
1950	4	YES	8	5
1950	4	NO	48	51
1950	3	YES	8	8
1950	3	NO	63	63
1951	9	YES	6	2
1951	9	NO	37	41
1951	8	YES	8	3
1951	8	NO	35	40
1951	7	YES	12	5
1951	7	NO	31	38
1951	6	YES	4	4
1951	6	NO	36	36
1951	5	YES	7	1
1951	5	NO	37	43
1951	4	YES	16	6
1951	4	NO	54	64
1951	3	YES	12	5
1951	3	NO	63	70
1951	2	YES	9	11
1951	2	NO	62	60
1952	9	YES	4	5
1952	9	NO	33	32
1952	8	YES	7	2
1952	8	NO	24	29
1952	7	YES	8	5
1952	7	NO	34	37
1952	6	YES	11	8
1952	6	NO	35	38
1952	5	YES	5	5
1952	5	NO	42	42
1952	4	YES	12	6
1952	4	NO	43	49
1952	3	YES	8	6
1952	3	NO	55	57
1952	2	YES	17	10
1952	2	NO	74	81
1952	1	YES	9	7
1952	1	NO	34	36

YEAR OF DEATH	AGE AT DEATH	X-RAYED	CASES	CONTROLS
1953	9	YES	3	5
1953	9	NO	36	34
1953	8	YES	2	5
1953	8	NO	33	30
1953	7	YES	7	2
1953	7	NO	25	30
1953	6	YES	6	8
1953	6	NO	47	45
1953	5	YES	5	1
1953	5	NO	44	48
1953	4	YES	11	13
1953	4	NO	64	62
1953	3	YES	14	9
1953	3	NO	50	55
1953	2	YES	13	11
1953	2	NO	56	58
1953	1	YES	8	9
1953	1	NO	56	55
1953	0	YES	6	4
1953	0	NO	43	45
1954	9	YES	4	4
1954	9	NO	25	25
1954	8	YES	8	8
1954	8	NO	32	32
1954	7	YES	4	6
1954	7	NO	23	21
1954	6	YES	8	8
1954	6	NO	40	40
1954	5	YES	7	6
1954	5	NO	36	37
1954	4	YES	15	8
1954	4	NO	46	53
1954	3	YES	15	14
1954	3	NO	62	63
1954	2	YES	9	6
1954	2	NO	46	49
1954	1	YES	9	5
1954	1	NO	51	55
1954	0	YES	5	5
1954	0	NO	41	41
1955	9	YES	6	2
1955	9	NO	22	26
1955	8	YES	3	4
1955	8	NO	30	29
1955	7	YES	9	2
1955	7	NO	23	30

YEAR OF DEATH	AGE AT DEATH	X-RAYED	CASES	CONTROLS
1955	6	YES	12	9
1955	6	NO	34	37
1955	5	YES	14	5
1955	5	NO	43	52
1955	4	YES	16	6
1955	4	NO	40	50
1955	3	YES	17	7
1955	3	NO	61	71
1955	2	YES	8	5
1955	2	NO	50	53
1955	1	YES	8	10
1955	1	NO	44	42
1955	0	YES	9	3
1955	0	NO	22	28
1956	8	YES	5	2
1956	8	NO	23	26
1956	7	YES	9	1
1956	7	NO	37	45
1956	6	YES	11	7
1956	6	NO	31	35
1956	5	YES	6	9
1956	5	NO	39	36
1956	4	YES	14	13
1956	4	NO	49	50
1956	3	YES	21	9
1956	3	NO	50	62
1956	2	YES	16	11
1956	2	NO	53	58
1956	1	YES	6	4
1956	1	NO	37	39
1956	0	YES	9	8
1956	0	NO	41	42
1957	7	YES	8	2
1957	7	NO	23	29
1957	6	YES	9	3
1957	6	NO	25	31
1957	5	YES	8	7
1957	5	NO	46	47
1957	4	YES	4	4
1957	4	NO	42	42
1957	3	YES	11	7
1957	3	NO	47	51
1957	2	YES	11	5
1957	2	NO	51	57
1957	1	YES	6	6
1957	1	NO	46	46
1957	0	YES	9	6
1957	0	NO	32	35

YEAR OF DEATH	AGE AT DEATH	X-RAYED	CASES	CONTROLS
1958	6	YES	4	5
1958	6	NO	30	29
1958	5	YES	4	6
1958	5	NO	48	46
1958	4	YES	9	9
1958	4	NO	54	54
1958	3	YES	9	7
1958	3	NO	50	52
1958	2	YES	10	7
1958	2	NO	78	81
1958	1	YES	14	7
1958	1	NO	48	55
1958	0	YES	6	4
1958	0	NO	41	43
1959	5	YES	3	2
1959	5	NO	50	51
1959	4	YES	4	3
1959	4	NO	53	54
1959	3	YES	6	4
1959	3	NO	68	70
1959	2	YES	10	10
1959	2	NO	58	58
1959	1	YES	4	3
1959	1	NO	57	58
1959	0	YES	3	4
1959	0	NO	42	41
1960	4	YES	3	2
1960	4	NO	42	43
1960	3	YES	10	10
1960	3	NO	52	52
1960	2	YES	4	5
1960	2	NO	69	68
1960	1	YES	10	4
1960	1	NO	43	49
1960	0	YES	5	5
1960	0	NO	34	34
1961	3	YES	4	4
1961	3	NO	41	41
1961	2	YES	3	6
1961	2	NO	48	45
1961	1	YES	13	5
1961	1	NO	42	50
1961	0	YES	1	3
1961	0	NO	40	38

YEAR OF DEATH	AGE AT DEATH	X-RAYED	CASES	CONTROLS
1962	2	YES	7	2
1962	2	NO	46	51
1962	1	YES	5	2
1962	1	NO	46	49
1962	0	YES	7	4
1962	0	NO	35	38
1963	1	YES	6	6
1963	1	NO	40	40
1963	0	YES	3	4
1963	0	NO	51	50
1964	0	YES	7	1
1964	0	NO	25	31

APPENDIX III:

MATCHED DATA FROM THE LOS ANGELES STUDY OF ENDOMETRIAL CANCER USED FOR ILLUSTRATION IN CHAPTERS 5 AND 7

CASE OR CONTROL	AGE	GALL BLADDER DISEASE	HYPER TENSION	OBESITY	ESTROGEN (ANY) USE	CONJUGATED DOSE (SEE CODE)	ESTROGEN DURATION (MONTHS)	NON ESTROGEN DRUG
CASE	74	NO	NO	YES	YES	3	96+	YES
CONTROL	75	NO	NO	UNK	NO	0	0	NO
CONTROL	74	NO	NO	UNK	NO	0	0	NO
CONTROL	74	NO	NO	UNK	NO	0	0	NO
CONTROL	75	NO	NO	YES	YES	1	48	YES
CASE	67	NO	NO	NO	YES	3	96+	YES
CONTROL	67	NO	NO	NO	YES	3	5	NO
CONTROL	67	NO	YES	YES	NO	0	0	YES
CONTROL	67	NO	NO	NO	YES	2	53	NO
CONTROL	68	NO	NO	NO	YES	2	45	YES
CASE	76	NO	YES	YES	YES	1	9	YES
CONTROL	76	NO	YES	YES	YES	2	96+	YES
CONTROL	76	NO	YES	NO	YES	1	3	YES
CONTROL	76	NO	YES	YES	YES	2	15	YES
CONTROL	77	NO	NO	NO	YES	1	36	YES
CASE	71	NO	NO	UNK	YES	UNK	96+	NO
CONTROL	70	YES	NO	NO	YES	2	7	YES
CONTROL	70	NO	NO	NO	YES	0	0	YES
CONTROL	71	NO	YES	YES	YES	2	7	YES
CONTROL	70	NO	NO	YES	YES	2	27	YES
CASE	69	YES	NO	YES	YES	2	36	YES
CONTROL	69	NO	YES	NO	YES	1	96+	YES
CONTROL	69	NO	NO	YES	YES	2	1	YES
CONTROL	69	NO	NO	NO	YES	0	0	YES
CONTROL	68	NO	NO	UNK	NO	0	0	NO
CASE	70	NO	YES	YES	YES	2	71	YES
CONTROL	71	NO	NO	NO	NO	0	0	NO
CONTROL	71	NO	YES	YES	YES	3	5	YES
CONTROL	70	NO	NO	YES	NO	0	0	NO
CONTROL	71	NO	NO	UNK	NO	0	0	NO
CASE	65	YES	NO	NO	YES	1	96+	YES
CONTROL	65	NO	NO	UNK	NO	0	0	NO
CONTROL	64	NO	NO	NO	YES	3	91	YES
CONTROL	64	NO	NO	NO	YES	2	96+	YES
CONTROL	65	NO	NO	YES	YES	2	60	NO
CASE	68	YES	YES	YES	YES	1	36	YES
CONTROL	68	NO	YES	UNK	NO	0	0	YES
CONTROL	68	NO	NO	YES	NO	0	0	YES
CONTROL	68	YES	NO	UNK	YES	0	0	NO

CASE OR CONTROL	AGE	GALL BLADDER DISEASE	HYPER TENSION	OBESITY	ESTROGEN (ANY) USE	CONJUGATED DOSE (SEE CODE)	ESTROGEN DURATION (MONTHS)	NON ESTROGEN DRUG
CONTROL	68	NO	NO	UNK	YES	1	1	YES
CASE	61	NO	NO	UNK	NO	0	0	YES
CONTROL	61	NO	NO	YES	NO	0	0	YES
CONTROL	61	NO	NO	NO	YES	1	24	YES
CONTROL	61	NO	NO	UNK	NO	0	0	YES
CONTROL	60	YES	NO	NO	NO	0	0	NO
CASE	64	NO	NO	YES	YES	1	54	YES
CONTROL	64	NO	NO	UNK	NO	0	0	NO
CONTROL	65	NO	YES	UNK	YES	3	2	YES
CONTROL	64	NO	YES	YES	YES	3	10	YES
CONTROL	65	NO	NO	UNK	NO	0	0	NO
CASE	68	YES	NO	YES	YES	3	96+	YES
CONTROL	69	NO	NO	UNK	NO	0	0	NO
CONTROL	69	NO	NO	YES	NO	0	0	YES
CONTROL	69	YES	YES	YES	YES	0	0	YES
CONTROL	69	YES	NO	YES	YES	1	35	NO
CASE	74	NO	NO	NO	YES	2	96+	YES
CONTROL	74	NO	YES	NO	YES	3	4	YES
CONTROL	73	NO	YES	NO	YES	2	11	YES
CONTROL	74	NO	NO	YES	YES	1	6	YES
CONTROL	74	NO	NO	YES	YES	1	12	NO
CASE	67	YES	NO	YES	YES	0	0	YES
CONTROL	68	NO	YES	NO	YES	0	0	YES
CONTROL	68	NO	YES	YES	YES	3	65	YES
CONTROL	68	NO	NO	UNK	NO	0	0	NO
CONTROL	68	NO	NO	YES	YES	2	96+	YES
CASE	62	YES	NO	NO	YES	1	UNK	YES
CONTROL	62	YES	NO	NO	NO	0	0	NO
CONTROL	63	NO	NO	YES	NO	0	0	NO
CONTROL	63	NO	NO	UNK	NO	0	0	NO
CONTROL	63	NO	NO	YES	YES	2	UNK	NO
CASE	71	YES	NO	YES	YES	2	59	YES
CONTROL	70	NO	YES	YES	NO	0	0	YES
CONTROL	71	NO	NO	YES	YES	UNK	UNK	YES
CONTROL	71	NO	YES	YES	NO	0	0	YES
CONTROL	71	NO	YES	YES	YES	2	84	YES
CASE	83	NO	YES	YES	YES	3	96+	YES
CONTROL	82	NO	NO	YES	NO	0	0	NO
CONTROL	82	NO	YES	NO	YES	3	4	YES
CONTROL	82	NO	YES	NO	NO	0	0	YES
CONTROL	82	NO	NO	UNK	NO	0	0	NO
CASE	70	NO	NO	YES	NO	0	0	YES
CONTROL	70	YES	YES	YES	YES	2	55	YES
CONTROL	70	NO	YES	YES	YES	2	14	YES
CONTROL	70	NO	YES	YES	YES	1	39	YES

CASE OR CONTROL	AGE	GALL BLADDER DISEASE	HYPER TENSION	OBESITY	ESTROGEN (ANY) USE	CONJUGATED DOSE (SEE CODE)	ESTROGEN DURATION (MONTHS)	NON ESTROGEN DRUG
CONTROL	70	NO	YES	YES	NO	0	0	YES
CASE	74	NO	NO	NO	YES	0	0	YES
CONTROL	75	YES	YES	NO	YES	2	6	YES
CONTROL	74	NO	NO	YES	NO	0	0	YES
CONTROL	74	NO	YES	NO	YES	2	46	YES
CONTROL	75	NO	NO	UNK	NO	0	0	NO
CASE	70	NO	NO	UNK	YES	0	0	YES
CONTROL	70	NO	YES	NO	YES	1	96+	YES
CONTROL	70	NO	NO	UNK	NO	0	0	NO
CONTROL	70	NO	NO	UNK	NO	0	0	YES
CONTROL	70	NO	NO	UNK	NO	0	0	NO
CASE	66	NO	YES	YES	YES	3	48	YES
CONTROL	66	NO	NO	UNK	YES	1	96+	YES
CONTROL	66	NO	NO	UNK	NO	0	0	YES
CONTROL	66	NO	NO	YES	NO	0	0	NO
CONTROL	66	NO	YES	YES	YES	1	12	YES
CASE	77	NO	NO	YES	YES	3	4	YES
CONTROL	77	YES	YES	YES	YES	0	0	YES
CONTROL	77	NO	YES	NO	YES	2	24	YES
CONTROL	77	NO	NO	YES	NO	0	0	NO
CONTROL	78	NO	YES	YES	YES	2	9	YES
CASE	66	NO	YES	NO	YES	3	29	YES
CONTROL	67	NO	YES	NO	NO	0	0	YES
CONTROL	66	NO	NO	YES	NO	0	0	YES
CONTROL	67	NO	NO	YES	NO	0	0	YES
CONTROL	69	NO	YES	YES	YES	2	10	YES
CASE	71	NO	YES	YES	YES	1	96+	NO
CONTROL	72	NO	NO	UNK	NO	0	0	NO
CONTROL	72	NO	NO	NO	NO	0	0	YES
CONTROL	71	NO	NO	UNK	NO	0	0	NO
CONTROL	71	NO	YES	YES	NO	0	0	YES
CASE	80	NO	NO	NO	YES	2	UNK	YES
CONTROL	79	NO	NO	UNK	NO	0	0	NO
CONTROL	79	NO	NO	NO	NO	0	0	NO
CONTROL	79	NO	NO	YES	NO	0	0	NO
CONTROL	80	NO	NO	NO	NO	0	0	NO
CASE	64	NO	NO	YES	YES	2	UNK	YES
CONTROL	64	NO	NO	NO	YES	0	0	YES
CONTROL	63	NO	NO	YES	YES	1	60	YES
CONTROL	64	NO	YES	NO	YES	1	6	YES
CONTROL	66	NO	YES	YES	YES	1	UNK	YES
CASE	63	NO	NO	NO	YES	1	60	YES
CONTROL	63	NO	YES	NO	YES	1	96+	YES
CONTROL	65	NO	NO	NO	YES	1	25	NO
CONTROL	65	NO	NO	NO	NO	0	0	YES
CONTROL	64	NO	NO	NO	YES	1	96+	YES

CASE OR CONTROL	AGE	GALL BLADDER DISEASE	HYPER TENSION	OBESITY	ESTROGEN (ANY) USE	CONJUGATED DOSE (SEE CODE)	ESTROGEN DURATION (MONTHS)	NON ESTROGEN DRUG
CASE	72	YES	NO	YES	NO	0	0	YES
CONTROL	72	NO	YES	UNK	NO	0	0	NO
CONTROL	72	NO	YES	YES	NO	0	0	YES
CONTROL	72	NO	YES	NO	YES	1	48	YES
CONTROL	72	NO	YES	YES	YES	0	0	YES
CASE	57	NO	NO	NO	YES	3	12	NO
CONTROL	57	NO	YES	YES	YES	0	0	YES
CONTROL	58	NO	NO	YES	YES	1	36	YES
CONTROL	57	NO	NO	NO	YES	1	36	NO
CONTROL	57	NO	NO	NO	YES	0	0	NO
CASE	74	YES	NO	YES	NO	0	0	YES
CONTROL	74	NO	NO	YES	NO	0	0	YES
CONTROL	73	NO	NO	YES	YES	2	2	YES
CONTROL	75	NO	NO	YES	NO	0	0	YES
CONTROL	75	NO	NO	UNK	NO	0	0	NO
CASE	62	NO	YES	YES	YES	2	6	YES
CONTROL	62	NO	NO	YES	YES	2	37	YES
CONTROL	62	NO	NO	YES	YES	2	63	YES
CONTROL	63	NO	NO	UNK	NO	0	0	NO
CONTROL	61	YES	YES	YES	YES	3	96+	YES
CASE	73	NO	YES	YES	YES	1	4	YES
CONTROL	72	NO	NO	NO	YES	2	90	YES
CONTROL	73	NO	NO	NO	YES	3	5	YES
CONTROL	73	NO	YES	NO	YES	1	15	YES
CONTROL	73	NO	YES	NO	NO	0	0	NO
CASE	71	NO	YES	YES	YES	1	UNK	YES
CONTROL	71	NO	NO	UNK	NO	0	0	NO
CONTROL	71	NO	NO	NO	NO	0	0	YES
CONTROL	71	NO	NO	NO	NO	0	0	YES
CONTROL	71	NO	YES	NO	YES	UNK	UNK	YES
CASE	64	NO	YES	YES	NO	0	0	YES
CONTROL	65	NO	NO	YES	YES	3	96+	YES
CONTROL	64	NO	NO	YES	YES	3	96+	YES
CONTROL	64	NO	NO	YES	YES	2	36	YES
CONTROL	64	NO	NO	YES	YES	3	96+	NO
CASE	63	NO	NO	NO	YES	UNK	96+	YES
CONTROL	64	NO	NO	YES	NO	0	0	YES
CONTROL	62	NO	NO	YES	NO	0	0	YES
CONTROL	64	YES	NO	NO	YES	1	18	NO
CONTROL	64	NO	YES	YES	YES	3	UNK	YES
CASE	79	YES	YES	YES	YES	1	96+	YES
CONTROL	78	YES	YES	YES	YES	1	96+	YES
CONTROL	79	NO	NO	YES	NO	0	0	YES
CONTROL	79	NO	YES	NO	YES	0	0	YES
CONTROL	78	NO	NO	YES	YES	1	24	YES

CASE OR CONTROL	AGE	GALL BLADDER DISEASE	HYPER TENSION	OBESITY	ESTROGEN (ANY) USE	CONJUGATED DOSE (SEE CODE)	ESTROGEN DURATION (MONTHS)	NON ESTROGEN DRUG
CASE	80	NO	NO	YES	YES	1	15	YES
CONTROL	81	NO	YES	YES	NO	0	0	YES
CONTROL	81	NO	YES	NO	YES	1	18	YES
CONTROL	80	NO	NO	YES	YES	2	74	YES
CONTROL	80	NO	YES	YES	NO	0	0	YES
CASE	82	NO	YES	YES	YES	2	6	YES
CONTROL	82	NO	NO	YES	NO	0	0	YES
CONTROL	81	NO	YES	UNK	NO	0	0	YES
CONTROL	81	NO	YES	YES	YES	1	12	YES
CONTROL	82	NO	YES	YES	YES	2	13	YES
CASE	71	NO	YES	NO	YES	UNK	84	YES
CONTROL	71	NO	YES	YES	NO	0	0	YES
CONTROL	71	YES	NO	YES	NO	0	0	YES
CONTROL	71	YES	NO	YES	YES	1	96+	YES
CONTROL	71	NO	NO	NO	YES	1	30	YES
CASE	83	NO	YES	YES	YES	3	14	YES
CONTROL	83	NO	YES	YES	NO	0	0	YES
CONTROL	83	NO	NO	NO	NO	0	0	YES
CONTROL	83	NO	YES	YES	YES	2	16	YES
CONTROL	83	NO	NO	NO	NO	0	0	YES
CASE	61	NO	YES	NO	YES	3	96+	YES
CONTROL	60	NO	NO	NO	NO	0	0	YES
CONTROL	61	NO	NO	NO	YES	1	24	YES
CONTROL	62	NO	NO	YES	NO	0	0	YES
CONTROL	61	NO	NO	NO	YES	0	0	YES
CASE	71	NO	NO	NO	YES	1	96+	YES
CONTROL	71	NO	NO	YES	NO	0	0	NO
CONTROL	71	NO	YES	YES	NO	0	0	NO
CONTROL	70	NO	NO	NO	NO	0	0	NO
CONTROL	71	NO	YES	YES	YES	1	3	YES
CASE	69	NO	YES	YES	YES	2	40	YES
CONTROL	69	YES	NO	YES	NO	0	0	YES
CONTROL	70	NO	YES	NO	YES	0	0	YES
CONTROL	70	NO	YES	NO	YES	1	32	YES
CONTROL	70	NO	NO	YES	YES	UNK	UNK	YES
CASE	77	NO	NO	YES	YES	3	73	YES
CONTROL	76	NO	YES	NO	YES	0	0	YES
CONTROL	76	NO	YES	YES	YES	0	0	YES
CONTROL	77	YES	YES	YES	YES	0	0	YES
CONTROL	77	NO	YES	NO	NO	0	0	YES
CASE	64	NO	NO	YES	YES	1	37	NO
CONTROL	64	NO	NO	YES	YES	3	6	NO
CONTROL	63	YES	NO	YES	NO	0	0	NO
CONTROL	63	NO	YES	NO	YES	UNK	UNK	YES
CONTROL	63	NO	YES	YES	NO	0	0	YES

CASE OR CONTROL	AGE	GALL BLADDER DISEASE	HYPER TENSION	OBESITY	ESTROGEN (ANY) USE	CONJUGATED DOSE (SEE CODE)	ESTROGEN DURATION (MONTHS)	NON ESTROGEN DRUG
CASE	79	YES	NO	NO	NO	0	0	NO
CONTROL	82	NO	NO	YES	YES	1	UNK	YES
CONTROL	78	NO	NO	NO	NO	0	0	NO
CONTROL	80	NO	NO	YES	NO	0	0	NO
CONTROL	81	NO	NO	NO	NO	0	0	NO
CASE	72	NO	NO	NO	YES	0	0	YES
CONTROL	72	NO	NO	YES	YES	2	57	YES
CONTROL	73	NO	NO	UNK	NO	0	0	NO
CONTROL	73	YES	YES	NO	YES	2	96+	YES
CONTROL	73	NO	NO	NO	NO	0	0	YES
CASE	82	YES	YES	YES	YES	3	96+	YES
CONTROL	81	NO	NO	UNK	NO	0	0	NO
CONTROL	81	NO	NO	YES	NO	0	0	NO
CONTROL	81	NO	NO	YES	YES	0	0	YES
CONTROL	81	NO	YES	YES	NO	0	0	YES
CASE	73	NO	YES	YES	YES	2	60	YES
CONTROL	74	NO	NO	YES	YES	1	1	YES
CONTROL	75	NO	NO	NO	NO	0	0	YES
CONTROL	75	NO	YES	YES	YES	1	96+	YES
CONTROL	74	NO	NO	NO	NO	0	0	NO
CASE	69	NO	NO	UNK	YES	UNK	UNK	YES
CONTROL	68	NO	NO	NO	NO	0	0	YES
CONTROL	68	NO	NO	YES	YES	2	48	YES
CONTROL	68	NO	NO	NO	YES	1	96+	NO
CONTROL	70	NO	NO	NO	NO	0	0	NO
CASE	79	NO	YES	YES	YES	1	67	YES
CONTROL	79	NO	YES	YES	NO	0	0	YES
CONTROL	79	NO	YES	YES	NO	0	0	YES
CONTROL	78	YES	NO	YES	YES	1	UNK	YES
CONTROL	79	NO	NO	YES	NO	0	0	YES
CASE	72	NO	NO	YES	YES	3	60	NO
CONTROL	71	NO	NO	NO	YES	0	0	YES
CONTROL	72	NO	NO	NO	NO	0	0	YES
CONTROL	72	NO	YES	YES	YES	3	96+	YES
CONTROL	71	NO	YES	YES	YES	3	12	YES
CASE	72	NO	YES	YES	YES	1	27	YES
CONTROL	72	NO	YES	YES	YES	1	3	YES
CONTROL	71	NO	NO	UNK	NO	0	0	NO
CONTROL	72	NO	YES	YES	NO	0	0	YES
CONTROL	72	NO	YES	YES	NO	0	0	YES
CASE	65	NO	YES	YES	YES	2	16	YES
CONTROL	67	NO	NO	NO	NO	0	0	NO
CONTROL	67	NO	NO	UNK	NO	0	0	NO
CONTROL	66	NO	NO	YES	NO	0	0	YES
CONTROL	66	NO	NO	NO	YES	2	3	NO

CASE OR CONTROL	AGE	GALL BLADDER DISEASE	HYPER TENSION	OBESITY	ESTROGEN (ANY) USE	CONJUGATED DOSE (SEE CODE)	ESTROGEN DURATION (MONTHS)	NON ESTROGEN DRUG
CASE	67	NO	YES	YES	YES	2	96+	YES
CONTROL	66	NO	NO	YES	YES	2	56	YES
CONTROL	66	NO	NO	YES	NO	0	0	NO
CONTROL	67	NO	NO	YES	YES	1	UNK	YES
CONTROL	67	NO	NO	YES	YES	2	34	YES
CASE	64	YES	NO	YES	YES	3	96+	YES
CONTROL	63	NO	NO	YES	NO	0	0	YES
CONTROL	64	NO	NO	YES	YES	1	4	YES
CONTROL	63	NO	NO	YES	NO	0	0	YES
CONTROL	65	NO	NO	UNK	NO	0	0	NO
CASE	62	NO	NO	UNK	YES	2	36	NO
CONTROL	63	NO	NO	YES	NO	0	0	NO
CONTROL	62	NO	NO	NO	NO	0	0	YES
CONTROL	62	NO	NO	UNK	YES	3	UNK	NO
CONTROL	62	NO	NO	UNK	NO	0	0	NO
CASE	83	YES	YES	UNK	NO	0	0	YES
CONTROL	83	YES	NO	UNK	NO	0	0	NO
CONTROL	82	NO	NO	NO	YES	2	6	YES
CONTROL	83	NO	NO	UNK	NO	0	0	YES
CONTROL	83	YES	NO	UNK	NO	0	0	YES
CASE	81	NO	NO	YES	YES	0	0	YES
CONTROL	79	NO	NO	UNK	NO	0	0	NO
CONTROL	80	NO	NO	YES	NO	0	0	YES
CONTROL	82	NO	NO	YES	NO	0	0	YES
CONTROL	80	NO	NO	NO	NO	0	0	NO
CASE	67	NO	NO	YES	YES	2	96+	YES
CONTROL	66	NO	NO	YES	YES	2	40	YES
CONTROL	68	NO	NO	UNK	NO	0	0	YES
CONTROL	65	NO	NO	NO	NO	0	0	YES
CONTROL	66	NO	YES	YES	YES	1	96+	YES
CASE	73	YES	YES	YES	YES	1	UNK	YES
CONTROL	72	NO	NO	YES	YES	1	12	YES
CONTROL	71	NO	NO	YES	YES	1	96+	YES
CONTROL	73	YES	NO	NO	YES	2	96+	YES
CONTROL	72	NO	NO	YES	NO	0	0	YES
CASE	67	YES	NO	NO	YES	3	96+	YES
CONTROL	67	YES	NO	YES	YES	2	96+	YES
CONTROL	68	NO	NO	YES	NO	0	0	NO
CONTROL	67	NO	NO	YES	NO	0	0	NO
CONTROL	67	NO	NO	YES	NO	0	0	YES
CASE	74	NO	YES	YES	YES	2	9	YES
CONTROL	75	NO	NO	NO	NO	0	0	YES
CONTROL	75	NO	NO	UNK	NO	0	0	NO
CONTROL	75	YES	YES	NO	NO	0	0	YES
CONTROL	75	NO	NO	NO	YES	2	41	YES
CASE	68	YES	NO	YES	YES	3	18	YES
CONTROL	69	NO	NO	YES	YES	2	96+	YES
CONTROL	70	NO	NO	UNK	NO	0	0	NO
CONTROL	69	NO	YES	YES	YES	2	92	YES
CONTROL	69	NO	YES	NO	YES	3	59	YES

APPENDIX IV
LISTING OF PROGRAM MATCH

The following main program and subroutine perform the conditional logistic regression analysis for matched sets consisting of a single case and a variable number of controls, as described in § 7.4. To illustrate how the program works we have input the data from the Los Angeles endometrial cancer study shown in Appendix III. Four different models were fit in hierarchical fashion using the variables GALL, OB, EST and GALL × EST (see Table 7.2). The last two of these correspond precisely to Models 4 and 8 of Table 7.7. Note the use of the SCORE statistic, calculated at the first iteration of each fit with the estimated regression coefficients from the previous model, to test the significance of the added variable(s).

The subprogram calls the IBM scientific subroutine SINV for inversion of symmetric matrices.

MAIN PROGRAM

(READS DATA, SETS UP RISK VARIABLES, CALLS SUBROUTINE)

```
C       MASTER MAIN
        DIMENSION NR(63),IVAR(6),W(6),EZB(6),
     *  Z(6,5,63),B(6),SCORE(6),COV(21),COVI(21)
C
C       DIMENSION IVAR(NM),NCA(NS),NCT(NS),IP(NMAX2),W(NM),WW(NM),
C     *Z(NM,NRMAX,NS),B(NM),SCORE(NM),COV(NM1),COVI(NM1)
C       SEE SUBROUTINE FOR DEFINITIONS
C
        DATA NR/63*5/,B/6*0.0/,IVAR/1,2,3,4,5,6/,NP/6/
        DATA NM,NRMAX,NIT,EPS/6,5,10,0.0001/
        NM1=NM*(NM+1)/2
        I-0
        READ(1,100) GALL,OB,EST
 1000   CONTINUE
 100    FORMAT(10X,F5.0,5X,F5.0,15X,F5.0)
C
C    I IS THE ORDER NUMBER OF THE SET
C
        I=I+1
        K=0
        DO 6 KK-1,5
        K=K+1
        Z(1,K,I)=2-GALL
        IF (OB.EQ.9)  OB=2
        Z(2,K,I)=2-OB
        Z(3,K,I)=2-EST
        Z(4,K,I)=(2-GALL)*(2-EST)
        Z(5,K,I)=(2-OB)*(2-EST)
        Z(6,K,I)=(2-GALL)*(2-OB)
        READ(1,100,END=2000) GALL,OB,EST
 6      CONTINUE
        GOTO 1000
 2000   CONTINUE
        NS = I
        DO 2 I=1,NP
        B(I)=0.0
 2      CALL MATCH(NS,NR,NRMAX,NM,I,NIT,B,Z,SCORE,COVI,COV,
     *  EZB,IVAR,NM1,EPS,W)
        STOP
        END
```

SUBPROGRAM MATCH

```
C
C     REFERENCES:
C     N. E. BRESLOW,N.E. DAY,K. T. HALVORSEN, R. L. PRENTICE,C. SABAI :
C       ESTIMATION OF MULTIPLE RELATIVE RISK FUNCTIONS IN MATCHED
C       CASE-CONTROL STUDIES. AMERICAN JOURNAL OF EPIDEMIOLOGY
C       VOL108,NO4, P 299-307 , 1978
C
C     THIS SUBROUTINE COMPUTES A LINEAR LOGISTIC REGRESSION ANALYSIS FOR
C     MATCHED SETS OF 1  CASE A VARIABLE NO. OF CONTROLS PER CASE
C     THE VARIABLES APPEARING IN THE CALL STATEMENT ARE DEFINED AS FOLLO
C     NS  NUMBER OF MATCHED SETS
C     NR  VECTOR OF NO. OF CONTROLS IN EACH SET + 1
C     NRMAX  (MAX NO. OF CONTROLS PER CASE)+1
C     NM  MAXIMUM NUMBER OF VARIABLES TO BE ANALYZED
C     NP  NUMBER OF VARIABLES ANALYZED IN THIS RUN
C     NIT   MAXIMUM NUMBER OF ITERATIONS OF THE NEWTON-RAPHSON TYPE
C     B  PARAMETER VECTOR OF LENGTH NM
C     Z  NM BY NRMAX BY NS MATRIX CONTAINING COVARIATES
C     SCORE FIRST DERIVATIVE OF THE LN-LIKELIHOOD OF LENGTH NM
C     COVI INFORMATION MATRIX(2ND DERIVATIVE OF LN-LIKELIHOOD)
C     COV INVERSE INFORMATION MATRIX(ESTIMATED COVARIANCE MATRIX)
C     EZB WORKING VECTOR OF LENGTH NRMAX
C     IVAR VECTOR OF VARIABLES USED IN THIS RUN (DIMENSION NM)
C     NM1 = NM*(NM+1)/2 DIMENSION OF COVI AND COV
C     EPS    CHANGE IN LIKELIHOOD BELOW WHICH ITERATION STOPS
C     W  WORKING VECTOR OF LENGTH NM
C
C     NOTE(Z,J,K,I) IS THE VALUE OF THE JTH COVARIATE FOR THE KTH
C     MEMBER IN THE ITH SET.IT IS ASSUMED THAT THE FIRST MEMBER IS THE
C     CASE AND THAT THE REMAINING NR(I)-1 MEMBERS ARE CONTROLS.
C
C     NOTE(Z MUST BE DIMENSIONED TO HAVE NM ROWS,NRMAX COLUMNS
C     AND AT LEAST NS SLICES IN THE MAIN PROGRAM,
C     COVI AND COV ARE ARRAYS OF LENGTH NM*(NM+1)/2 SINCE THEY USE
C     THE SYMMETRIC STORAGE MODE.
C
      SUBROUTINE MATCH(NS,NR,NRMAX,NM,NP,NIT,B,Z,SCORE,COVI,COV,
     * EZB,IVAR,NM1,EPS,W)
      DIMENSION Z(NM,NRMAX,NS),B(NM),EZB(NRMAX),SCORE(NM),COV(NM1),
     * COVI(NM1),IVAR(NM),NR(NS),W(NM)
      REAL LOGLIK
      DATA TEST/1.0/,ISUB/1/
      WRITE(6,100)
100   FORMAT(///' LOGISTIC REGRESSION ANALYSIS FOR MATCHED SETS',/)
      WRITE(6,101)NS
101   FORMAT(1H ,'NUMBER OF MATCHED SETS',I4)
      WRITE(6,102)((I,NR(I)),I=1,NS)
102   FORMAT(1H ,'SET NUMBER AND NUMBER OF MEMBERS',
     *' IN EACH SET,(INCLUDING CASE)',/,50(1X,10(I4,I3),/))
      WRITE(6,103)NP,(IVAR(J),J=1,NP)
```

```
103    FORMAT(1H ,'NUMBER OF VARIABLES IN THIS ANALYSIS=',I3,
      */,' THESE VARIABLES ARE NUMBERS',30I3)
       WRITE(6,104)NIT
104    FORMAT(1H ,'MAXIMUM NUMBER OF ITERATIONS',I4)
       WRITE(6,106)
106    FORMAT(' ITER  LOG-LIKELIHOOD   SCORE',8X,'PARAMETER ESTIMATES')
       ITS=0
       IF(ISUB.NE.1)GOTO 1
C      SUBTRACT VALUE OF COVARIATES FOR THE CASE  FROM THOSE OF CONTROLS
C      THIS ONLY NEEDS TO BE DONE AT THE FIRST CALL OF THE SUBROUTINE
       L=1
       DO 99 I=1,NS
       NRI=NR(I)
       DO 99 J=2,NRI
       DO 99 K=1,NM
       Z(K,J,I)=Z(K,J,I)-Z(K,L,I)
99     CONTINUE
       ISUB=0
1      CONTINUE
       ITS= ITS+1
C   CLEAR ARRAYS PRIOR TO NEXT ITERATION
       LOGLIK=0.0
       K=0
       DO 2 J=1,NP
       SCORE(J)=0.0
       DO 2 JJ=J,NP
       K=K+1
2      COVI(K)=0.0
C   CALCULATE LOGLIK,SCORE,COVI
       DO 7 I=1,NS
       DENOM=0.0
       NRI=NR(I)
       DO 4 K=2,NRI
       ZB=0.0
       DO 3 J=1,NP
       L=IVAR(J)
3      ZB=ZB+B(J)*Z(L,K,I)
       EZB(K)=EXP(ZB)
4      DENOM=DENOM+EZB(K)
       DENOM=1.0+DENOM
       LOGLIK=LOGLIK-ALOG(DENOM)
       KJ=0
       DO 7 J=1,NP
       L=IVAR(J)
       EZJ=0.0
       NRI=NR(I)
       DO 5 K=2,NRI
5      EZJ=EZJ+EZB(K)*Z(L,K,I)
       SCORE(J)=SCORE(J)-EZJ/DENOM
```

```
        DO 7 JJ=1,J
        LL=IVAR(JJ)
        EZJJ=0.0
        EZZ=0.0
        NRI=NR(I)
        DO 6 K=2,NRI
        EZJJ=EZJJ+EZB(K)*Z(LL,K,I)
6       EZZ=EZB(K)*Z(L,K,I)*Z(LL,K,I)+EZZ
        KJ=KJ+1
        COVI(KJ)=COVI(KJ)+(EZZ/DENOM)-EZJ*EZJJ/(DENOM*DENOM)
7       CONTINUE
        DO 500 I=1,NM1
        COV(I)=COVI(I)
500     CONTINUE
        CALL SINV(COV,NP,EPS,IER)
        IF (IER.NE.0) WRITE (6,501)IER
501     FORMAT(" IER = ',I3)
        TEMP=0.0
        K=0
        DO 51 J=1,NP
        DO 51 JJ=1,J
        K=K+1
        G=1.0
        IF (J.NE.JJ) G=2.0
        TEMP=TEMP+G*SCORE(J)*SCORE(JJ)*COV(K)
 51     CONTINUE
C  WRITE OUT ITERATION NUMBER AND LOG-LIKELIHOOD AND B'S
        WRITE(6,107)ITS,LOGLIK,TEMP,(B(J),J=1,NP)
107     FORMAT(1X,I4,F14.4,F11.3,2X,8F12.4,20(/,21X,8F12.4)
C  TEST FOR CONVERGENCE
        TEST=ABS(TEST-LOGLIK)
        IF(TEST.LE.EPS.OR.ITS.GE.NIT)GO TO 9
        TEST=LOGLIK
C  CALCULATE NEW VALUE OF PARAMETER ESTIMATE AND REPEAT
C       CALL SYMINV(COVI,NP,COV,W,NULLTY,IFAULT,NM1)
        DO 180 I=1,NP
        W(I)=0.0
        DO 181 J=1,I
        K=I*(I-1)/2+J
181     W(I)=W(I)+SCORE(J)*COV(K)
        I1=I+1
        IF(I1.GT.NP)GOTO 180
        DO 182 K=I1,NP
        J=K*(K-1)/2+I
182     W(I)=W(I)+SCORE(K)*COV(J)
180     CONTINUE
        DO 183 I=1,NP
183     SCORE(I)=W(I)
        DO 8 J=1,NP
8       B(J)=B(J)+SCORE(J)
```

```
C   UPON CONVERGENCE OF MAXIMUM ITERATIONS WRITE OUT RESULTS
        GO TO 1
9       WRITE(6,108)(B(J),J=1,NP)
108     FORMAT(' ESTIMATED PARAMETER VECTOR',(/1X,10F12.6))
        WRITE(6,109)(SCORE(J),J=1,NP)
109     FORMAT(' FIRST DERIVATIVE LOG-LIKELIHOOD',(/1X,10F12.6))
        WRITE(6,110)
110     FORMAT(' INFORMATION MATRIX')
        DO 10 J=1,NP
        K=J*(J-1)/2+1
        JJ=J*(J+1)/2
10      WRITE(6,111) (COVI(I),I=K,JJ)
111     FORMAT(1X,10F12.6)
C   INVERT INFORMATION MATRIX AND WRITE OUT
C       CALL SYMINV(COVI,NP,COV,W,NULLTY,IFAULT,NM1)
        DO 600 I=1,NM1
        COV(I)=COVI(I)
600     CONTINUE
        CALL SINV(COV,NP,EPS,IER)
        IF (IER.NE.0) WRITE (6,501)IER
        WRITE(6,112)
112     FORMAT(' ESTIMATED COVARIANCE MATRIX')
        DO 11 J=1,NP
        K=J*(J-1)/2+1
        JJ=J*(J+1)/2
        SCORE(J)=B(J)/SQRT(COV(JJ))
11      WRITE(6,111)(COV(I),I=K,JJ)
        WRITE(6,113)(SCORE(J),J=1,NP)
113     FORMAT(' STANDARDIZED REGRESSION COEFFICIENTS',(/1X,100F12.6))
        RETURN
        END
```

MODEL WITH SINGLE VARIABLE: GALL

LOGISTIC REGRESSION ANALYSIS FOR MATCHED SETS

NUMBER OF MATCHED SETS 63
SET NUMBER AND NUMBER OF MEMBERS IN EACH SET,(INCLUDING CASE)

1	5	2	5	3	5	4	5	5	5	6	5	7	5	8	5	9	5	10	5
11	5	12	5	13	5	14	5	15	5	16	5	17	5	18	5	19	5	20	5
21	5	22	5	23	5	24	5	25	5	26	5	27	5	28	5	29	5	30	5
31	5	32	5	33	5	34	5	35	5	36	5	37	5	38	5	39	5	40	5
41	5	42	5	43	5	44	5	45	5	46	5	47	5	48	5	49	5	50	5
51	5	52	5	53	5	54	5	55	5	56	5	57	5	58	5	59	5	60	5
61	5	62	5	63	5														

NUMBER OF VARIABLES IN THIS ANALYSIS = 1
THESE VARIABLES ARE NUMBERS   1
MAXIMUM NUMBER OF ITERATIONS 10

ITER	LOG-LIKELIHOOD	SCORE	PARAMETER ESTIMATES
1	-101.3945	13.829	0.0
2	-95.6566	0.512	1.5714
3	-95.4043	0.000	1.3011
4	-95.4043	0.000	1.3061

ESTIMATED PARAMETER VECTOR
     1.306142
FIRST DERIVATIVE LOG-LIKELIHOOD
     0.000010
INFORMATION MATRIX
     7.232518
ESTIMATED COVARIANCE MATRIX
     0.138264
STANDARDIZED REGRESSION COEFFICIENTS
     3.512652

MODEL WITH 2 VARIABLES: GALL + OB

LOGISTIC REGRESSION ANALYSIS FOR MATCHED SETS

NUMBER OF MATCHED SETS 63
SET NUMBER AND NUMBER OF MEMBERS IN EACH SET,(INCLUDING CASE)

1	5	2	5	3	5	4	5	5	5	6	5	7	5	8	5	9	5	10	5
11	5	12	5	13	5	14	5	15	5	16	5	17	5	18	5	19	5	20	5
21	5	22	5	23	5	24	5	25	5	26	5	27	5	28	5	29	5	30	5
31	5	32	5	33	5	34	5	35	5	36	5	37	5	38	5	39	5	40	5
41	5	42	5	43	5	44	5	45	5	46	5	47	5	48	5	49	5	50	5
51	5	52	5	53	5	54	5	55	5	56	5	57	5	58	5	59	5	60	5
61	5	62	5	63	5														

NUMBER OF VARIABLES IN THIS ANALYSIS = 2
THESE VARIABLES ARE NUMBERS 1 2
MAXIMUM NUMBER OF ITERATIONS 10

ITER	LOG-LIKELIHOOD	SCORE	PARAMETER ESTIMATES	
1	−95.4043	5.031	1.3061	0.0
2	−92.8562	0.016	1.2673	0.7044
3	−92.8483	0.000	1.3085	0.7254
4	−92.8484	0.000	1.3086	0.7255

ESTIMATED PARAMETER VECTOR
    1.308584   0.725526
FIRST DERIVATIVE LOG-LIKELIHOOD
    −0.000000   0.000001
INFORMATION MATRIX
    7.115846
    −0.413175   9.369903
ESTIMATED COVARIANCE MATRIX
    0.140892
    0.006213   0.106999
STANDARDIZED REGRESSION COEFFICIENTS
    3.486248   2.218012

MODEL WITH 3 VARIABLES: GALL + OB + EST
(model 4, Table 7.7)

LOGISTIC REGRESSION ANALYSIS FOR MATCHED SETS

NUMBER OF MATCHED SETS 63
SET NUMBER AND NUMBER OF MEMBERS IN EACH SET,(INCLUDING CASE)

1	5	2	5	3	5	4	5	5	5	6	5	7	5	8	5	9	5	10	5
11	5	12	5	13	5	14	5	15	5	16	5	17	5	18	5	19	5	20	5
21	5	22	5	23	5	24	5	25	5	26	5	27	5	28	5	29	5	30	5
31	5	32	5	33	5	34	5	35	5	36	5	37	5	38	5	39	5	40	5
41	5	42	5	43	5	44	5	45	5	46	5	47	5	48	5	49	5	50	5
51	5	52	5	53	5	54	5	55	5	56	5	57	5	58	5	59	5	60	5
61	5	62	5	63	5														

NUMBER OF VARIABLES IN THIS ANALYSIS = 3
THESE VARIABLES ARE NUMBERS 1 2 3
MAXIMUM NUMBER OF ITERATIONS 10

ITER	LOG-LIKELIHOOD	SCORE	PARAMETER ESTIMATES		
1	-92.8484	26.837	1.3086	0.7255	0.0
2	-78.4750	1.213	1.0256	0.4851	1.6166
3	-77.8264	0.017	1.2543	0.5086	1.9860
4	-77.8179	0.000	1.2746	0.5113	2.0394
5	-77.8179	0.000	1.2748	0.5113	2.0403

ESTIMATED PARAMETER VECTOR
    1.274839   0.511342   2.040298
FIRST DERIVATIVE LOG-LIKELIHOOD
    0.000004   0.000002   0.000004
INFORMATION MATRIX
    5.996700
   -0.295261   7.917870
   -0.581349   0.554122   5.222640
ESTIMATED COVARIANCE MATRIX
    0.168775
    0.005016   0.127390
    0.018255   -0.012958   0.194881
STANDARDIZED REGRESSION COEFFICIENTS
    3.103139   1.432659   4.621776

MODEL WITH 4 VARIABLES: GALL + OB + EST + GALL×EST

(model 8, Table 7.5)

LOGISTIC REGRESSION ANALYSIS FOR MATCHED SETS

NUMBER OF MATCHED SETS   63
SET NUMBER AND NUMBER OF MEMBERS IN EACH SET,(INCLUDING CASE)

1	5	2	5	3	5	4	5	5	5	6	5	7	5	8	5	9	5	10	5
11	5	12	5	13	5	14	5	15	5	16	5	17	5	18	5	19	5	20	5
21	5	22	5	23	5	24	5	25	5	26	5	27	5	28	5	29	5	30	5
31	5	32	5	33	5	34	5	35	5	36	5	37	5	38	5	39	5	40	5
41	5	42	5	43	5	44	5	45	5	46	5	47	5	48	5	49	5	50	5
51	5	52	5	53	5	54	5	55	5	56	5	57	5	58	5	59	5	60	5
61	5	62	5	63	5														

NUMBER OF VARIABLES IN THIS ANALYSIS = 4
THESE VARIABLES ARE NUMBERS   1   2   3   4
MAXIMUM NUMBER OF ITERATIONS   10

ITER	LOG-LIKELIHOOD	SCORE	PARAMETER ESTIMATES			
1	−77.8179	4.392	1.2748	0.5113	2.0403	0.0
2	−75.9031	0.221	3.0331	0.4859	2.5096	−2.2027
3	−75.7909	0.000	2.8467	0.4901	2.6172	−2.0003
4	−75.7910	0.000	2.8446	0.4901	2.6206	−1.9975

ESTIMATED PARAMETER VECTOR
     2.844563   0.490130   2.620620   −1.997451
FIRST DERIVATIVE LOG-LIKELIHOOD
    −0.000001   0.000004   0.000020   0.000006
INFORMATION MATRIX
      6.692919
     −0.287091   7.667604
     −1.389089   0.432648   4.504435
      4.758762   −0.133908   0.584442   4.981014
ESTIMATED COVARIANCE MATRIX
      0.774399
     −0.003830   0.131275
      0.340368   −0.014950   0.376377
     −0.779885   0.008943   −0.369744   0.989473
STANDARDIZED REGRESSION COEFFICIENTS
      3.232460   1.352757   4.271620   −2.008047

APPENDIX V
LISTING OF PROGRAM STRAT

The following main program and subroutine perform the conditional logistic regression analysis for matched sets consisting of a variable number of cases and a variable number of controls, using the general likelihood (7.1). It was written by Mr Peter Smith as a generalization of the program MATCH. To illustrate its operation we have used exactly the same data as used with MATCH, namely those corresponding to several of the models in Table 7.7. Slight differences in the numerical output are due to the use of different computing formulae.

The program is completely self-contained, with the subroutines SYMINV, CHOL, and TWIDL which it calls being listed also.

APPENDIX V

MAIN PROGRAM

```
      DIMENSION NCT(63),NCA(63),IVAR(6),IP(7),W(20),WW(20),
     : Z(6,5,63)   ,B(6),SCORE(6),COV(21),COVI(21)
      DATA NCA/63*1/,NCT/63*4/,NS,NM,NMAX,NIT,EPS/63,6,5,10,0.0001/
      DATA B/6*0.0/,IVAR/1,2,3,4,5,6/,NP/6/
      NMAX2=NMAX+2
      NM1=NM*(NM+1)/2
      DO 6 I=1,NS
      N=NCT(I)+NCA(I)
      DO 6 J=1,N
      L=N+1-J
      READ(1,100) GALL,OB,EST
 100  FORMAT(10X,F5.0,5X,F5.0,15X,F5.0)
      Z(1,L,I)=2-GALL
      IF (OB.EQ.9) OB=2
      Z(2,L,I)=2-OB
      Z(3,L,I)=2-EST
      Z(4,L,I)=(2-GALL)*(2-EST)
      Z(5,L,I)=(2-OB)*(2-EST)
      Z(6,L,I)=(2-GALL)*(2-OB)
 6    CONTINUE
      DO 2 I=1,NP
      B(I)=0.0
 2    CALL STRAT(NS,NCA,NCT,NMAX,NM,I,NIT,B,Z,SCORE,COVI,COV,
     :IVAR,EPS,NM1,W,WW,IP,NMAX2)
 99   STOP
      END
```

SUBPROGRAM STRAT

```
      SUBROUTINE STRAT(NS,NCA,NCT,NMAX,NM,NP,NIT,B,Z,SCORE,COVI,COV,
     *IVAR,EPS,NM1,W,WW,IP,NMAX2)
C     THIS SUBROUTINE COMPUTES A LINEAR LOGISTIC REGRESSION ANALYSIS
C     FOR STRATIFIED SETS CONSISTING OF NCA(I) CASES AND NCT(I) CONTROLS
C     THE ITH STRATUM
C     THE VARIABLES APPEARING INTHE CALL STATEMENT ARE DEFINED AS FOLLO
C     NS   NUMBER OF STRATA
C     NCA  VECTOR OF THE NUMBER OF CASES IN EACH STRATUM
C     NCT  VECTOR OF THE NUMBER OF CONTROLS IN EACH STRATUM
C     NMAX MAXIMUM NUMBER OF CASES + CONTROLS IN ANY STRATUM
C     NM   MAXIMUM NUMBER OF VARIABLES TO BE ANALYSED
C     NP   NUMBER OF VARIABLES TO BE ANALYSED IN THIS RUN
C     NIT  MAXIMUM NUMBER OF ITERATIONS OF THE NEWTON-RAPHSON TYPE
C     B    PARAMETER VECTOR OF LENGTH NM
C     Z    NM BY NMAX BY NS MATRIX CONTAINING COVARIATES
C     SCORE FIRST DERIVATIVE OF THE LN-LIKELIHOOD OF LENGTH NM
C     COVI INFORMATION MATRIX (2ND DERIVATIVE OF LN-LIKELIHOOD)
C     COV  INVERSE INFORMATION MATRIX : ESTIMATED COVARIANCE MATRIX
C     IVAR VECTOR OF VARIABLE NUMBERS USED IN THIS RUN
C     EPS  CHANGE IN LIKELIHOOD BELOW WHICH ITERATION STOPS
C     NM1  NM*(NM+1)/2
C     WW   WORKING VECTOR OF LENGTH NM
C     IP   WORKING VECTOR OF LENGTH NMAX2
C     NMAX2 NMAX+2
C     NOTE: IN THE ARRAY Z INDIVIDUALS ARE INDEXED BY THE 2ND
C     SUBSCRIPT,WITHIN EACH STRATUM DATA ON CONTROLS MUST BE STORED
C     FIRST FOLLOWED BY THOSE ON CASES.
```

```
C   REFERENCES:
C    N. E.BRESLOW, N.E. DAY, K. T. HALVORSEN,R. L. PRENTICE,C. SABAI:
C       ESTIMATION OF MULTIPLE RELATIVE RISK FUNCTIONS IN MATCHED
C          CASE CONTROL STUDIES . AM. J EPIDEMIOL 108:299-307, 1978
        DIMENSION Z(NM,NMAX,NS),B(NM),SCORE(NM),COV(NM1),COVI(NM1)
       *,IVAR(NM),NCA(NS),NCT(NS),W(NM),WW(NM),IP(NMAX2)
        REAL LOGLIK
        DATA TEST/1.0/
        WRITE(6,100)
100     FORMAT(1H1,///' LOGISTIC REGRESSION ANALYSIS IN STRATA',/)
        WRITE(6,101)NS
101     FORMAT(1H ,'NUMBER OF STRATA',I4)
        WRITE(6,102)(I,NCA(I),NCT(I),I=1,NS)
102     FORMAT(1H ,'STRATUM NUMBER AND NUMBERS OF CASES AND CONTROLS',
       *50(1X,10(I4,I3,I3),/))
        WRITE(6,103)NP,(IVAR(J),J=1,NP)
103     FORMAT(1H ,'NUMBER OF VARIABLES IN THIS ANALYSIS',I3,/,
       *' THESE VARIABLES ARE',30I3)
        WRITE(6,104)NIT
104     FORMAT(1H ,'MAXIMUM NUMBER OF ITERATIONS',I4)
        WRITE(6,106)
106     FORMAT(1H ,'ITER LOG-LIKELIHOOD  SCORE   PARAMETER ESTIMATES')
        ITS=0
1       ITS=ITS+1
        LOGLIK=0.0
        K=0
        DO 2 J=1,NP
        SCORE(J)=0.0
        DO 2 JJ=1,J
        K=K+1
2       COVI(K)=0.0
C       CALCULATE LOGLIK,SCORE AND COVI
        DO 27 I=1,NS
        IFG=0
        SX=0.0
        K=0
        DO 8 J=1,NP
        W(J)=0.0
        WW(J)=0.0
        DO 8 JJ=1,J
        K=K+1
8       COV(K)=0.0
        M=NCA(I)
        N=M+NCT(I)
        XX=1.0
        X=0.0
        IP(1)=N+1
        IP(N+2)=-2
        NMX=N-M+1
        DO 30 J=2,NMX
```

```
30      IP(J)=0
        DO 31 J=1,M
31      IP(NMX+J)=J
        KK=N-M+1
        DO 12 J=KK,N
        DO 12 K=1,NP
        L=IVAR(K)
        W(K)=W(K)+Z(L,J,I)
12      X=X+B(K)*Z(L,J,I)
11      XX=EXP(X)
        SX=SX+XX
        IF(IFG.NE.0)GOTO 13
        LOGLIK=LOGLIK+ALOG(SX)
        DO 17 K=1,NP
17      SCORE(K)=SCORE(K)+W(K)
        IFG=1
13      L=0
        DO 14 K=1,NP
        WW(K)=WW(K)+XX*W(K)
        DO 14 KK=1,K
        L=L+1
14      COV(L)=COV(L)+XX*W(K)*W(KK)
        ID=0
        CALL TWIDL(IPS,IM,IZ,ID,IP,NMAX2)
        IF(ID.EQ.1)GOTO 20
        DO 15 K=1,NP
        L=IVAR(K)
        ZC=Z(L,IPS,I)-Z(L,IM,I)
        W(K)=W(K)+ZC
15      X=X+B(K)*ZC
        GOTO 11
20      LOGLIK=LOGLIK-ALOG(SX)
        L=0
        DO 21 J=1,NP
        SCORE(J)=SCORE(J)-WW(J)/SX
        DO 21 K=1,J
        L=L+1
21      COVI(L)=COVI(L)+(SX*COV(L)-WW(J)*WW(K))/SX**2
27      CONTINUE
```

```
        CALL SYMINV(COVI,NP,COV,W,NULLTY,IFAULT,NM1)
        TEMP=0 .0
        K=0
        DO 51 J=1,NP
        DO 51 JJ=1,J
        K=K+1
        G=1.0
        IF (J.NE.JJ) G=2.0
        TEMP=TEMP+G*SCORE(J)*SCORE(JJ)*COV(K)
51      CONTINUE
C       WRITE OUT ITERATION NUMBER AND LOG-LIKELIHOOD AND B'S
        WRITE (6,107)ITS,LOGLIK,TEMP,(B(J),J=1,NP)
107     FORMAT(1X,I4,F14.4,F11.3,2X,8F12.4,20(/,21X,8F12.4))
C       TEST FOR CONVERGENCE
        TEST=ABS(TEST-LOGLIK)
        IF (TEST.LE.EPS.OR.ITS.GE.NIT)GOTO 9
        TEST=LOGLIK
C       CALCULATE NEW VALUE OF PARAMETER ESTIMATE AND REPEAT
        DO 180 I=1,NP
        W(I)=0.0
        DO 181 J=1,I
        K=I*(I-1)/2+J
181     W(I)=W(I)+SCORE(J)*COV(K)
        I1=I+1
        IF(I1.GT.NP)GOTO 180
        DO 182 K=I1,NP
        J=K*(K-1)/2+I
182     W(I)=W(I)+SCORE(K)*COV(J)
180     CONTINUE
        DO 183 I=1,NP
183     SCORE(I)=W(I)
        DO 18 J=1,NP
18      B(J)=B(J)+SCORE(J)
C       UPON CONVERGENCE OR MAXIMUM ITERATIONS WRITE OUT RESULTS
        GOTO 1
9       WRITE(6,108)(B(J),J=1,NP)
108     FORMAT(1H0,'ESTIMATED PARAMETER VECTOR',(/1X,10F12.6))
        WRITE(6,109)(SCORE(J),J=1,NP)
109     FORMAT(1H0,'FIRST DERIVATIVE LOG-LIKELIHOOD',(/1X,10F12.6))
        WRITE(6,110)
110     FORMAT(1H0,'INFORMATION MATRIX')
        DO 10 J=1,NP
        K=J*(J-1)/2+1
        JJ=J*(J+1)/2
10      WRITE (6,111) (COVI(I),I=K,JJ)
111     FORMAT(1X,10F12.6)
C       INVERT INFORMATION MATRIX AND WRITE OUT
        CALL SYMINV(COVI,NP,COV,W,NULLTY,IFAULT,NM1)
        WRITE(6,112)
```

```
112     FORMAT(1H0,'ESTIMATED COVARIANCE MATRIX')
        DO 19 J=1,NP
        K=J*(J-1)/2+1
        JJ=J*(J+1)/2
        SCORE(J)=B(J)/SQRT(COV(JJ))
19      WRITE(6,111)(COV(I),I=K,JJ)
        WRITE(6,113)(SCORE(J),J=1,NP)
113     FORMAT(1H0,'STNDIZED REGRESSION COEFFICIENTS',(/1X,100F12.6))
        RETURN
        END
```

```
        SUBROUTINE SYMINV(A,N,C,W,NULLTY,IFAULT,NFAC)
        DIMENSION A(NFAC),C(NFAC),W(N)
C
C       ALGORITHM AS7 J.R. STATIST.SOC.C.(1968) VOL.17,NO.2
C
        NROW=N
        IFAULT=1
        IF(NROW.LE.0)GOTO 100
        IFAULT=0
        CALL CHOL(A,NROW,C,NULLTY,IFAULT,NFAC)
        IF(IFAULT.NE.0)GOTO 100
        NN=(NROW*(NROW+1))/2
        IROW=NROW
        NDIAG=NN
16      IF(C(NDIAG).EQ.090)GOTO 11
        L=NDIAG
        DO 10 I=IROW,NROW
        W(I)=C(L)
        L=L+1
10      CONTINUE
        ICOL=NROW
        JCOL=NN
        MDIAG=NN
15      L=JCOL
        X=0.0
        IF(ICOL.EQ.IROW)X=1.0/W(IROW)
        K=NROW
13      IF(K.EQ.IROW)GOTO12
        X=X-W(K)*C(L)
        K=K-1
        L=L-1
        IF(L.GT.MDIAG)L=L-K+1
        GOTO 13
12      C(L)=X/W(IROW)
        IF(ICOL.EQ.IROW)GOTO 14
        MDIAG=MDIAG-ICOL
        ICOL=ICOL-1
        JCOL=JCOL-1
        GOTO 15
11      L=NDIAG
        DO 17 J=IROW,NROW
        C(L)=0.0
        L=L+J
17      CONTINUE
14      NDIAG=NDIAG-IROW
        IROW=IROW-1
        IF(IROW.NE.0)GOTO 16
100     RETURN
        END
```

```
      SUBROUTINE CHOL(A,N,U,NULLTY,IFAULT,NFAC)
      DIMENSION A(NFAC),U(NFAC)
      REAL ETA
      DATA ETA/0.000001/
C
C     ALGORITHM AS6 J.R.STATIS. SOC. C. (1968). VOL.17, NO.2
C
      IFAULT=1
      IF(N.LE.0)GOTO 100
      IFAULT=2
      NULLTY=0
      J=1
      K=0
      DO 10 ICOL=1,N
      L=0
      DO 11 IROW=1,ICOL
      K=K+1
      W=A(K)
      M=J
      DO 12 I=1,IROW
      L=L+1
      IF(I.EQ.IROW-GOTO 13
      W=W-U(L)::U(M)
      M=M+1
12    CONTINUE
13    IF(IROW.EQ.ICOL)GOTO 14
      IF(U(L).EQ.0.0)GOTO 21
      U(K)=W/U(L)
      GOTO 11
21    U(K)=0.0
11    CONTINUE
14    IF(ABS(W).LT.ABS(ETA::A(K))) GOTO 20
      IF(W.LT.0.0)GOTO 100
      U(K)=SQRT(W)
      GOTO 15
20    U(K)=0.0
      NULLTY=NULLTY+1
15    J=J+ICOL
10    CONTINUE
      IFAULT=0
100   RETURN
      END
```

```
      SUBROUTINE TWIDL(X,Y,Z,DONE,P,N2)
      INTEGER X,Y,Z,DONE,N2,P(N2)
C
C     THIS SUBROUTINE IS A FORTRAN VERSION OF CACM 382
C     FOR SELECTING ALL POSSIBLE COMBINATIONS OF M THINGS
C     OUT OF N OBJECTS.OUTSIDE OF THE SUBROUTINE
C     INITIALLY SET P(1)=N+1,P(N+2)=-2,P(2) TO
C     P(N-M+1-)0,P(N-M+2) TO P(N+1)=1 TO M
C     RESPECTIVELY.IF M=0,P(2)=1
C     INITIALLY SET DONE =0 AND THE S/R SETS THIS TO
C     1 WHEN ALL COMBINATIONS HAVE BEEN SELECTED
C     SUPPOSE THE N OBJECTS ARE IN A(1:N) AND
C     SUCCESSIVE COMBINATIONS ARE STORED IN C(1:M)
C     INITIALLY SET C(1) TO C(M)=A(N-M+1) TO A(N)
C     THEN CALL TWIDL IF DONE=1 ALL COMBINATIONS
C     HAVE BEEN GENERATED,OTHERWISE SET C(Z)=A(X)
C     ALTERNATIVELY STORE (N-M) 0'S AND M 1'S IN
C     B(1:N) IN THAT ORDER THEN CALL TWIDL.
C     IF DONE.NE.1 SET B(X)=1 AND B(Y)=0
C     AND CONTINUE IN THIS WAY UNTIL DONE=1
C
      J=0
1     J=J+1
      IF(P(J+1).LE.0)GOTO 1
      IF(P(J).NE.0)GOTO 5
      J1=J-1
      IF(J1.LT.2)GOTO 6
      DO 7 I=2,J1
      K=J1-I+2
7     P(K+1)=-1
6     P(J+1)=0
      P(2)=1
      X=1
      Z=1
      Y=J
      GOTO 4
5     CONTINUE
      IF(J.GT.1)P(J)=0
2     J=J+1
      IF(P(J+1).GT.0)GOTO 2
      I=J-1
      K=J-1
3     I=I+1
      IF(P(I+1).NE.0)GOTO 8
      P(I+1)=-1
      GOTO 3
8     CONTINUE
```

```
        IF(P(I+1).NE.-1)GOTO 9
        P(I+1)=P(K+1)
        Z=P(K+1)
        X=I
        Y=K
        P(K+1)=-1
        GOTO 4
9       CONTINUE
        IF(I.NE.P(1)) GOTO 10
        DONE=1
        GOTO 4
10      Z=P(I+1)
        P(J+1)=Z
        P(I+1)=0
        X=J
        Y=I
4       RETURN
        END
```

MODEL WITH SINGLE VARIABLE: GALL

LOGISTIC REGRESSION ANALYSIS IN STRATA

NUMBER OF STRATA 63
STRATUM NUMBER AND NUMBERS OF CASES AND CONTROLS

1	1	4	2	1	4	3	1	4	4	1	4	5	1	4	6	1	4	7	1	4	8	1	4
9	1	4	10	1	4	11	1	4	12	1	4	13	1	4	14	1	4	15	1	4	16	1	4
17	1	4	18	1	4	19	1	4	20	1	4	21	1	4	22	1	4	23	1	4	24	1	4
25	1	4	26	1	4	27	1	4	28	1	4	29	1	4	30	1	4	31	1	4	32	1	4
33	1	4	34	1	4	35	1	4	36	1	4	37	1	4	38	1	4	39	1	4	40	1	4
41	1	4	42	1	4	43	1	4	44	1	4	45	1	4	46	1	4	47	1	4	48	1	4
49	1	4	50	1	4	51	1	4	52	1	4	53	1	4	54	1	4	55	1	4	56	1	4
57	1	4	58	1	4	59	1	4	60	1	4	61	1	4	62	1	4	63	1	4			

NUMBER OF VARIABLES IN THIS ANALYSIS 1
THESE VARIABLES ARE 1
MAXIMUM NUMBER OF ITERATIONS 10

ITER	LOG-LIKELIHOOD	SCORE	PARAMETER ESTIMATES
1	-101.3945	13.829	0.0
2	-95.6567	0.512	1.5714
3	-95.4042	0.000	1.3011
4	-95.4041	0.000	1.3061
5	-95.4041	0.000	1.3061

ESTIMATED PARAMETER VECTOR
    1.306143
FIRST DERIVATIVE LOG-LIKELIHOOD
    0.000002
INFORMATION MATRIX
    7.232529
ESTIMATED COVARIANCE MATRIX
    0.138264
STNDIZED REGRESSION COEFFICIENTS
    3.512656

MODEL WITH 2 VARIABLES: GALL + OB

LOGISTIC REGRESSION ANALYSIS IN STRATA

NUMBER OF STRATA 63
STRATUM NUMBER AND NUMBERS OF CASES AND CONTROLS
```
 1  1  4   2  1  4   3  1  4   4  1  4   5  1  4   6  1  4   7  1  4   8  1  4
 9  1  4  10  1  4  11  1  4  12  1  4  13  1  4  14  1  4  15  1  4  16  1  4
17  1  4  18  1  4  19  1  4  20  1  4  21  1  4  22  1  4  23  1  4  24  1  4
25  1  4  26  1  4  27  1  4  28  1  4  29  1  4  30  1  4  31  1  4  32  1  4
33  1  4  34  1  4  35  1  4  36  1  4  37  1  4  38  1  4  39  1  4  40  1  4
41  1  4  42  1  4  43  1  4  44  1  4  45  1  4  46  1  4  47  1  4  48  1  4
49  1  4  50  1  4  51  1  4  52  1  4  53  1  4  54  1  4  55  1  4  56  1  4
57  1  4  58  1  4  59  1  4  60  1  4  61  1  4  62  1  4  63  1  4
```
NUMBER OF VARIABLES IN THIS ANALYSIS 2
THESE VARIABLES ARE 1 2
MAXIMUM NUMBER OF ITERATIONS 10

ITER	LOG-LIKELIHOOD	SCORE	PARAMETER ESTIMATES	
1	-95.4041	5.031	1.3061	0.0
2	-92.8559	0.016	1.2673	0.7044
3	-92.8481	0.000	1.3085	0.7254
4	-92.8483	0.000	1.3086	0.7255
5	-92.8483	0.000	1.3086	0.7255

ESTIMATED PARAMETER VECTOR
     1.308584   0.725525
FIRST DERIVATIVE LOG-LIKELIHOOD
    -0.000006   0.000004
INFORMATION MATRIX
     7.115862
    -0.413175   9.369920
ESTIMATED COVARIANCE MATRIX
     0.140892
     0.006213   0.106998
STNDIZED REGRESSION COEFFICIENTS
     3.486253   2.218013

MODEL WITH 3 VARIABLES: GALL + OB + EST

(Model 4, Table 7.7)

LOGISTIC REGRESSION ANALYSIS IN STRATA

NUMBER OF STRATA 63
STRATUM NUMBER AND NUMBERS OF CASES AND CONTROLS
```
  1  1  4    2  1  4    3  1  4    4  1  4    5  1  4    6  1  4    7  1  4    8  1  4
  9  1  4   10  1  4   11  1  4   12  1  4   13  1  4   14  1  4   15  1  4   16  1  4
 17  1  4   18  1  4   19  1  4   20  1  4   21  1  4   22  1  4   23  1  4   24  1  4
 25  1  4   26  1  4   27  1  4   28  1  4   29  1  4   30  1  4   31  1  4   32  1  4
 33  1  4   34  1  4   35  1  4   36  1  4   37  1  4   38  1  4   39  1  4   40  1  4
 41  1  4   42  1  4   43  1  4   44  1  4   45  1  4   46  1  4   47  1  4   48  1  4
 49  1  4   50  1  4   51  1  4   52  1  4   53  1  4   54  1  4   55  1  4   56  1  4
 57  1  4   58  1  4   59  1  4   60  1  4   61  1  4   62  1  4   63  1  4
```
NUMBER OF VARIABLES IN THIS ANALYSIS 3
THESE VARIABLES ARE   1 2 3
MAXIMUM NUMBER OF ITERATIONS   10
```
ITER   LOG-LIKELIHOOD   SCORE    PARAMETER ESTIMATES
  1       -92.8483      26.837    1.3086    0.7255    0.0
  2       -78.4745       1.213    1.0256    0.4851    1.6166
  3       -77.8259       0.017    1.2543    0.5085    1.9860
  4       -77.8176       0.000    1.2746    0.5113    2.0394
  5       -77.8177       0.000    1.2748    0.5113    2.0403
  6       -77.8178       0.000    1.2748    0.5113    2.0403
```
ESTIMATED PARAMETER VECTOR
     1.274838   0.511341   2.040295
FIRST DERIVATIVE LOG-LIKELIHOOD
    -0.000002   -0.000016   -0.000012
INFORMATION MATRIX
     5.996716
    -0.295262   7.917883
    -0.581353   0.554115   5.222651
ESTIMATED COVARIANCE MATRIX
     0.168775
     0.005016   0.127390
     0.018255   -0.012958   0.194880
STNDIZED REGRESSION COEFFICIENTS
     3.103141   1.432656   4.621776

MODEL WITH 4 VARIABLES: GALL + OB + EST + GALL×EST

(Model 8, Table 7.7)

LOGISTIC REGRESSION ANALYSIS IN STRATA

NUMBER OF STRATA   63
STRATUM NUMBER AND NUMBERS OF CASES AND CONTROLS

1	1	4	2	1	4	3	1	4	4	1	4	5	1	4	6	1	4	7	1	4	8	1	4
9	1	4	10	1	4	11	1	4	12	1	4	13	1	4	14	1	4	15	1	4	16	1	4
17	1	4	18	1	4	19	1	4	20	1	4	21	1	4	22	1	4	23	1	4	24	1	4
25	1	4	26	1	4	27	1	4	28	1	4	29	1	4	30	1	4	31	1	4	32	1	4
33	1	4	34	1	4	35	1	4	36	1	4	37	1	4	38	1	4	39	1	4	40	1	4
41	1	4	42	1	4	43	1	4	44	1	4	45	1	4	46	1	4	47	1	4	48	1	4
49	1	4	50	1	4	51	1	4	52	1	4	53	1	4	54	1	4	55	1	4	56	1	4
57	1	4	58	1	4	59	1	4	60	1	4	61	1	4	62	1	4	63	1	4			

NUMBER OF VARIABLES IN THIS ANALYSIS   4
THESE VARIABLES ARE NUMBERS   1   2   3   4
MAXIMUM NUMBER OF ITERATIONS   10

ITER	LOG-LIKELIHOOD	SCORE	PARAMETER ESTIMATES			
1	−77.8178	4.392	1.2748	0.5113	2.0403	0.0
2	−75.9028	0.221	3.0330	0.4859	2.5096	−2.2027
3	−75.7904	0.000	2.8467	0.4901	2.6172	−2.0003
4	−75.7906	0.000	2.8446	0.4901	2.6206	−1.9974
5	−75.7907	0.000	2.8446	0.4901	2.6206	−1.9974
6	−75.7904	0.000	2.8446	0.4901	2.6206	−1.9975
7	−75.7906	0.000	2.8446	0.4901	2.6206	−1.9974
8	−75.7906	0.000	2.8446	0.4901	2.6206	−1.9974

ESTIMATED PARAMETER VECTOR
$$2.844558 \quad 0.490128 \quad 2.620618 \quad -1.997445$$

FIRST DERIVATIVE LOG-LIKELIHOOD
$$0.000001 \quad -0.000002 \quad 0.000000 \quad 0.000002$$

INFORMATION MATRIX

6.692031			
−0.287092	7.667618		
−1.389091	0.432643	4.504441	
4.758771	−0.133909	0.584442	4.981022

ESTIMATED COVARIANCE MATRIX

0.774393			
−0.003830	0.131275		
0.340365	−0.014950	0.376375	
−0.779880	0.008943	−0.369741	0.989468

STNDIZED REGRESSION COEFFICIENTS
$$3.232466 \quad 1.352753 \quad 4.271628 \quad -2.008047$$

APPENDIX VI

LISTING OF PROGRAM LOGODD

The following main program and subroutine perform the regression analysis of a set of 2×2 tables as described in § 7.5. For illustration we have used the data from the Oxford Childhood Cancer Survey published by Kneale (1971) and listed in Appendix II. Two different models were fit, the first with just the coefficient β representing the overall log relative risk for radiation, and the second with both β and the coefficient γ_1 representing the linear change in the log relative risk with year. The option for an 'exact' analysis was selected, giving numerical results as shown in § 7.5. (The last line in Table 6.17 shows the results which are obtained using the option for an 'approximate' analysis.) Following the fitting of the two parameter model, the programme was instructed (IPRINT = 1) to print out the observed and fitted entries for each table, the variance associated with that table (equation 4.13), the contribution it makes to the log likelihood, the estimated value of the odds ratio, and the associated covariates of which the first is the constant term and the second the coded year.

MAIN PROGRAM

```
      INTEGER P
      DOUBLE PRECISION INFO(10,10),LOGLIK,B(10),SCORE(10),SCORE1(10)
      DOUBLE PRECISION Z(10,120),T(4,120),PROB,E,V,DETER,CHIS,ULL
      REAL FMT(60),RT(4),RZ(10)
      DIMENSION IVAR(10)
      DATA NM/10/
      EQUIVALENCE(P,NP)
      EPS=1. E-4
 1000 READ(5,150,END=900) P,NFORMT,ITS,ITAPE,IME,IBETA,IPRINT
  150 FORMAT(15I5)
  999 INF=20*INFORMT
      READ(5,155) (FMT(I),I=1,INF)
  155 FORMAT(20A4)
      IF(P.GT.10.OR.P.LT.1.OR.ITS.GT.20.OR.NFORMT.GT.3)GO TO 996
C NOW READ DATA ONE TABLE AND ASSOCIATED COVARIATES PER LINE
      K=0
    7 K=K+1
      READ(ITAPE,FMT,END=10)(RT(I),I=1,4)Z1,Z2
      RZ(1)=Z1
      RZ(2)=Z2
   86 IF(K.GT.120)GO TO 9
      IF(RT(1).EQ.0.0.AND.RT(2).EQ.0.0.AND.RT(3).EQ.0.0.AND.RT(4).EQ.0.0
     A)GO TO 10
      DO 8 I=1,4
    8 T(I,K)=RT(I)
      DO 85 I=1,2
   85 Z(I,K)=RZ(I)
      GO TO 7
    9 WRITE(6,154)
  154 FORMAT('0DATA EXCEEDS MAXIMUM OF 120 TABLES')
      GO TO 900
   10 NTAB = K-1
      NP=1
      DO 14 K=1,NP
   14 B(K)=0.0
      IVAR(1)=1
      JPRINT=0
      CALL LOGODD(NM,NP,NTAB,B,SCORE,ITS,EPS,IME,JPRINT,Z,INFO,T,IVAR,
     *SCORE1)
      IVAR(1)=1
      IVAR(2)=2
      NP=2
      CALL LOGODD(NM,NP,NTAB,B,SCORE,ITS,EPS,IME,IPRINT,Z,INFO,T,IVAR,
     *SCORE1)
  900 CONTINUE
  996 STOP
      END
```

SUBPROGRAM LOGODD

```
      SUBROUTINE LOGODD(NM,NP,NTAB,B,SCORE,ITS,EPS,IME,IPRINT,Z,INFO,T,
     * IVAR,SCORE1)
C    PROGRAM FOR THE REGRESSION ANALYSIS OF THE LOG ODDS RATIO
      DOUBLE PRECISION INFO(NM,1),LOGLIK,B(1),SCORE(1)
      DOUBLE PRECISION Z(NM,1),T(4,1),PROB,E,V,DETER,CHIS,ULL
      DOUBLE PRECISION TEMP,SCORE1(1)
      DIMENSION IVAR(1)
C    ITS = MAXIMUM NUMBER OF ITERATIONS
C    IME = 1 IF WANT EXACT CALCULATIONS
C    IME = 2 IF WANT APPROXIMATE CALCULATIONS
C    IPRINT = 1 IF WANT OBSERVED AND FITTED TABLES
C    PRINTED OUT AT IST AND LAST ITERATIONS
      WRITE(6,149)
  149 FORMAT('1REGRESSION ANALYSIS OF LOG ODDS RATIO'/)
      WRITE(6,151)NTAB
  151 FORMAT(' NUMBER OF TABLES = ',I3)
      IF(IME.EQ.1)WRITE(6,152)
      IF(IME.EQ.2)WRITE(6,153)
  152 FORMAT(' EXACT ANALYSIS')
  153 FORMAT(' APPROXIMATE ANALYSIS')
      WRITE(6,150)NP,(IVAR(K),K=1,NP)
  150 FORMAT(' NUMBER OF VARIABLES IN THIS ANALYSIS =',I3,
     */,' THESE VARIABLES ARE NUMBERS',30I3)
      WRITE(6,154)ITS
  154 FORMAT(' MAXIMUM NUMBER OF ITERATIONS',I4)
C INITIALIZE BETA TO ZERO
   15 NFLAG=0
      DO 60 II=1,ITS
      IF(II.EQ.ITS)NFLAG=1
        I1=0
      CALL CALC(NTAB,NP,NM,IME,I1,SCORE,INFO,LOGLIK,B,CHIS,ULL,Z,T,IVAR)
      TEST=0.0
      DO 20 K=1,NP
      S=SNGL(SCORE(K))
      SCORE1(K)=SCORE(K)
   20 TEST=TEST+ABS(S)
      IF(TEST.LT.EPS)NFLAG=1
      IF(NFLAG.EQ.1) GOTO 47
   48 CALL INVR(INFO,NP,SCORE,1,DETER,NM,NP)
      TEMP=0.0
      DO 10 I=1,NP
      TEMP=TEMP+SCORE(I)*SCORE1(I)
   10 CONTINUE
      IF(II.EQ.1)WRITE(6,116)
  116 FORMAT(' ITER    LOG-LIKELIHOOD    SCORE         PARAMETER ESTIMA
     *TES')
   47 CONTINUE
```

```
      WRITE(6,107)II,LOGLIK,TEMP,(B(J),J=1,NP)
107   FORMAT(1X,I4,F17.4,F13.4,2X,8F12.4,20(/,36X,8F12.4))
      IF(NFLAG.EQ.1)GO TO 99
CALCULATE NEW VALUE OF BETA
  52  CONTINUE
      DO 55 K=1,NP
  55  B(K)=B(K)-SCORE(K)
  60  CONTINUE
  99  CONTINUE
      WRITE(6,101)(B(J),J=1,NP)
101   FORMAT(' ESTIMATED PARAMETER VECTOR'/,(1X,10F12.6)
      WRITE(6,102)(SCORE(J),J=1,NP)
102   FORMAT(' FIRST DERIVATIVE LOG-LIKELIHOOD'/,(1X,10F12.6))
      WRITE(6,103)
103   FORMAT(' INFORMATION MATRIX')
      DO 11 I=1,NP
      WRITE(6,104)(INFO(I,J),J=1,I)
 11   CONTINUE
104   FORMAT(1X,10F12.6)
      CALL INVR(INFO,NP,SCORE,1,DETER,NM,NP)
      WRITE(6,105)
105   FORMAT(' ESTIMATED COVARIANCE MATRIX')
      DO 12 I=1,NP
      SCORE1(I)=B(I)/DSQRT(INFO(I,I))
C   SCORE1 IS USED TO CALCULATE STANDARDISED COEFFICIENTS
      WRITE(6,104)(INFO(I,J),J=1,I)
 12   CONTINUE
      WRITE(6,106)(SCORE1(I),I=1,NP)
106   FORMAT('0STANDARDISED REGRESSION COEFFICIENTS'/(1X,10F12.6))
 4    CONTINUE
      WRITE(6,156)CHIS
156   FORMAT('0CHI-SQUARE GOODNESS OF FIT ',F12.4)
      WRITE(6,157)ULL
157   FORMAT('02XLR RATIO GOODNESS OF FIT ',F12.4)
      I=NTAB-NP
      WRITE(6,158)I
158   FORMAT('0DEGREES OF FREEDOM ',I5)
      IF(IPRINT.NE.1)GO TO 899
      WRITE(6,290)(B(J),J=1,NP)
290   FORMAT('1 FITTED VALUES EACH TABLE FOR BETA VALUES :', 9F9.4/(43X,
     :: 9F9.4))
      CALL CALC(NTAB,NP,NM,IME,1,SCORE,INFO,LOGLIK,B,CHIS,ULL,Z,T,IVAR)
899   CONTINUE
900   WRITE(6,667)
667   FORMAT('0'//'0RUN TERMINATES SUCCESSFULLY')
      RETURN
      END
```

```
      SUBROUTINE CALC(NTAB,P,NM,IME,IPRINT,SCORE,INFO,LOGLIK,B,CHIS,ULL
     :: Z,T,IVAR)
      DOUBLE PRECISION SCORE(1),INFO(NM,1),LOGLIK,Z(NM,1)B(1)
      DOUBLE PRECISION T(4,1),SUM,PROB,E,V,CHIS,ULL,T1,T2,T3,T4,T5,
     ::T6,T7,T8
      DIMENSION IVAR(1)
      INTEGER P
      CHIS=0.0
      LOGLIK=0.0
      ULL=0.0
      IF(IPRINT.NE.1) GOTO 1
      WRITE(6,290)
290   FORMAT(//'0 TABLE',5X,'A',11X,'B',11X,'C',11X,'D', 8X,'VARIANCE   L
     ::OG-LIKE',4X,  'PSI      COVARIATES'/6X,4(4X,'0',4X,'E',2X))
1     CONTINUE
      DO 5 K=1,P
      SCORE(K)=0.0
      DO 5 KK=1,P
5     INFO(K,KK)=0.0
      DO 20 I=1,NTAB
      SUM=0.0
      DO 10 K=1,P
      L=IVAR(K)
10    SUM=SUM-Z(L,I)::B(K)
      CALL MYST(T(1,I),SUM,PROB,E,V,P,IME)
      PROB=DLOG(PROB)
      LOGLIK=LOGLIK+PROB
      CHIS=CHIS+((T(2,I)-E)::(T(2,I)-E))/V
      DO 15 K=1,P
      L=IVAR(K)
      SCORE(K)=SCORE(K)+Z(L,I)::(T(2,I)-E)
      DO 15 KK=1,P
      LL=IVAR(KK)
15    INFO(K,KK)=INFO(K,KK)+Z(L,I)::Z(LL,I)::V
      T1=T(1,I)
      T2=T(2,I)
      T3=T(3,I)
      T4=T(4,I)
      T6=E
      T5=T(1,I)+T(2,I)-T6
      T7=T(1,I)+T(3,I)-T5
      T8=T(3,I)  +T(4,I)-T7
      IF(T1.GT.0.0)ULL=ULL+T1::DLOG(T5/T1)
      IF(T2.GT.0.0)ULL=ULL+T2::DLOG(T6/T2)
      IF(T3.GT.0.0)ULL=ULL+T3::DLOG(T7/T3)
      IF(T4.GT.0.0)ULL=ULL+T4::DLOG(T8/T4)
      IF(IPRINT.EQ.1)GO TO 21
      GO TO 20
21    CONTINUE
```

```
      I1=T1
      I2=T2
      I3=T3
      I4=T4
      WRITE(6,291) I,I1,T5,I2,T6,I3,T7,I4,T8,V,PROB,SUM,(Z(IVAR(K),I),K=
     *1,P)
  291 FORMAT(I4,2X,4(1X,I4,F7.2),3F10.3,8F6.2,20(/,84X,8F6.2))
   20 CONTINUE
      ULL=-2.0*ULL
      RETURN
      END
```

```
      SUBROUTINE MYST(T,SUM,PROB,E,V,P,IME)
C    THE EXTERNALS :::QUAD::: AND :::BINCOF::: ARE NECESSARY TO USE THIS
C                                                           SUBROUTINE
      INTEGER P
      DOUBLE PRECISION T,PROB,E,V,TOT,BINCOF,PI
      DIMENSION T(4)
      DOUBLE PRECISION SUM,EM,EN,TEE ,ENMT,A,B,C,U,G,H,HH
      PI= 3.14159 26535 89793 23846 26433
      U=0.
      H=0.
      G=0.
      HH=0.
      EM   = T(1) + T(3)
      EN   = T(2) + T(4)
      TEE = T(1) + T(2)
      ENMT = T(3) + T(4)
C    VARIABLE :IME: IS THE FLAT TO DETERMINE EXACT OR ASYMPTOTIC COMP
C    IME = 1 GIVES EXACT
C    IME = 2 GIVES ASYMPTOTIC
      IF(IME.LT.2) GO TO 100
      GO TO 101
C   EXACT CALCULATIONS
  100 SAP=SNGL(DEXP(SUM))
      IF(SAP .EQ.1.0)GO TO 403
      A=BINCOF (EM,TEE-T(2))
      B=BINCOF (EN,T(2))
      C = DEXP(T(2) :: SUM)
      FNUM  = A::B::C
      KK = IDINT(TEE + 1.)
      DO 14 J=1,KK
      A=BINCOF(EM,TEE-U)
      B=BINCOF(EN,U)
      C =DEXP(U::SUM)
      H = A :: B ::C + H
      G = A::B::C::U + G
      HH = A::B::C::U:::2 + HH
   14 U = U + 1.
      PROB= FNUM/H
      E = G/H
      V = HH/H - E:::2
      SUM=DEXP(SUM)
      GO TO 677
  403 A=BINCOF(TEE,T(2))
      B=BINCOF(ENMT,T(4))
      TOT = ENMT + TEE
      C = BINCOF(TOT,EN)
      PROB = (A::B)/C
      EN   = T(2) + T(4)
      E = TEE :: (EN/(TOT))
      V = (EM::EN::TEE::ENMT)/(TOT::TOT::(TOT-1))
      SUM=DEXP(SUM)
      GO TO 677
```

```
C    ASYMPTOTIC METHOD
  101 SUM =DEXP(SUM)
      SAP =SNGL(SUM)
      IF(SAP-1.0)16,15,16
   15 E = TEE * (EN/(ENMT + TEE))
      GO TO 102
   16 A = (1. - SUM)
      B = EM - TEE + (SUM*TEE) + (SUM*EN)
      C = -(SUM*TEE*EN)
      E = QUAD(A,B,C,TEE,EN)
  102 V = 1./((1./E) + (1./(TEE-E)) + (1./(EN-E)) + (1./(EM-TEE+E)))
      PROB= 1./(DSQRT(2.*PI*V))
      PROB=PROB*DEXP(-(0.50* ((T(2) - E)**2/V)))
  677 CONTINUE
      RETURN
      END
```

```
      DOUBLE PRECISION FUNCTION QUAD(A,B,C,TEE,EN)
      DOUBLE PRECISION A,B,C,TEE,EN
      C =        B**2 - (4.*A*C)
      GA = SNGL(TEE)
      GB = SNGL(EN)
      G = SNGL(C)
      IF(G) 32,40,40
   40 C = DSQRT(C)
      QUAD = ((-B) -C)/(2. * A)
      G = SNGL(QUAD)
      IF(G.GT.0.0.AND.G.LT.AMIN1(GA,GB)) RETURN
      QUAD = ((-B) + C)/(2. * A)
      G = SNGL(QUAD)
      IF(G.GT.0.0.AND.G.LT.AMIN1(GA,GB)) RETURN
   32 WRITE(6,100)
  100 FORMAT(' ERROR IN QUAD COMPLEX SOLUTION')
      STOP
      END



      DOUBLE PRECISION FUNCTION BINCOF(X,Y)
      DOUBLE PRECISION UPPER,BELOW,X,Y
      UUPER=X
      BELOW=Y
      BINCOF=0.
      A = SNGL(UPPER)
      B = SNGL(BELOW)
      IF(A-B.LT.B) BELOW= UPPER - BELOW
      K = IDINT(BELOW)
      IF(K.LT.0)GO TO 2
      BINCOF = 1.
      IF(K.EQ.0)GO TO 2
      DO 41 I=1,K
      BINCOF =(UPPER/BELOW) * BINCOF
      UPPER = UPPER - 1.
   41 BELOW = BELOW - 1.
    2 RETURN
      END
```

```
      SUBROUTINE INVR(A,N,B,M,DETERM,ISIZE,JSIZE)
      DIMENSION IPIVOT(100),INDEX(100,2)
      DOUBLE PRECISION A(ISIZE,JSIZE),B(ISIZE,M),PIVOT(100),AMAX,T
     ASWAP,DETERM
      EQUIVALENCE (IROW,JROW),(ICOLUM,JCOLUM),(AMAX,T,SWAP)
C
   10 DETERM=1.0
   15 DO 20 J=1,N
   20 IPIVOT(J)=0
   30 DO 550 I=1,N
C
C     SEARCH FOR PIVOT ELEMENT
C
   40 AMAX=0.0
   45 DO 105 J=1,N
   50 IF (IPIVOT(J)-1) 60, 105, 60
   60 DO 100 K=1,N
   70 IF (IPIVOT(K)-L) 80, 100, 740
   80 IF(DABS(AMAX)-DABS(A(J,K)))85,100,100
   85 IROW=J
   90 ICOLUM=K
   95 AMAX=A(J,K)
  100 CONTINUE
  105 CONTINUE
  110 IPIVOT(ICOLUM)=IPIVOT(ICOLUM)+1
C
C     INTERCHANGE ROWS TO PUT PIVOT ELEMENT ON DIAGONAL
C
  130 IF (IROW-ICOLUM) 140, 260, 140
  140 DETERM=-DETERM
  150 DO 200 L=1,N
  160 SWAP=A(IROW,L)
  170 A(IROW,L)=A(ICOLUM,L)
  200 A(ICOLUM,L)=SWAP
  205 IF(M) 260, 260, 210
  210 DO 250 L=1, M
  220 SWAP=B(IROW,L)
  230 B(IROW,L)=B(ICOLUM,L)
  250 B(ICOLUM,L)=SWAP
  260 INDEX(I,1)=IROW
  270 INDEX(I,2)=ICOLUM
  310 PIVOT(I)=A(ICOLUM,ICOLUM)
  320 DETERM-DETERM*PIVOT(I)
C
C     DIVIDE PIVOT ROW BY PIVOT ELEMENT
C
  330 A(ICOLUM,ICOLUM)=1.0
  340 DO 350 L=1,N
  350 A(ICOLUM,L)=A(ICOLUM,L)/PIVOT(I)
  355 IF(M) 380, 380, 360
  360 DO 370 L=1,M
  370 B(ICOLUM,L)=B(ICOLUM,L)/PIVOT(I)
```

```
C
C      REDUCE NON-PIVOT ROWS
C
  380 DO 550 L1=1,N
  390 IF(L1-ICOLUM) 400, 550, 400
  400 T=A(L1,ICOLUM)
  420 A(L1,ICOLUM=0.0
  430 DO 450 L=1,N
  450 A(L1,L)=A(L1,L)-A(ICOLUM,L)*T
  455 IF(M) 550, 550, 460
  460 DO 500 L=1,M
  500 B(L1,L)=B(L1,L)-B(ICOLUM,L)*T
  550 CONTINUE
C
C      INTERCHANGE COLUMNS
C
  600 DO 710 I=1,N
  610 L=N+1-I
  620 IF (INDEX(L,I)-INDEX(L,2)) 630, 710, 630
  630 JROW=INDEX(L,1)
  640 JCOLUM=INDEX(L,2)
  650 DO 705 K=1,N
  660 SWAP=A(K,JROW)
  670 A(K,JROW)=A(K,JCOLUM)
  700 A(K,JCOLUM)=SWAP
  705 CONTINUE
  710 CONTINUE
  740 RETURN
      END
```

MODEL WITH CONSTANT TERM ONLY

REGRESSION ANALYSIS OF LOG ODDS RATIO

NUMBER OF TABLES = 120
EXACT ANALYSIS
NUMBER OF VARIABLES IN THIS ANALYSIS = 1
THESE VARIABLES ARE NUMBERS   1
MAXIMUM NUMBER OF ITERATIONS   15

ITER	LOG-LIKELIHOOD	SCORE	PARAMETER ESTIMATES
1	−261.4516	82.1955	0.0
2	−220.0785	0.0152	0.4982
3	−220.0708	0.0000	0.5051
4	−220.0708	0.0000	0.5051

ESTIMATED PARAMETER VECTOR
   0.505080
FIRST DERIVATIVE LOG-LIKELIHOOD
  −0.000000
INFORMATION MATRIX
 313.718469
ESTIMATED COVARIANCE MATRIX
   0.003147
STANDARDISED REGRESSION COEFFICIENTS
   9.002886
CHI-SQUARE GOODNESS OF FIT   117.3498
2XLR RATIO GOODNESS OF FIT   124.1829
DEGREES OF FREEDOM   119

MODEL WITH LINEAR EFFECT OF YEAR

REGRESSION ANALYSIS OF LOG ODDS RATIO

NUMBER OF TABLES = 120
EXACT ANALYSIS
NUMBER OF VARIABLES IN THIS ANALYSIS = 2
THESE VARIABLES ARE NUMBERS 1 2
MAXIMUM NUMBER OF ITERATIONS 15

ITER	LOG-LIKELIHOOD	SCORE	PARAMETER ESTIMATES	
1	-220.0708	7.2135	0.5051	0.0
2	-216.4595	0.0013	0.5144	-0.0384
3	-216.4588	0.0000	0.5165	-0.0385
4	-216.4588	0.0000	0.5165	-0.0385

ESTIMATED PARAMETER VECTOR
    0.516496   -0.038542
FIRST DERIVATIVE LOG-LIKELIHOOD
  -0.000000   0.000000
INFORMATION MATRIX
  316.476245
 110.182468 4876.820615
ESTIMATED COVARIANCE MATRIX
   0.003185
  -0.000072   0.000207
STANDARDISED REGRESSION COEFFICIENTS
    9.152142   -2.680950
CHI-SQUARE GOODNESS OF FIT   111.2280
2XLR RATIO GOODNESS OF FIT   116.8751
DEGREES OF FREEDOM   118

OBSERVED AND EXPECTED VALUES FOR MODEL 2

FITTED VALUES EACH TABLE FOR BETA VALUES : 0.5165 -0.0385

TABLE	A O	A E	B O	B E	C O	C E	D O	D E	VARIANCE	LOG-LIKE	PSI	COVARIATES
1	3	2.11	0	0.89	25	25.89	28	27.11	0.605	-1.068	2.464	1.00 -10.00
2	5	4.74	2	2.26	16	16.26	19	18.74	1.331	-1.094	2.371	1.00 -9.00
3	2	2.78	2	1.22	30	29.22	30	30.78	0.813	-1.295	2.371	1.00 -9.00
4	7	5.42	1	2.58	28	29.58	34	32.42	1.590	-1.816	2.281	1.00 -8.00
5	7	6.08	2	2.92	28	28.92	33	32.08	1.770	-1.390	2.281	1.00 -8.00
6	2	1.39	0	0.61	36	36.61	38	37.39	0.421	-0.738	2.281	1.00 -8.00
7	5	4.04	1	1.96	25	25.96	29	28.04	1.221	-1.304	2.195	1.00 -7.00
8	3	2.73	1	1.27	40	40.27	42	41.73	0.842	-0.892	2.195	1.00 -7.00
9	5	4.07	1	1.93	44	44.93	48	47.07	1.250	-1.280	2.195	1.00 -7.00
10	11	8.69	2	4.31	42	44.31	51	48.69	2.587	-2.357	2.195	1.00 -7.00
11	6	6.55	4	3.45	25	24.45	27	27.55	1.955	-1.375	2.112	1.00 -6.00
12	6	6.58	4	3.42	29	28.42	31	31.58	1.984	-1.392	2.112	1.00 -6.00
13	11	8.55	2	4.45	35	37.45	44	41.55	2.576	-2.498	2.112	1.00 -6.00
14	4	3.36	1	1.64	49	49.64	52	51.36	1.064	-1.084	2.112	1.00 -6.00
15	4	7.32	7	3.68	57	53.68	54	57.32	2.267	-3.633	2.112	1.00 -6.00
16	2	3.96	4	2.04	38	36.04	36	37.96	1.269	-2.495	2.112	1.00 -6.00
17	8	7.07	3	3.93	21	21.93	26	25.07	2.113	-1.466	2.032	1.00 -5.00
18	8	8.43	5	4.57	36	35.57	39	39.43	2.585	-1.462	2.032	1.00 -5.00
19	6	5.93	3	3.07	46	46.07	49	48.93	1.882	-1.259	2.032	1.00 -5.00
20	5	4.63	2	2.37	50	50.37	53	52.63	1.489	-1.163	2.032	1.00 -5.00
21	15	12.30	4	6.70	46	48.70	57	54.30	3.741	-2.509	2.032	1.00 -5.00
22	4	3.26	1	1.74	27	27.74	30	29.26	1.067	-1.145	1.956	1.00 -4.00
23	9	8.36	4	4.64	39	39.64	44	43.36	2.635	-1.469	1.956	1.00 -4.00
24	9	8.95	5	5.05	35	35.05	39	38.95	2.778	-1.443	1.956	1.00 -4.00
25	4	3.92	2	2.08	38	38.08	40	39.92	1.285	-1.081	1.956	1.00 -4.00
26	12	12.08	7	6.92	41	40.92	46	46.08	3.691	-1.585	1.956	1.00 -4.00
27	8	8.39	5	4.61	48	47.61	51	51.39	2.677	-1.472	1.956	1.00 -4.00
28	8	10.33	8	5.67	63	60.67	65	65.33	3.300	-2.361	1.882	1.00 -3.00
29	6	5.13	2	2.87	37	37.87	41	40.13	1.700	-1.364	1.882	1.00 -3.00
30	8	7.00	3	4.00	35	36.00	40	39.00	2.266	-1.514	1.882	1.00 -3.00

TABLE	A O	A E	B O	B E	C O	C E	D O	D E	VARIANCE	LOG-LIKE	PSI	COVARIATES
31	12	10.64	5	6.36	31	32.36	38	36.64	3.269	-1.765	1.882	1.00 -3.00
32	4	5.12	4	2.88	36	34.88	36	37.12	1.691	-1.604	1.882	1.00 -3.00
33	7	5.13	1	2.87	37	38.87	43	41.13	1.703	-2.107	1.882	1.00 -3.00
34	16	13.89	6	8.11	54	56.11	64	61.89	4.392	-2.127	1.882	1.00 -3.00
35	12	10.84	5	6.16	63	64.16	70	68.84	3.534	-1.713	1.882	1.00 -3.00
36	9	12.68	11	7.32	62	58.32	60	63.68	4.055	-3.259	1.882	1.00 -3.00
37	4	5.64	2	3.33	33	31.33	32	33.67	1.883	-1.991	1.810	1.00 -2.00
38	7	5.64	5	3.36	24	25.36	29	27.64	1.846	-1.666	1.810	1.00 -2.00
39	8	8.12	8	4.88	34	33.88	37	37.12	2.631	-1.425	1.810	1.00 -2.00
40	11	11.73	5	7.27	35	34.27	38	38.73	3.639	-1.659	1.810	1.00 -2.00
41	5	6.31	6	3.69	42	40.69	42	43.31	2.117	-1.740	1.810	1.00 -2.00
42	12	11.22	6	6.78	43	43.78	49	48.22	3.602	-1.635	1.810	1.00 -2.00
43	8	8.82	6	5.18	55	54.18	57	57.82	2.944	-1.609	1.810	1.00 -2.00
44	17	16.87	10	10.13	74	74.13	81	80.87	5.469	-1.775	1.810	1.00 -2.00
45	9	9.92	7	6.08	34	33.08	36	36.92	3.135	-1.653	1.742	1.00 -1.00
46	3	4.99	5	3.01	36	34.01	34	35.99	1.717	-2.327	1.742	1.00 -1.00
47	2	4.37	5	2.63	33	30.63	30	32.37	1.507	-2.902	1.742	1.00 -1.00
48	7	5.57	2	3.43	25	26.43	30	28.57	1.867	-1.716	1.742	1.00 -1.00
49	6	8.67	8	5.33	47	44.33	45	47.67	2.912	-2.671	1.742	1.00 -1.00
50	5	3.77	1	2.23	44	45.23	48	46.77	1.333	-1.528	1.742	1.00 -1.00
51	11	14.77	13	9.23	64	60.23	62	65.77	4.842	-3.165	1.742	1.00 -1.00
52	14	14.10	9	8.90	50	49.90	55	55.10	4.550	-1.687	1.742	1.00 -1.00
53	13	14.73	11	9.27	56	54.27	58	59.73	4.775	-2.036	1.742	1.00 -1.00
54	8	10.53	9	6.47	56	53.47	55	57.53	3.529	-2.463	1.742	1.00 -1.00
55	6	6.24	4	3.76	43	42.76	45	45.24	2.142	-1.344	1.676	1.00 0.0
56	4	4.89	4	3.11	25	24.11	25	25.89	1.678	-1.455	1.676	1.00 0.0
57	8	9.65	8	6.35	32	30.35	32	33.65	3.127	-1.947	1.676	1.00 0.0
58	4	6.06	6	3.94	23	20.94	21	23.06	1.998	-2.319	1.676	1.00 0.0
59	8	9.72	8	6.28	40	38.28	40	41.72	3.237	-1.983	1.676	1.00 0.0
60	7	7.92	6	5.08	36	35.08	37	37.92	2.676	-1.600	1.676	1.00 0.0

TABLE	A O	A E	B O	B E	C O	C E	D O	D E	VARIANCE	LOG-LIKE	PSI	COVARIATES	
61	15	13.90	8	9.10	46	47.10	53	51.90	4.535	-1.797	1.676	1.00	0.0
62	15	17.52	14	11.48	62	59.48	63	65.52	5.710	-2.362	1.676	1.00	0.0
63	9	9.16	6	5.84	46	45.84	49	49.16	3.127	-1.511	1.676	1.00	0.0
64	9	8.59	5	5.41	51	51.41	55	54.59	2.975	-1.495	1.676	1.00	0.0
65	5	6.14	5	3.86	41	39.86	41	42.14	2.146	-1.643	1.676	1.00	0.0
66	6	4.82	2	3.18	22	23.18	26	24.82	1.681	-1.542	1.613	1.00	1.00
67	3	4.25	4	2.75	30	28.75	29	30.25	1.522	-1.669	1.613	1.00	1.00
68	9	6.59	2	4.41	23	25.41	30	27.59	2.236	-2.569	1.613	1.00	1.00
69	12	12.44	9	8.56	34	33.56	37	37.44	3.985	-1.648	1.613	1.00	1.00
70	14	11.39	5	7.61	43	45.61	52	49.39	3.860	-2.443	1.613	1.00	1.00
71	16	13.11	6	8.89	40	42.89	50	47.11	4.325	-2.588	1.613	1.00	1.00
72	17	14.41	7	9.59	61	63.59	71	68.41	4.932	-2.365	1.613	1.00	1.00
73	8	7.87	5	5.13	50	50.13	53	52.87	2.794	-1.448	1.613	1.00	1.00
74	8	10.78	10	7.22	44	41.22	42	44.78	3.634	-2.623	1.613	1.00	1.00
75	9	7.16	3	4.84	22	23.84	28	26.16	2.383	-2.017	1.613	1.00	1.00
76	5	4.18	2	2.82	23	23.82	26	25.18	1.507	-1.322	1.552	1.00	2.00
77	9	5.98	1	4.02	37	40.02	45	41.98	2.175	-3.416	1.552	1.00	2.00
78	11	10.56	7	7.44	31	31.44	35	34.56	3.492	-1.574	1.552	1.00	2.00
79	6	8.88	9	6.12	39	36.12	36	38.88	3.070	-2.810	1.552	1.00	2.00
80	14	15.83	13	11.17	49	47.17	50	51.83	5.218	-2.080	1.552	1.00	2.00
81	21	17.60	9	12.40	50	53.40	62	58.60	5.813	-2.775	1.552	1.00	2.00
82	16	15.88	11	11.12	53	53.12	58	57.88	5.329	-1.762	1.552	1.00	2.00
83	6	5.97	4	4.03	37	37.03	39	38.97	2.160	-1.324	1.552	1.00	2.00
84	9	10.05	8	6.95	41	39.95	42	43.05	3.463	-1.721	1.552	1.00	2.00
85	8	5.85	2	4.15	23	25.15	29	26.85	2.079	-2.346	1.493	1.00	3.00
86	9	7.00	3	5.00	25	27.00	31	29.00	2.449	-2.142	1.493	1.00	3.00
87	8	8.80	7	6.20	46	45.20	47	47.80	3.175	-1.619	1.493	1.00	3.00
88	4	4.73	4	3.27	42	41.27	42	42.73	1.789	-1.399	1.493	1.00	3.00
89	11	10.52	7	7.48	47	47.48	51	50.52	3.741	-1.611	1.493	1.00	3.00
90	11	9.40	5	6.60	51	52.60	57	55.40	3.418	-1.883	1.493	1.00	3.00

TABLE	A O	A E	B O	B E	C O	C E	D O	D E	VARIANCE	LOG-LIKE	PSI	COVARIATES	
91	6	7.06	6	4.94	46	44.94	46	47.06	2.604	−1.642	1.493	1.00	3.00
92	9	8.73	6	6.27	32	32.27	35	34.73	3.032	−1.492	1.493	1.00	3.00
93	4	5.21	5	3.79	30	28.79	29	30.21	1.938	−1.651	1.437	1.00	4.00
94	4	5.82	6	4.18	48	46.18	46	47.82	2.226	−2.067	1.437	1.00	4.00
95	9	10.40	9	7.60	54	52.60	54	55.40	3.807	−1.862	1.437	1.00	4.00
96	9	9.25	7	6.75	50	49.75	52	52.25	3.412	−1.558	1.437	1.00	4.00
97	10	9.89	7	7.11	78	78.11	81	80.89	3.768	−1.594	1.437	1.00	4.00
98	14	12.08	7	8.92	48	49.92	55	53.08	4.312	−2.055	1.437	1.00	4.00
99	6	5.81	4	4.19	41	41.19	43	42.81	2.204	−1.337	1.437	1.00	4.00
100	3	2.89	2	2.11	50	50.11	51	50.89	1.175	−1.194	1.382	1.00	5.00
101	4	4.03	3	2.97	53	52.97	54	54.03	1.621	−1.363	1.382	1.00	5.00
102	6	5.75	4	4.25	68	68.25	70	69.75	2.297	−1.882	1.382	1.00	5.00
103	10	11.38	10	8.62	58	56.62	58	59.38	4.225	−1.197	1.382	1.00	5.00
104	4	4.03	3	2.97	57	56.97	58	58.03	1.626	−1.510	1.382	1.00	5.00
105	3	4.02	4	2.98	42	40.98	41	42.02	1.598	−1.046	1.382	1.00	5.00
106	3	2.84	2	2.16	42	42.16	43	42.84	1.173	−1.820	1.330	1.00	6.00
107	10	11.20	10	8.80	52	50.80	52	53.20	4.176	−1.603	1.330	1.00	6.00
108	4	5.10	5	3.90	69	67.90	68	69.10	2.090	−2.187	1.330	1.00	6.00
109	10	7.87	4	6.13	43	45.13	49	46.87	3.025	−1.424	1.330	1.00	6.00
110	5	5.63	5	4.37	34	33.37	34	34.63	2.177	−1.306	1.330	1.00	6.00
111	4	4.45	4	3.55	41	40.55	41	41.45	1.821	−2.245	1.280	1.00	7.00
112	3	5.01	6	3.99	48	45.99	45	47.01	2.047	−2.24⊂	1.280	1.00	7.00
113	13	9.93	5	8.07	42	45.07	50	46.93	3.764	−2.805	1.280	1.00	7.00
114	1	2.24	3	1.76	40	38.76	38	39.24	0.950	−1.663	1.280	1.00	7.00
115	7	4.93	2	4.07	46	48.07	51	48.93	2.061	−2.263	1.280	1.00	7.00
116	5	3.84	4	3.16	46	47.16	49	47.84	1.631	−1.542	1.231	1.00	8.00
117	7	6.00	6	5.00	35	36.00	38	37.00	2.401	−1.557	1.231	1.00	8.00
118	6	6.45	6	5.55	40	39.55	40	40.45	2.625	−1.457	1.231	1.00	8.00
119	3	3.78	4	3.22	51	50.22	50	50.78	1.642	−1.377	1.185	1.00	9.00
120	7	4.23	1	3.77	25	27.77	31	28.23	1.772	−3.338	1.140	1.00	10.00

SUBJECT INDEX TO VOLUMES I AND II

A

Additive effect, I.55
Additive models, I.55, I.58, II.122–31
  choice between additive and multiplicative
    models, II.142–46
Age-incidence curves, II.55
Age-specific rates, II.49–51, II.193–95
Age-specific ratios, II.61, II.72
Age standardization, I.254
  of mortality rates, II.51–70
Age-standardized death rates, II.91
Age-standardized mortality ratios. *See*
    Standardized mortality ratios
    (SMRs)
Age/stratum-specific rates, II.61
Age-time specific comparisons, II.48
Alcohol consumption
  in relation to oesophageal cancer, I.216,
    I.218–20, I.223–24, I.227–35
  in relation to oral cancer, I.66, I.67, I.86,
    I.109, I.110
Alternative explanation of observed
    relationships, I.89
AMFIT program, II.175
Analysis of variance, multiplicative model
    for SMRs, II.158
Animal models, I.236
Ankylosing spondylitis, irradiation for, I.62
Annual incidence rates, I.43, I.47
Armitage–Doll model, II.256, II.264
  see also Multistage models of
    carcinogenesis
Asbestos exposure, I.21, I.90, II.31–34,
    II.38, II.103
  and lung cancer, II.242–44, II.262
  and mesothelioma, II.237–39, II.261

combined with cigarette smoking, I.66–68,
    II.352–53
Association. *See* Disease association
Association strength, I.88–89
Asymptotic normality, II.133–35
Atomic bomb survivors, I.62, II.22
  life-span study, II.340–44
Attained significance level, I.128
Attributable risk, I.73–78, II.21
  for exposed persons, I.74
  population risk, I.74
  relative attributable risk, I.,76

B

Background rates
  incorporation into multiplicative model,
    II.151–53
  non-parametric estimation of,
    II.192–99
Bandwidth, choice of kernel estimates,
    II.193–95
Benzene exposure, risk of leukaemia, I.87
Benzidine exposure and bladder cancer,
    II.252
Benzo[*a*]pyrene, and incidence of skin
    tumours, I.237
Bermuda Case-Control Symposium, I.19
Bernoulli distribution, II.132
Biases, I.22, I.35, I.73, I.84–85, I.89, I.105,
    I.113, II.9, II.16, II.73
  arising from unconditional analysis of
    matched data, I.249–51
  due to errors of measurement, II.41–42
  see also Recall bias; Selection bias
Binomial coefficient, definition, I.125
Binomial distribution, definition, I.125

Biological monitoring, II.20
Birth cohort analysis, I.48
Bladder cancer, II.21, II.30
    and benzidine exposure, II.252
    in chemical industry, II.11
Bone tumours, and radiation exposure,
        II.249–50
Boston Drug Surveillance Program, I.22,
        I.115
Breast cancer, II.21
    age at first birth, I.64–66, I.77, I.86
    age-specific incidence rates, I.49, I.50,
        I.59, I.60, II.129
    and radiation exposure, II.247–49, II.262
    bilateral, I.87
    cohort analysis of Icelandic data, II.126–31
    comparison of indirect standardization and
        multiplicative model fitting, II.130
    example of negative confounding, I.93–94
    influence of reproductive factors, I.66
    irradiation-induced, I.62
    relative risks for, I.92
    reproductive experience in, I.17, I.66
Breast disease, benign, II.187
British doctors study, II.27, II.28, II.101,
        II.163–65, II.168–70, II.236,
        II.336–39

C

Calendar period-specific rates, II.49–51
Calendar time, I.43
Carcinogenesis, multistage models of,
        II.256–60
Case-control sampling, II.205, II.289–302
    see also Risk set sampling
Case-control studies
    applicability, I.21
    as related to cohort studies, II.3–22,
        II.35–36, II.42, II.44
    chi-squared test statistic
        1 D.F. test for trend, I.147–50
        combination of 2 × K table, I.149
        goodness-of-fit, I.209–10
        in logistic regression, I.208–10
            goodness-of-fit, I.208, I.222, I.273
        matched pairs (McNemar test), I.165,
            I.184
            for homogeneity of relative risk,

            I.166–69, I.185
            1 D.F. test for trend, I.184
        matched samples (1:M), I.171, I.177
            for homogeneity and trend in relative
                risk, I.173–76
        series of 2 × 2 tables (Mantel–Haenszel
            statistic), I.138
            for homogeneity of relative risk,
                I.142, I.143
            for trend in relative risk, I.142
        series of 2 × K tables, I.149
            trend test, I.149
        summary chi-squared for combination of
            2 × 2 table (Mantel–Haenszel
            statistic), I.138
        test of homogeneity, I.166–69
        2 × 2 table, I.131–32
        2 × K table, I.147
    contradictory results, I.19
    definition, I.14–16
    design considerations, II.272, II.289–302
        choice of case, I.23–25
        choice of control, I.25–28
        efficiency of, I.21
        future role of, I.18
        general considerations, I.14–40
        history, I.17
        limitations, I.22
        low cost of, I.21
        major strengths of, I.20–22
        objectives of, I.17, I.19–20
        planning, I.23–32
        present significance, I.17–19
        status of cases, I.24
        unmatched design considerations,
            II.289–94, II.302–4
Causality, I.84–85
    criteria, I.36–37, I.86–90
    evidence of, I.90
Chi-squared test statistic. See under Case-
        control studies; Cohort studies
Childhood cancers, I.239–42
Chronological age, I.43
Cigarette smoking. See Tobacco
        consumption
Classification errors, I.114
Coding of disease, II.30
Coffee drinking, lack of dose response for
        bladder cancer, I.86,

Cohort studies
    chi-squared test statistic, II.68, II.94, II.137
        comparison of two SMRs, II.94
        for SMR, II.68, II.69
        goodness-of-fit test for grouped data, II.129
        heterogeneity of SMR, II.96
        1 d.f. test for trend of SMR, II.96
        summary test for equality of relative risk, II.108, II.113
        test for heterogeneity of relative risk, II.112
        test for trend in relative risk, II.112
    definition, II.2
    design and execution, II.22
    design considerations, II.271–88
    further information from, II.28–29
    general considerations, II.2–46
    historical, II.2, II.5–11, II.19, II.21, II.32, II.33, II.35, II.37, II.42
    identification of cancer cases, II.28
    implementation, II.22–36
    interpretation, II.36–45
    limitations of, II.20–22
    present significance of, II.11–20
    problems in interpretation of, II.39–45
    prospective, II.2, II.20, II.33, II.35, II.37
    retrospective. See historical (above)
    sample size for
        comparison with external standard, 2.273–79
        comparison with internal control group, 2.279–85
    specific strengths of, 2.11–20
Combined exposures, I.66–68
    see also Joint effects
Comparative mortality figure (CMF), II.48, II.61–63, II.90, II.125, II.126
    instability of, II.63
    standard error of, II.64
    versus SMR, II.72
Comparison groups, choice of, II.33–34, II.39–40, II.61
Comparisons with several disease or control groups, I.111–12
Composite variables, I.105
Computer programs, II.175, II.192, II.206
    AMFIT, II.175

GLIM. See GLIM
    LOGODDS, I.322–38, II.189
    MATCH, I.297–306
    PECAN, II.206
Conditional analysis, I.249
Conditional distribution
    for 2 × 2 table, I.125
    for series of 2 × 2 tables, I.138
Conditional likelihood, I.204, I.209, I.248, I.251, I.253, I.255, I.270
Conditional logistic regression analysis for matched sets, I.248–79, I.297–306
Conditional maximum likelihood estimate for 2 × 2 table, I.127
Confidence coefficient, definition, I.128
Confidence intervals, I.134, I.165–67, I.182
    definition, I.128–29
    for common odds ratio in series of 2 × 2 tables, I.141–42
    for odds ratio in 2 × 2 table
        Cornfield, I.133–34
        exact, I.129
        logit, 1.134
        test based, I.134
    for ratio of SMR, II.95
    for relative risk in matched pairs, I.163–67
    for relative risk in matched sets (1:M), I.172–76, I.182
    for the SMR, II.69–71
    logistic regression parameters. See Covariance matrix of logistic regression parameters
    test based, I.134, I.135
    see also Standard error of Mantel-Haenszel estimate
Confounding, residual, I.100, I.101
Confounding effects, I.84–85, I.93–108, II.87
    and misclassification, I.106
    control of, I.29–30, I.36, I.111, I.136–56, I.162, I.166
    effect of study design on, I.101–3
    negative, I.95
    of nuisance factors, I.225–26
    on sample size requirements, II.304–6
    statistical aspects of, I.94–97
    see also Logistic model and logistic regression; Standardized mortality ratios (SMRs), bias in the ratio of Stratification

Confounding risk ratio, I.76, I.96–97,
    I.99–101, II.33
Confounding score index, I.101
Conjugated oestrogen dose, I.178
Continuity correction, I.131–34, II.296,
    II.301
Continuous data, fitting models to
    II.178–229
Continuous data analysis, I.227–33
  choice of basic time variable, II.180–81
  comparison with grouped data analysis,
    II.211–12
  construction of exposure functions,
    II.181–82
  external standard rates, II.183–84
  fundamentals of, II.179–84
  in matched studies, I.265–68
  model equations, II.182–83
  of Montana smelter workers, II.206–18
  of South Wales nickel refiners – nasal sinus
    cancer, II.218–29
Continuous variables, I.92
Contour plot of deviances, II.169
Controls
  choice of control series, I.25–28
  selection procedure, II.205–6
  see also Case-control studies; Matching;
    Risk set sampling
Cornfield's limits, I.133–34
Coronary disease among British male
    doctors, II.112, II.145, II.146
Corrected chi-squared statistic, I.131
Covariance matrix of logistic regression
    parameters, I.207
Cross-classification. See Stratification
Cross-sectional analysis of incidence rates,
    I.48
Cross-tabulation. See Stratification
Cumulative background rates, estimation of,
    II.192–97, II.204–5
Cumulative incidence rates, I.49–53
Cumulative rate, II.57–58
  standard error, II.58–61
Cumulative ratio, kernel estimation of,
    II.193–95
Cumulative relative rates, II.204–5
Cumulative standardized mortality ratio,
    II.207

D

Data acquisition, II.36
Data collection, II.35, II.42
Data points, influence of, II.139–40
Death rates, US national, II.358–61
Denominator information, II.26–28
Design considerations. See under Case-
    control studies; Cohort studies;
    Matching
Deviances
  contour plot of, II.169
  see also Likelihood inference
Dichotomous exposure
  1:M matching, I.169–76
  in unmatched studies, I.124–46
  matched pairs, I.164–76
  variable number of controls, I.176–82
Dichotomous variables, I.91, I.94–97
Directly standardized rate, I.50, II.52–57,
    II.89–91
  standard error, II.58–61
  see also Comparative mortality figure
    (CMF)
Disease association models, I.53–59
Disease occurrence, measures of, I.42–47
Dose metameter selection, II.98–99
Dose-response analysis, II.105, II.115–18
  see also Logistic model and logistic
    regression; Regression analysis;
    Trend tests
Dose-response relationship, I.86, I.88, II.37,
    II.41, II.42, II.82, II.83, II.88,
    II.97, II.96, II.159, II.232
  multistage models, 2.262–63
  see also Joint effects
Dose-time relationships, II.233–55
Dose-time-response relationships, II.120
Dose transformations, II.159
Dummy variables for logistic regression
    models, I.196, I.214

E

Ecological studies, II.4
Effect modification. See Interaction
    (modifying) effects

Efficiency calculations for matched designs, II.302–4
Empirical odds ratio, I.127
Endometrial cancer, I.24, I.29, I.90, I.104, I.265
  Los Angeles study of, I.162–63, I.185, I.253, I.255, I.258, I.260, I.261, I.263, I.264, I.266, I.290–96
Endometrial hyperplasia, I.30
Epithelial tumours, age-specific rates and latent period, I.60, I.62, I.89
Errors of classification and of measurement, I.114, II.41–42, II.265–66
generating confounding, I.106
Estimation of odds ratio
  combination of 2×2 table
    logit estimate, I.139
    Mantel-Haenszel estimate, I.140, I.141
    maximum likelihood estimate, I.140
  2×2 table
    asymptotic maximum likelihood, I.130
    exact conditional maximum likelihood, I.124
  see also Logistic regression
Excess mortality ratio (EMR), II.174, II.175, II.268
Excess risk, I.55, I.58, I.64, I.84, II.45
Excess risk model
  fitting to grouped data, II.171–76
  see also Additive models
Exponential distribution, II.132
Exponential survival times, II.131–32
Exposure functions, II.181–82
Exposure index, II.172–73
Exposure information, II.30–33, II.37
Exposure probability, I.71
Exposure variables, lagging of, II.48, II.87
External standard rates, II.212–14
Extra Poisson variability, II.99–100

F

Familial risk, I.87
Fisher's exact test, I.128, I.129, I.133
Fitted values in 2×2 table, I.130
Follow-up losses, II.40–41, II.49
Follow-up mechanisms, II.17, II.25–29
Follow-up period, II.288–89

Follow-up schema, II.50
Force of morbidity, I.45
Force of mortality, I.45
Forerunners of disease, II.44

G

Gall-bladder disease, I.22, I.168, I.254–59, I.262, I.264, I.265
Gastric cancer, age-specific incidence rates, I.62
GLIM computer program, I.206, I.208, I.214, I.253, II.128, II.136–37, II.139, II.141–143, II.160, II.162, II.163, II.167, II.174, II.175
Global statistic for homogeneity test, I.142
Global test, I.153
Goodness-of-fit, I.142, II.161, II.190, II.199
  analysis of residuals, II.138–39, II.144–46
  in logistic regression, I.208, I.222, I.273
  influential data points, II.139–40, II.144–46
  multiplicative models, II.148, II.149
  statistics, II.141, II.144
  summary of measures of, II.137–38
  see also Case-control studies, chi-squared test statistic; Cohort studies, chi-squared test statistic
Greenwood's formula, II.192
Group-matching, I.122
Grouped data, fitting models to, II.120–76
Grouped data analysis
  case-control studies, I.122–59
    goodness-of-fit in logistic regression, I.208, I.222, I.273
    Ille-et-Vilaine study of oesophageal cancer, I.281–83
    Oxford Childhood Cancer Survey, I.284–89
    qualitative analysis of, I.213–19
    quantitative analysis of, I.221–24
  cohort studies, II.106–15
    comparison with continuous data analysis, II.211–12
    conservatism of indirect standardization, II.114–15
    extensions to $K > 2$ exposure classes, II.113–114

Grouped data analysis—contd.
  cohort studies—contd.
    heterogeneity of relative risk, II.110–13
    Mantel-Haenszel estimate, II.109–13
    Montana cohort, II.146–50, II.155–59
    restrictions on, II.178
    summary test of significance, II.108
    two dose levels, exposed versus
        unexposed, II.107–8
  maximum likelihood estimate, II.108–13

H

Hat matrix in residual analysis, II.138–40
Hazard rate, I.45
Hazards, proportional, I.201
Healthy worker effect, II.17, II.39–40, II.87,
    II.98
Heterogeneity, II.75–76
  see also Case-control studies, chi-squared
      test statistic; Cohort studies, chi-
      squared statistic
Historical cohort studies, II.2, II.19
HLA antigen A2 and leukaemia, association
      with survival, I.25
HLA antigens and multiple comparison,
      I.115
Hodgkin's disease and tonsillectomy, I.16,
      I.31

Homogeneity of relative risk
  in matched pairs, I.166–67
  in matched sets (1:M), I.173–74
  in series of 2×2 tables, I.137, I.142–43
  tests for homogeneity, see under Case-
      control studies; Cohort studies
Homogeneity test, global statistic for, I.142
Hypergeometric distribution
  central, definition, I.127
  K-dimensional, I.147
  non-central, definition, I.127
Hypertension, I.168, I.169, I.254–59

I

Ille-et-Vilaine study of oesophageal cancer,
      I.122–24, I.162, I.210, I.213–33,
      I.238, I.281–83
Implementation
  in case-control studies, I.32–35

in cohort studies, II.22–36
Incidence cohorts, II.25
Incidence rates, I.43, I.66, I.71
  age-specific, I.44, I.47–48, I.59–61
  calculation of, I.44
  cumulative, I.49–53
  directly standardized, I.50
  estimation of, I.45
  logarithmic transformation of, I.57
  overall, I.76
  time-specific, I.47–48
  variations in, I.55
Indicator variables. See Dummy variables
Indirect standardization, II.48
  see also Standardized mortality ratios
      (SMRs)
Influence of individual data points,
      II.139–40, II.144–46
Information matrix, I.207
Initial treatment of data, I.90–93
Instantaneous rate, I.45
Insulation workers, 2.103
Interaction (modifying) effects, I.108–11,
      I.167, II.110–13
  definition of, I.108–11
  effect on sample size requirement and
      matching, II.308–10
  in conditional logit analysis, I.262–68,
      I.273
  in logistic model
      definition of, I.196–200
      test for, I.221–24
  in series of 2×2 tables, I.238–42
  negative, I.196
  see also Case-control studies; Cohort
      studies
Interaction parameter
  in logistic regression, I.196
Internally standardized mortality ratios,
      II.103–6
International Classification of Diseases
      (ICD), II.30, II.355–57
Interpretation, basic considerations, I.35–37,
      I.112–15
Interviews, I.33–34
  questionnaires, I.34
Iran, oesophageal cancer in Caspian littoral
      of, I.275, I.276
Irradiation
  obstetric, and associated cancer risk,

I.239–42
risk of cancer following, I.62–63
Ischaemic heart disease, and cigarette
  smoking, I.68

J

Joint distribution, I.99
Joint effects of multiple exposures, I.66–68,
  I.99, I.111, I.154–56, I.227,
  II.266–67
  see also Interaction (modifying) effects

K

Kernael estimation of cumulative ratio,
  II.193–95

L

Lagging of exposure variables, II.48, II.87
Large strata, unconditional logistic
  regression for, I.192–246
Latency function, II.181–82, II.216–17,
  II.264–66
Latent period, I.89
Least-squares analyses, II.161
Least-squares linear regression analysis,
  II.99–103
Leukaemia, and radiation exposure,
  II.244–47
Likelihood inference: outline of I.205–10
  likelihood ratio statistic, I.209
  likelihood ratio test, I.207
  log-likelihood analysis, I.206
  log-likelihood function, I.206, II.134,
    II.184–92, II.202–3
  see also Partial likelihood
  log-likelihood statistic, I.206
  log-normal distribution, II.181
Log-linear models, definition, I.57
Log odds. See Logit transform
Log relative risks as logistic regression
  parameters, I.196
Logistic model and logistic regression, I.142
  case-control studies, I.202–5
  general definition of, I.200–2

introduction to, I.193–200
  results of fitting several versions of, I.212
Logistic regression model, II.153–54
  dummy variable for, I.196, I.214
Logit confidence limits from combination of
    2×2 tables, I.134
Logit estimate, I.139
Logit limits, I.141
Logit transform, I.194, I.196
LOGODDS program listing, I.322–38,
    II.189
Longitudinal studies, II.2
Los Angeles study of endometrial cancer,
    I.162–63, I.185, I.253, I.255, I.258,
    I.260, I.261, I.263, I.264, I.266,
    I.290–96
Losses to follow-up, II.40–41, II.49
Lost-to-follow-up subjects, II.49
Lung cancer, II.38, II.39, II.43, II.100,
    II.103
  age- and year-specific death rates,
    II.391–94
  and asbestos exposure, II.242–44, II.262
  and uranium miners, II.253–55
  British male doctors, II.163–65, II.168,
    II.169, II.170
  in relation to tobacco consumption, I.17,
    I.55, I.58, I.64, I.66–69, I.75,
    I.86–93, I.100, I.101, I.104, I.166,
    I.193, II.5–9, II.15, II.234–36,
    II.261
  combined with asbestos exposure,
    I.66–68
  relative risk of, II.235
  South Wales nickel refiners, II.171, II.174,
    II.268, II.347–48

M

McNemar's test, I.165
Mantel test for trend, I.148
Mantel-Haenszel analysis, II.82
  estimate for cohort studies, II.109–113,
    II.147, II.285
  for case-control studies, I.138–42, I.144,
    I.165, I.171, I.172, I.174, I.177,
    I.179, I.181, I.192, I.195–96
  test for cohort studies, II.189
Mantel-Haenszel statistic, I.138
MATCH program listing, I.297–306

Matched case-control studies, II.297
  design
    comparison with unmatched design,
      II.306
    number of controls per case, II.304
    sample size requirements for
      dichotomous exposure, II.294–302
Matched data analysis, I.162–89
  conditional logistic regression analysis for,
    I.248–79, I.297–306
  conditional logistic regression, I.248–79,
    I.297–306
  dichotomous variables
    1:1 matching, I.164–69
    1:M matching, I.169–76
    variable number of controls, I.176–82
  polytomous variables, I.182–87
Matched designs, efficiency calculations for,
    I.270–76, II.302–4
Matched versus unmatched analyses,
    I.102–6, I.249–51, I.270–76
Matching
  by strata, I.30–31
  in choice of controls, I.28–32
  problems associated with, I.31
Maximum likelihood estimate (MLE). See
    Estimation of odds ratio;
    Likelihood inference
Mesothelioma
  and asbestos exposure, II.237–39, II.261
  of the pleura, I.21
Misclassification, I.114
  see also Biases; Errors of classification and
    of measurement
Misclassification rates, II.42
  see also Biases, due to errors of
    measurement
Missing data, I.113–14
Model selection, II.203–4
  biological basis for, II.125
Modelling risk, I.111
Models, disease association, I.53–59
Modifying effect. See Interaction
Montana smelter workers
  cohort studies, II.18, II.23, II.32, II.37,
    II.52, II.53, II.60, II.78, II.79,
    II.86–99, II.105, II.114, II.148,
    II.149, II.152, II.154, II.206–18,
    II.232, II.349–50

grouped data analyses, II.146–50,
    II.155–59, II.363–65
multiplicative models, II.146–50, II.211,
    II.213,
numbers alive and under observation,
    II.202
regression analyses, II.157–59
respiratory cancer, II.157, II.158
Mortality, proportional, II.45–46, II.76,
    II.115–18
Mortality rates, I.43
  age-specific, I.65
  age standardization of, II.51–70
  estimation of, I.45
Mortality ratios, standardized. See
    Standardized mortality ratios
Mouth cancer. See Oral cancer
Multiple comparison, I.115, II.43–44
Multiple exposure levels, I.189
  matched studies, I.146–54, I.182–87
  see also Logistic model and logistic
    regression
Multiplicative models, I.57, I.58, I.67,
    II.122–31, II.135–42
  choice between additive and multiplicative
    models, II.142–46
  comparison with indirect standardization,
    II.125–31
  estimating base line rates under, II.195–99
  fitting of, II.148
  general form of, II.136
  goodness-of-fit, II.148, II.149
  incorporating external standard rates,
    II.151–53
  Montana smelter workers, II.146–50,
    II.211, II.213
  nasal sinus cancer in South Wales nickel
    workers, II.223, II.224, II.226,
    II.227
  partial likelihood for, II.185–86
  regression coefficients, II.158
Multistage models of carcinogenesis,
    II.256–60
  dose-response relationship, II,262–63
  interpretation of epidemiological data in
    terms of, II.261–62
  metameters of dose when dose levels vary,
    II.263–65
  Welsh nickel refinery data, II.267–70

Multivariate analysis. *See* Logistic model and logistic regression
Multivariate normality, I.204

N

Nasal sinus cancer in South Wales nickel refinery workers, II.105, II.106, II.142, II.172, II.218–29, II.268, II.367, II.369–74
  age- and year-specific death rates, II.391–94
  fitting relative and excess risk models to grouped data, II.171–76
  multiplicative model, II.223, II.224, II.226, II.227
  see also Continuous data analysis
Negative confounding, I.95
Negative interaction, I.196
Negative results, II.44–45
Nested hierarchy of models, I.207
Nickel workers. *See* South Wales nickel refiners
Non-central hypergeometric distribution, definition, I.127
Non-identifiability problem, II.128
Non-multiplicative models and partial likelihood, II.191
Non-oestrogen drug use, I.262, I.264, I.265
Non-parametric estimation
  background rates, II.192–99
  relative mortality functions, II.197–99
Normal approximation to exact distribution for 2×2 table, I.129
Nuisance factors, confounding effects of, I.225–26
Nuisance parameters, I.205

O

Obesity and risk of endometrial cancer, I.262, I.265
Obstetric radiation and associated risk of cancer, I.239–42
Odds ratio, I.70, I.73, I.94–96, I.99, I.102, I.103, I.106, I.108, I.130–31, I.135, I.139, I.140, I.196, I.250–10, I.241, I.252
  empirical, I.172
  equivalence to relative risk, I.70–72
  estimation of. *See* Estimation of odds ratio
  test for consistency, I.185–87
  test for homogeneity, I.142–46, I.167
Oesophageal cancer, II.36, II.45, II.159
  among Singapore Chinese, I.274
  dose-response, II.263
  Ille-et-Vilaine study of, I.222–24, I.162, I.210, I.213–33, I.238, I.281–83
  in Caspian littoral of Iran, 1.275, I.276
  in relation to alcohol consumption, I.216, I.218–20, I.223–24, I.227–35
  in relation to tobacco consumption, I.154, I.155, I.217–19, I.221, I.223–24, I.227–35, II.266
  log relative risk, I.216, I.217, I.220, I.221
Oestrogen use, I.24, I.29, I.90, I.93, I.104, I.254–59, I.262, I.264, I.265
Oral cancer in relation to alcohol and tobacco consumption, I.66, I.67, I.86, I.109, I.110
Oral contraceptives, I.22
Overmatching, I.104–6
Oxford Childhood Cancer Survey, I.239–42, I.270, I.284–89, I.322

P

p-values as measure of degree of evidence, I.128
Partial likelihood, II.186, II.188, II.189
  for multiplicative models, II.185–86
Partial likelihood analysis, II.200, II.212–14, II.212
PECAN program, II.206
Person-years, algorithm for exact calculation, II.362
Person-years allocation, II.49–51, II.83, II.85–86, II.88
  to time-dependent exposure categories, II.82–86
Point prevalence I.42
Poisson distribution, II.68, II.69, II.70, II.274
Poisson models
  and the Poisson assumption, II.131–35
  for grouped data, II.185
Poisson rates, fitting general models to, II.160–67

Poisson variability, II.99, II.100
Poolability of data. *See* Matched data
    analysis
Population attributable risk, I.74, II.21
Population controls, I.276
Portsmouth (USA) Naval Shipyard workers,
    II.99
Positive confounding, I.95, I.101
Positive interaction, I.196
Potential confounding, I.107
Power considerations, II.34–35
    see also Case-control studies, design
        considerations; Cohort studies,
        design considerations
Power to detect interaction, II.308–10
Prevalence, point, I.42
Prevalence cohorts, II.25
Proportional hazards, I.201
Proportional mortality, II.45–46, II.76,
    II.115–18
    analysis II.153–55, II.216
    incorporating standard rates, II.154–55
    risk functions for, II.168–71
Proportionality assumption, II.93
Prospective cohort studies, II.2

Q

Questionnaires, I.34
    information management, I.34–35

R

Radiation exposure
    and bone tumours, II.249–50
    and breast cancer, II.247–49, II.262
    and cigarette smoking, II.254
    and leukaemia, II.244–47
Rate of occurrence, I.43
Rates and rate standardization, II.48–79
    cumulative rate, II.57–58
    directly standardized rate, II.52–57
    standard error of cumulative or directly
        standardized rate, II.58–61
    standardized to world population, II.55–57
    summary measures, II.51
    see also Incidence rates; Mortality rate;
        Standardized mortality ratios
        (SMRs)
Recall bias, I.22, I.35, I.84–85, I.113, II.16

Regression adjustment for confounders,
    I.225–26
Regression analysis, I.232, II.91, II.99,
    II.100
    Montana smelter workers, II.157–59
    see also Logistic model and logistic
        regression
Regression coefficients, I.197, I.215, I.218,
    I.224, I.274, II.140, II.142
    interpretation of, I.233–36
    multiplicative model, II.158
    standardized, I.208
Regression diagnostics, II.138–42, II.146,
    II.161, II.203–4
Regression models, I.214, I.215, I.222, I.240
Regression variables, I.239, I.254–59
Relative attributable risk (RAR), I.76
Relative mortality functions, nonparametric
    estimation, II.197–99
Relative mortality index (RMI), II.75
Relative risk, I.57–67, I.69–73, I.77, I.84,
    I.87–89, I.110, I.113, II.106–14,
    II.142
    additive, II.160
    see also Odds ratio
Relative risk estimation, II.94–95, II.108–10,
    II.147
    general models of, II.159–71
    incorporating external standard rates,
        II.167
    see also Estimation of odds ratio; Mantel-
        Haenszel analysis
Relative standardized mortality ratio
    (RSMR), II.77–78
Reproductive factors in breast cancer, I.66
Residual analysis, Hat matrix in, II.138–40
Residual confounding, I.100, I.101
Residuals, standardized, I.213
Respiratory cancer, II.60, II.105, II.207
    standard death rates, II.88
    standard proportion of deaths due to,
        II.155
Retirement, II.27
Risk, 1.51, 1.53
    see also Excess risk; Relative risk
Risk-dose-time relationship, modelling,
    II.232–70
Risk factors, I.25, I.53, I.55, I.56, I.58, I.66,
    I.76, I.123, I.128
    binary, I.263

constellation of, I.199
joint effects of, I.154–56
more than two levels, I.198
Risk ratio. *See* Relative risk; Odds ratio
Risk set sampling, II.199–206, II.214–16,
    II.302–4
Risk specificity
    disease subgroups, I.86–87
    exposure subcategories, I.87
Risk variables, I.123
    transforming continuous, I.236–38
Rule of 5, I.139

S

Sample size. *See* Case-control studies, design
    considerations; Cohort studies,
    design considerations; Confounding
    effects; Interaction; Matching
Sampling requirements, I.72
Score statistic, I.207
Second order interaction, I.199
Selection bias, I.22, I.35, I.85, I.89, I.113,
    II.17, II.49
Serial measurements, II.20
Significance level
    attained, I.218
    two-sided, I.133
Significance tests, I.127, I.131–33
Single-tail test, I.133
Skin cancer, case-control study of, I.200
Skin tumours, I.236
    estimated cumulative incidence rates, I.237
    in mice, I.46, I.53, I.54
South Wales nickel refiners, II.23–25, II.32,
    II.37, II.142, II.143, II.218–29,
    II.233
    continuous data II.374–90
    lung cancer in II.171, II.174, II.268,
        II.347–48
    mortality experiences, II.171
    multistage models, II.267–70
    nasal sinus cancer, II.268, II.365–67,
        II.369–74
Spurious associations, I.89
Standard error
    of CMF, 2.64
    of Mantel-Haenszel estimate, II.109
    of SMR, II.67

Standard populations, II.54–55
Standardized mortality ratios (SMRs), II.49,
    II.65–68, II.83, II.88, II.125, II.126,
    II.128, II.151, II.152, II.157, II.158,
    II.173, II.175, II.197–98, II.268
    advantages over CMF, II.65–66
    approximate limits for, II.70
    bias in the ratio of, II.72–75, II.92
    by years since first employed, II.217–18
    comparison of II.91–103
    confidence intervals for, II.69–72
    testing for heterogeneity and trend in,
        II.96–97
    testing significance of, II.68–69
    versus CMF, II.72
Standardized regression coefficient, I.208
Standardized residuals, I.213
Statistical inference, I.124–29, I.206
    approximate methods of, I.129
    see also Likelihood inference
Statistical interaction, definition, I.56
Statistical modelling, advantages and
        limitations of, II.120
Stomach cancer, age-specific incidence rates,
        I.60, I.61
STRAT program listing, I.307–21
Strata matching, I.30–31
Stratification, I.89, I.105, I.111, I.122, I.225,
        I.242
    see also Confounding, control of
Stratification degree, I.99–101
Summary chi-squared test for combination of
        2 × 2 tables. *See* under Case-control
        studies; Cohort studies
Summary measures
    of goodness-of-fit, II.137–38
    of rates, II.51–61
Survival rates, I.43
Survival times, II.131–32

T

Tail probabilities, I.27
Time-dependent exposure categories,
        person-years allocation to, II.82–86
Time on study, I.43
Time relationships, II.37–39
Tobacco consumption, II.43, II.46, II.88,
        II.101, II.103

Tobacco consumption—contd.
  and mortality, II.6
  and radiation exposure, II.254
  in relation to lung cancer, I.17, I.55, I.58,
    I.64, I.66–69, I.75, I.86–93, I.100,
    I.101, I.104, I.166, I.193, II.5–9,
    II.15, II.234–36, II.261
    combined with asbestos exposure,
      I.66–68, II.352–53
  in relation to oesophageal cancer, I.154,
    I.155, I.217–19, I.221, I.223–24,
    I.227–35, II.266
  in relation to oral cancer, I.66–69, I.86,
    I.110
Tonsillectomy and Hodgkin's disease, I.16,
  I.31
Trend tests
  for exposure effect versus trend test for
    dose-response, II.97–98
  see also under Case-control studies,
    chi-squared test statistic; Cohort
    studies, chi-squared test statistic
2 × 2 table, I.126, I.146, I.148, I.154, I.169
  approximate statistical inference for,
    I.129–44
  combining results from, I.136–56,
    I.210–13
  combining sets of, I.268–70
  conditional distribution for, I.125, I.138
  conditional maximum likelihood estimate
    for, I.127
  equivalence of odds ratio and relative risk,
    I.70–72
  exact statistical inference, I.124–29
  interaction in, I.238–42
  odds ratio in, I.248
2 × K table, I.146–54
Two-sided significance level, I.133
Two-sided test, I.128

U

Unconditional analysis of matched data, bias
  arising from, I.249–51
Unconditional likelihood for logistic
  regression, I.209, I.253
Unconditional likelihood function, I.269
Unconditional logistic regression, I.269
  for large strata, I.192–46
Unconditional model, I.269
Unknown parameters, I.125
Unmatched analysis, I.271–76
Unmatched case-control studies, design
  considerations, II.289–94, II.302–4
Unstratified analysis, I.146–47
Uranium miners, and lung cancer, II.253–55
Urinary tract tumour, I.52, I.86
US national death rates, II.358–61
Uterine bleeding, I.104
Uterine cancer, I.27

V

Vaginal adenocarcinoma, I.89

W

Weighted least squares regression, I.60
Welsh nickel refiners. See South Wales nickel
  refiners
Woolf estimate. See Logit estimate

Y

Yates correction. See Continuity correction

PUBLICATIONS OF THE INTERNATIONAL AGENCY FOR RESEARCH ON CANCER

Scientific Publications Series

(Available from Oxford University Press through local bookshops)

No. 1 Liver Cancer
1971; 176 pages (*out of print*)

No. 2 Oncogenesis and Herpesviruses
Edited by P.M. Biggs, G. de-Thé and L.N. Payne
1972; 515 pages (*out of print*)

No. 3 N-Nitroso Compounds: Analysis and Formation
Edited by P. Bogovski, R. Preussman and E.A. Walker
1972; 140 pages (*out of print*)

No. 4 Transplacental Carcinogenesis
Edited by L. Tomatis and U. Mohr
1973; 181 pages (*out of print*)

No. 5/6 Pathology of Tumours in Laboratory Animals, Volume 1, Tumours of the Rat
Edited by V.S. Turusov
1973/1976; 533 pages (*out of print*)

No. 7 Host Environment Interactions in the Etiology of Cancer in Man
Edited by R. Doll and I. Vodopija
1973; 464 pages (*out of print*)

No. 8 Biological Effects of Asbestos
Edited by P. Bogovski, J.C. Gilson, V. Timbrell and J.C. Wagner
1973; 346 pages (*out of print*)

No. 9 N-Nitroso Compounds in the Environment
Edited by P. Bogovski and E.A. Walker
1974; 243 pages (*out of print*)

No. 10 Chemical Carcinogenesis Essays
Edited by R. Montesano and L. Tomatis
1974; 230 pages (*out of print*)

No. 11 Oncogenesis and Herpesviruses II
Edited by G. de-Thé, M.A. Epstein and H. zur Hausen
1975; Part I: 511 pages
Part II: 403 pages (*out of print*)

No. 12 Screening Tests in Chemical Carcinogenesis
Edited by R. Montesano, H. Bartsch and L. Tomatis
1976; 666 pages (*out of print*)

No. 13 Environmental Pollution and Carcinogenic Risks
Edited by C. Rosenfeld and W. Davis
1975; 441 pages (*out of print*)

No. 14 Environmental N-Nitroso Compounds. Analysis and Formation
Edited by E.A. Walker, P. Bogovski and L. Griciute
1976; 512 pages (*out of print*)

No. 15 Cancer Incidence in Five Continents, Volume III
Edited by J.A.H. Waterhouse, C. Muir, P. Correa and J. Powell
1976; 584 pages (*out of print*)

No. 16 Air Pollution and Cancer in Man
Edited by U. Mohr, D. Schmähl and L. Tomatis
1977; 328 pages (*out of print*)

No. 17 Directory of On-going Research in Cancer Epidemiology 1977
Edited by C.S. Muir and G. Wagner
1977; 599 pages (*out of print*)

No. 18 Environmental Carcinogens. Selected Methods of Analysis. Volume 1: Analysis of Volatile Nitrosamines in Food
Editor-in-Chief: H. Egan
1978; 212 pages (*out of print*)

No. 19 Environmental Aspects of N-Nitroso Compounds
Edited by E.A. Walker, M. Castegnaro, L. Griciute and R.E. Lyle
1978; 561 pages (*out of print*)

No. 20 Nasopharyngeal Carcinoma: Etiology and Control
Edited by G. de-Thé and Y. Ito
1978; 606 pages (*out of print*)

No. 21 Cancer Registration and its Techniques
Edited by R. MacLennan, C. Muir, R. Steinitz and A. Winkler
1978; 235 pages (*out of print*)

No. 22 Environmental Carcinogens. Selected Methods of Analysis. Volume 2: Methods for the Measurement of Vinyl Chloride in Poly(vinyl chloride), Air, Water and Foodstuffs
Editor-in-Chief: H. Egan
1978; 142 pages (*out of print*)

No. 23 Pathology of Tumours in Laboratory Animals. Volume II: Tumours of the Mouse
Editor-in-Chief: V.S. Turusov
1979; 669 pages (*out of print*)

No. 24 Oncogenesis and Herpesviruses III
Edited by G. de-Thé, W. Henle and F. Rapp
1978; Part I: 580 pages, Part II: 512 pages (*out of print*)

Prices, valid for February 1994 are subject to change without notice

No. 25 **Carcinogenic Risk. Strategies for Intervention**
Edited by W. Davis and C. Rosenfeld
1979; 280 pages (*out of print*)

No. 26 **Directory of On-going Research in Cancer Epidemiology 1978**
Edited by C.S. Muir and G. Wagner
1978; 550 pages (*out of print*)

No. 27 **Molecular and Cellular Aspects of Carcinogen Screening Tests**
Edited by R. Montesano, H. Bartsch and L. Tomatis
1980; 372 pages £30.00

No. 28 **Directory of On-going Research in Cancer Epidemiology 1979**
Edited by C.S. Muir and G. Wagner
1979; 672 pages (*out of print*)

No. 29 **Environmental Carcinogens. Selected Methods of Analysis. Volume 3: Analysis of Polycyclic Aromatic Hydrocarbons in Environmental Samples**
Editor-in-Chief: H. Egan
1979; 240 pages (*out of print*)

No. 30 **Biological Effects of Mineral Fibres**
Editor-in-Chief: J.C. Wagner
1980; **Volume 1:** 494 pages **Volume 2:** 513 pages (*out of print*)

No. 31 *N*-**Nitroso Compounds: Analysis, Formation and Occurrence**
Edited by E.A. Walker, L. Griciute, M. Castegnaro and M. Börzsönyi
1980; 835 pages (*out of print*)

No. 32 **Statistical Methods in Cancer Research. Volume 1. The Analysis of Case-control Studies**
By N.E. Breslow and N.E. Day
1980; 338 pages £18.00

No. 33 **Handling Chemical Carcinogens in the Laboratory**
Edited by R. Montesano *et al.*
1979; 32 pages (*out of print*)

No. 34 **Pathology of Tumours in Laboratory Animals. Volume III. Tumours of the Hamster**
Editor-in-Chief: V.S. Turusov
1982; 461 pages (*out of print*)

No. 35 **Directory of On-going Research in Cancer Epidemiology 1980**
Edited by C.S. Muir and G. Wagner
1980; 660 pages (*out of print*)

No. 36 **Cancer Mortality by Occupation and Social Class 1851-1971**
Edited by W.P.D. Logan
1982; 253 pages (*out of print*)

No. 37 **Laboratory Decontamination and Destruction of Aflatoxins B$_1$, B$_2$, G$_1$, G$_2$ in Laboratory Wastes**
Edited by M. Castegnaro *et al.*
1980; 56 pages (*out of print*)

No. 38 **Directory of On-going Research in Cancer Epidemiology 1981**
Edited by C.S. Muir and G. Wagner
1981; 696 pages (*out of print*)

No. 39 **Host Factors in Human Carcinogenesis**
Edited by H. Bartsch and B. Armstrong
1982; 583 pages (*out of print*)

No. 40 **Environmental Carcinogens. Selected Methods of Analysis. Volume 4: Some Aromatic Amines and Azo Dyes in the General and Industrial Environment**
Edited by L. Fishbein, M. Castegnaro, I.K. O'Neill and H. Bartsch
1981; 347 pages (*out of print*)

No. 41 *N*-**Nitroso Compounds: Occurrence and Biological Effects**
Edited by H. Bartsch, I.K. O'Neill, M. Castegnaro and M. Okada
1982; 755 pages £50.00

No. 42 **Cancer Incidence in Five Continents, Volume IV**
Edited by J. Waterhouse, C. Muir, K. Shanmugaratnam and J. Powell
1982; 811 pages (*out of print*)

No. 43 **Laboratory Decontamination and Destruction of Carcinogens in Laboratory Wastes: Some *N*-Nitrosamines**
Edited by M. Castegnaro *et al.*
1982; 73 pages £7.50

No. 44 **Environmental Carcinogens. Selected Methods of Analysis. Volume 5: Some Mycotoxins**
Edited by L. Stoloff, M. Castegnaro, P. Scott, I.K. O'Neill and H. Bartsch
1983; 455 pages £32.50

No. 45 **Environmental Carcinogens. Selected Methods of Analysis. Volume 6: *N*-Nitroso Compounds**
Edited by R. Preussmann, I.K. O'Neill, G. Eisenbrand, B. Spiegelhalder and H. Bartsch
1983; 508 pages £32.50

No. 46 **Directory of On-going Research in Cancer Epidemiology 1982**
Edited by C.S. Muir and G. Wagner
1982; 722 pages (*out of print*)

No. 47 **Cancer Incidence in Singapore 1968–1977**
Edited by K. Shanmugaratnam, H.P. Lee and N.E. Day
1983; 171 pages (*out of print*)

No. 48 **Cancer Incidence in the USSR (2nd Revised Edition)**
Edited by N.P. Napalkov, G.F. Tserkovny, V.M. Merabishvili, D.M. Parkin, M. Smans and C.S. Muir
1983; 75 pages (*out of print*)

No. 49 **Laboratory Decontamination and Destruction of Carcinogens in Laboratory Wastes: Some Polycyclic Aromatic Hydrocarbons**
Edited by M. Castegnaro *et al.*
1983; 87 pages (*out of print*)

No. 50 **Directory of On-going Research in Cancer Epidemiology 1983**
Edited by C.S. Muir and G. Wagner
1983; 731 pages (*out of print*)

No. 51 **Modulators of Experimental Carcinogenesis**
Edited by V. Turusov and R. Montesano
1983; 307 pages (*out of print*)

List of IARC Publications

No. 52 **Second Cancers in Relation to Radiation Treatment for Cervical Cancer: Results of a Cancer Registry Collaboration**
Edited by N.E. Day and J.C. Boice, Jr
1984; 207 pages (*out of print*)

No. 53 **Nickel in the Human Environment**
Editor-in-Chief: F.W. Sunderman, Jr
1984; 529 pages (*out of print*)

No. 54 **Laboratory Decontamination and Destruction of Carcinogens in Laboratory Wastes: Some Hydrazines**
Edited by M. Castegnaro *et al.*
1983; 87 pages (*out of print*)

No. 55 **Laboratory Decontamination and Destruction of Carcinogens in Laboratory Wastes: Some N-Nitrosamides**
Edited by M. Castegnaro *et al.*
1984; 66 pages (*out of print*)

No. 56 **Models, Mechanisms and Etiology of Tumour Promotion**
Edited by M. Börzsönyi, N.E. Day, K. Lapis and H. Yamasaki
1984; 532 pages (*out of print*)

No. 57 **N-Nitroso Compounds: Occurrence, Biological Effects and Relevance to Human Cancer**
Edited by I.K. O'Neill, R.C. von Borstel, C.T. Miller, J. Long and H. Bartsch
1984; 1013 pages (*out of print*)

No. 58 **Age-related Factors in Carcinogenesis**
Edited by A. Likhachev, V. Anisimov and R. Montesano
1985; 288 pages (*out of print*)

No. 59 **Monitoring Human Exposure to Carcinogenic and Mutagenic Agents**
Edited by A. Berlin, M. Draper, K. Hemminki and H. Vainio
1984; 457 pages (*out of print*)

No. 60 **Burkitt's Lymphoma: A Human Cancer Model**
Edited by G. Lenoir, G. O'Conor and C.L.M. Olweny
1985; 484 pages (*out of print*)

No. 61 **Laboratory Decontamination and Destruction of Carcinogens in Laboratory Wastes: Some Haloethers**
Edited by M. Castegnaro *et al.*
1985; 55 pages (*out of print*)

No. 62 **Directory of On-going Research in Cancer Epidemiology 1984**
Edited by C.S. Muir and G. Wagner
1984; 717 pages (*out of print*)

No. 63 **Virus-associated Cancers in Africa**
Edited by A.O. Williams, G.T. O'Conor, G.B. de-Thé and C.A. Johnson
1984; 773 pages (*out of print*)

No. 64 **Laboratory Decontamination and Destruction of Carcinogens in Laboratory Wastes: Some Aromatic Amines and 4-Nitrobiphenyl**
Edited by M. Castegnaro *et al.*
1985; 84 pages (*out of print*)

No. 65 **Interpretation of Negative Epidemiological Evidence for Carcinogenicity**
Edited by N.J. Wald and R. Doll
1985; 232 pages (*out of print*)

No. 66 **The Role of the Registry in Cancer Control**
Edited by D.M. Parkin, G. Wagner and C.S. Muir
1985; 152 pages £10.00

No. 67 **Transformation Assay of Established Cell Lines: Mechanisms and Application**
Edited by T. Kakunaga and H. Yamasaki
1985; 225 pages (*out of print*)

No. 68 **Environmental Carcinogens. Selected Methods of Analysis. Volume 7. Some Volatile Halogenated Hydrocarbons**
Edited by L. Fishbein and I.K. O'Neill
1985; 479 pages (*out of print*)

No. 69 **Directory of On-going Research in Cancer Epidemiology 1985**
Edited by C.S. Muir and G. Wagner
1985; 745 pages (*out of print*)

No. 70 **The Role of Cyclic Nucleic Acid Adducts in Carcinogenesis and Mutagenesis**
Edited by B. Singer and H. Bartsch
1986; 467 pages (*out of print*)

No. 71 **Environmental Carcinogens. Selected Methods of Analysis. Volume 8: Some Metals: As, Be, Cd, Cr, Ni, Pb, Se, Zn**
Edited by I.K. O'Neill, P. Schuller and L. Fishbein
1986; 485 pages (*out of print*)

No. 72 **Atlas of Cancer in Scotland, 1975–1980. Incidence and Epidemiological Perspective**
Edited by I. Kemp, P. Boyle, M. Smans and C.S. Muir
1985; 285 pages (*out of print*)

No. 73 **Laboratory Decontamination and Destruction of Carcinogens in Laboratory Wastes: Some Antineoplastic Agents**
Edited by M. Castegnaro *et al.*
1985; 163 pages £12.50

No. 74 **Tobacco: A Major International Health Hazard**
Edited by D. Zaridze and R. Peto
1986; 324 pages £22.50

No. 75 **Cancer Occurrence in Developing Countries**
Edited by D.M. Parkin
1986; 339 pages £22.50

No. 76 **Screening for Cancer of the Uterine Cervix**
Edited by M. Hakama, A.B. Miller and N.E. Day
1986; 315 pages £30.00

No. 77 **Hexachlorobenzene: Proceedings of an International Symposium**
Edited by C.R. Morris and J.R.P. Cabral
1986; 668 pages (*out of print*)

No. 78 **Carcinogenicity of Alkylating Cytostatic Drugs**
Edited by D. Schmähl and J.M. Kaldor
1986; 337 pages (*out of print*)

No. 79 **Statistical Methods in Cancer Research. Volume III: The Design and Analysis of Long-term Animal Experiments**
By J.J. Gart, D. Krewski, P.N. Lee, R.E. Tarone and J. Wahrendorf
1986; 213 pages £22.00

No. 80 **Directory of On-going Research in Cancer Epidemiology 1986**
Edited by C.S. Muir and G. Wagner
1986; 805 pages (*out of print*)

No. 81 **Environmental Carcinogens: Methods of Analysis and Exposure Measurement. Volume 9: Passive Smoking**
Edited by I.K. O'Neill,
K.D. Brunnemann, B. Dodet and D. Hoffmann
1987; 383 pages £35.00

No. 82 **Statistical Methods in Cancer Research. Volume II: The Design and Analysis of Cohort Studies**
By N.E. Breslow and N.E. Day
1987; 404 pages £25.00

No. 83 **Long-term and Short-term Assays for Carcinogens: A Critical Appraisal**
Edited by R. Montesano,
H. Bartsch, H. Vainio, J. Wilbourn and H. Yamasaki
1986; 575 pages £35.00

No. 84 **The Relevance of *N*-Nitroso Compounds to Human Cancer: Exposure and Mechanisms**
Edited by H. Bartsch, I.K. O'Neill and R. Schulte-Hermann
1987; 671 pages (*out of print*)

No. 85 **Environmental Carcinogens: Methods of Analysis and Exposure Measurement. Volume 10: Benzene and Alkylated Benzenes**
Edited by L. Fishbein and
I.K. O'Neill
1988; 327 pages £40.00

No. 86 **Directory of On-going Research in Cancer Epidemiology 1987**
Edited by D.M. Parkin and
J. Wahrendorf
1987; 676 pages (*out of print*)

No. 87 **International Incidence of Childhood Cancer**
Edited by D.M. Parkin, C.A. Stiller,
C.A. Bieber, G.J. Draper,
B. Terracini and J.L. Young
1988; 401 pages £35.00

No. 88 **Cancer Incidence in Five Continents Volume V**
Edited by C. Muir, J. Waterhouse, T. Mack, J. Powell and S. Whelan
1987; 1004 pages £55.00

No. 89 **Method for Detecting DNA Damaging Agents in Humans: Applications in Cancer Epidemiology and Prevention**
Edited by H. Bartsch, K. Hemminki and I.K. O'Neill
1988; 518 pages £50.00

No. 90 **Non-occupational Exposure to Mineral Fibres**
Edited by J. Bignon, J. Peto and
R. Saracci
1989; 500 pages £50.00

No. 91 **Trends in Cancer Incidence in Singapore 1968—1982**
Edited by H.P. Lee , N.E. Day and K. Shanmugaratnam
1988; 160 pages (*out of print*)

No. 92 **Cell Differentiation, Genes and Cancer**
Edited by T. Kakunaga,
T. Sugimura, L. Tomatis and
H. Yamasaki
1988; 204 pages £27.50

No. 93 **Directory of On-going Research in Cancer Epidemiology 1988**
Edited by M. Coleman and
J. Wahrendorf
1988; 662 pages (*out of print*)

No. 94 **Human Papillomavirus and Cervical Cancer**
Edited by N. Muñoz, F.X. Bosch and O.M. Jensen
1989; 154 pages £22.50

No. 95 **Cancer Registration: Principles and Methods**
Edited by O.M. Jensen,
D.M. Parkin, R. MacLennan,
C.S. Muir and R. Skeet
1991; 288 pages £28.00

No. 96 **Perinatal and Multigeneration Carcinogenesis**
Edited by N.P. Napalkov,
J.M. Rice, L. Tomatis and
H. Yamasaki
1989; 436 pages £50.00

No. 97 **Occupational Exposure to Silica and Cancer Risk**
Edited by L. Simonato,
A.C. Fletcher, R. Saracci and
T. Thomas
1990; 124 pages £22.50

No. 98 **Cancer Incidence in Jewish Migrants to Israel, 1961—1981**
Edited by R. Steinitz, D.M. Parkin,
J.L. Young, C.A. Bieber and
L. Katz
1989; 320 pages £35.00

No. 99 **Pathology of Tumours in Laboratory Animals, Second Edition, Volume 1, Tumours of the Rat**
Edited by V.S. Turusov and
U. Mohr
740 pages £85.00

No. 100 **Cancer: Causes, Occurrence and Control**
Editor-in-Chief L. Tomatis
1990; 352 pages £24.00

No. 101 **Directory of On-going Research in Cancer Epidemiology 1989/90**
Edited by M. Coleman and
J. Wahrendorf
1989; 818 pages £40.00

No. 102 **Patterns of Cancer in Five Continents**
Edited by S.L. Whelan, D.M. Parkin & E. Masuyer
1990; 162 pages £25.00

No. 103 **Evaluating Effectiveness of Primary Prevention of Cancer**
Edited by M. Hakama, V. Beral, J.W. Cullen and D.M. Parkin
1990; 250 pages £32.00

No. 104 **Complex Mixtures and Cancer Risk**
Edited by H. Vainio, M. Sorsa and
A.J. McMichael
1990; 442 pages £38.00

No. 105 **Relevance to Human Cancer of *N*-Nitroso Compounds, Tobacco Smoke and Mycotoxins**
Edited by I.K. O'Neill, J. Chen and
H. Bartsch
1991; 614 pages £70.00

No. 106 **Atlas of Cancer Incidence in the Former German Democratic Republic**
Edited by W.H. Mehnert, M. Smans,
C.S. Muir, M. Möhner & D. Schön
1992; 384 pages £55.00

No. 107 **Atlas of Cancer Mortality in the European Economic Community**
Edited by M. Smans, C.S. Muir and P. Boyle
1992; 280 pages £35.00

No. 108 **Environmental Carcinogens: Methods of Analysis and Exposure Measurement. Volume 11: Polychlorinated Dioxins and Dibenzofurans**
Edited by C. Rappe, H.R. Buser, B. Dodet and I.K. O'Neill
1991; 426 pages £45.00

No. 109 **Environmental Carcinogens: Methods of Analysis and Exposure Measurement. Volume 12: Indoor Air Contaminants**
Edited by B. Seifert, H. van de Wiel, B. Dodet and I.K. O'Neill
1993; 384 pages £45.00

No. 110 **Directory of On-going Research in Cancer Epidemiology 1991**
Edited by M. Coleman and J. Wahrendorf
1991; 753 pages £38.00

No. 111 **Pathology of Tumours in Laboratory Animals, Second Edition, Volume 2, Tumours of the Mouse**
Edited by V.S. Turusov and U. Mohr
1993; 776 pages; £90.00

No. 112 **Autopsy in Epidemiology and Medical Research**
Edited by E. Riboli and M. Delendi
1991; 288 pages £25.00

No. 113 **Laboratory Decontamination and Destruction of Carcinogens in Laboratory Wastes: Some Mycotoxins**
Edited by M. Castegnaro, J. Barek, J.–M. Frémy, M. Lafontaine, M. Miraglia, E.B. Sansone and G.M. Telling
1991; 64 pages £11.00

No. 114 **Laboratory Decontamination and Destruction of Carcinogens in Laboratory Wastes: Some Polycyclic Heterocyclic Hydrocarbons**
Edited by M. Castegnaro, J. Barek J. Jacob, U. Kirso, M. Lafontaine, E.B. Sansone, G.M. Telling and T. Vu Duc
1991; 50 pages £8.00

No. 115 **Mycotoxins, Endemic Nephropathy and Urinary Tract Tumours**
Edited by M. Castegnaro, R. Plestina, G. Dirheimer, I.N. Chernozemsky and H Bartsch
1991; 340 pages £45.00

No. 116 **Mechanisms of Carcinogenesis in Risk Identification**
Edited by H. Vainio, P.N. Magee, D.B. McGregor & A.J. McMichael
1992; 616 pages £65.00

No. 117 **Directory of On-going Research in Cancer Epidemiology 1992**
Edited by M. Coleman, J. Wahrendorf & E. Démaret
1992; 773 pages £42.00

No. 118 **Cadmium in the Human Environment: Toxicity and Carcinogenicity**
Edited by G.F. Nordberg, R.F.M. Herber & L. Alessio
1992; 470 pages £60.00

No. 119 **The Epidemiology of Cervical Cancer and Human Papillomavirus**
Edited by N. Muñoz, F.X. Bosch, K.V. Shah & A. Meheus
1992; 288 pages £28.00

No. 120 **Cancer Incidence in Five Continents, Volume VI**
Edited by D.M. Parkin, C.S. Muir, S.L. Whelan, Y.T. Gao, J. Ferlay & J.Powell
1992; 1080 pages £120.00

No. 121 **Trends in Cancer Incidence and Mortality**
M.P. Coleman, J. Estève, P. Damiecki, A. Arslan and H. Renard
1993; 806 pages, £120.00

No. 122 **International Classification of Rodent Tumours. Part 1. The Rat**
Editor-in-Chief: U. Mohr
1992/93; 10 fascicles of 60–100 pages, £120.00

No. 123 **Cancer in Italian Migrant Populations**
Edited by M. Geddes, D.M. Parkin, M. Khlat, D. Balzi and E. Buiatti
1993; 292 pages, £40.00

No. 124 **Postlabelling Methods for Detection of DNA Adducts**
Edited by D.H. Phillips, M. Castegnaro and H. Bartsch
1993; 392 pages; £46.00

No. 125 **DNA Adducts: Identification and Biological Significance**
Edited by K. Hemminki, A. Dipple, D. Shuker, F.F. Kadlubar, D. Segerbäck and H. Bartsch
1994; 480 pages; £52.00

No. 127 **Butadiene and Styrene: Assessment of Health Hazards.**
Edited by M. Sorsa, K. Peltonen, H. Vainio and K. Hemminki
1993; 412 pages; £54.00

No. 130 **Directory of On-going Research in Cancer Epidemiology 1994**
Edited by R. Sankaranarayanan, J. Wahrendorf and E. Démaret
1994; 792 pages, £46.00

IARC MONOGRAPHS ON THE EVALUATION OF CARCINOGENIC RISKS TO HUMANS

(Available from booksellers through the network of WHO Sales Agents)

Volume 1 Some Inorganic Substances, Chlorinated Hydrocarbons, Aromatic Amines, *N*-Nitroso Compounds, and Natural Products
1972; 184 pages *(out of print)*

Volume 2 Some Inorganic and Organometallic Compounds
1973; 181 pages *(out of print)*

Volume 3 Certain Polycyclic Aromatic Hydrocarbons and Heterocyclic Compounds
1973; 271 pages *(out of print)*

Volume 4 Some Aromatic Amines, Hydrazine and Related Substances, *N*-Nitroso Compounds and Miscellaneous Alkylating Agents
1974; 286 pages Sw. fr. 18.–

Volume 5 Some Organochlorine Pesticides
1974; 241 pages *(out of print)*

Volume 6 Sex Hormones
1974; 243 pages *(out of print)*

Volume 7 Some Anti-Thyroid and Related Substances, Nitrofurans and Industrial Chemicals
1974; 326 pages *(out of print)*

Volume 8 Some Aromatic Azo Compounds
1975; 357 pages Sw. fr. 44.–

Volume 9 Some Aziridines, *N*-, *S*- and *O*-Mustards and Selenium
1975; 268 pages Sw.fr. 33.–

Volume 10 Some Naturally Occurring Substances
1976; 353 pages *(out of print)*

Volume 11 Cadmium, Nickel, Some Epoxides, Miscellaneous Industrial Chemicals and General Considerations on Volatile Anaesthetics
1976; 306 pages *(out of print)*

Volume 12 Some Carbamates, Thiocarbamates and Carbazides
1976; 282 pages Sw. fr. 41.-

Volume 13 Some Miscellaneous Pharmaceutical Substances
1977; 255 pages Sw. fr. 36.–

Volume 14 Asbestos
1977; 106 pages *(out of print)*

Volume 15 Some Fumigants, The Herbicides 2,4-D and 2,4,5-T, Chlorinated Dibenzodioxins and Miscellaneous Industrial Chemicals
1977; 354 pages *(out of print)*

Volume 16 Some Aromatic Amines and Related Nitro Compounds - Hair Dyes, Colouring Agents and Miscellaneous Industrial Chemicals
1978; 400 pages Sw. fr. 60.–

Volume 17 Some *N*-Nitroso Compounds
1978; 365 pages Sw. fr. 60.–

Volume 18 Polychlorinated Biphenyls and Polybrominated Biphenyls
1978; 140 pages Sw. fr. 24.–

Volume 19 Some Monomers, Plastics and Synthetic Elastomers, and Acrolein
1979; 513 pages *(out of print)*

Volume 20 Some Halogenated Hydrocarbons
1979; 609 pages *(out of print)*

Volume 21 Sex Hormones (II)
1979; 583 pages Sw. fr. 72.–

Volume 22 Some Non-Nutritive Sweetening Agents
1980; 208 pages Sw. fr. 30.–

Volume 23 Some Metals and Metallic Compounds
1980; 438 pages *(out of print)*

Volume 24 Some Pharmaceutical Drugs
1980; 337 pages Sw. fr. 48.–

Volume 25 Wood, Leather and Some Associated Industries
1981; 412 pages Sw. fr. 72.–

Volume 26 Some Antineoplastic and Immunosuppressive Agents
1981; 411 pages Sw. fr. 75.–

Volume 27 Some Aromatic Amines, Anthraquinones and Nitroso Compounds, and Inorganic Fluorides Used in Drinking Water and Dental Preparations
1982; 341 pages Sw. fr. 48.–

Volume 28 The Rubber Industry
1982; 486 pages Sw. fr. 84.–

Volume 29 Some Industrial Chemicals and Dyestuffs
1982; 416 pages Sw. fr. 72.–

Volume 30 Miscellaneous Pesticides
1983; 424 pages Sw. fr. 72.–

Volume 31 Some Food Additives, Feed Additives and Naturally Occurring Substances
1983; 314 pages Sw. fr. 66.–

Volume 32 Polynuclear Aromatic Compounds, Part 1: Chemical, Environmental and Experimental Data
1983; 477 pages Sw. fr. 88.–

Volume 33 Polynuclear Aromatic Compounds, Part 2: Carbon Blacks, Mineral Oils and Some Nitroarenes
1984; 245 pages *(out of print)*

Volume 34 Polynuclear Aromatic Compounds, Part 3: Industrial Exposures in Aluminium Production Coal Gasification, Coke Production, and Iron and Steel Founding
1984; 219 pages Sw. fr. 53.–

Volume 35 Polynuclear Aromatic Compounds, Part 4: Bitumens, Coal-tars and Derived Products, Shale-oils and Soots
1985; 271 pages Sw. fr. 77.–

List of IARC Publications

Volume 36 Allyl Compounds, Aldehydes, Epoxides and Peroxides
1985; 369 pages Sw. fr. 77.—

Volume 37 Tobacco Habits Other than Smoking: Betel-quid and Areca-nut Chewing; and some Related Nitrosamines
1985; 291 pages Sw. fr. 77.—

Volume 38 Tobacco Smoking
1986; 421 pages Sw. fr. 83.—

Volume 39 Some Chemicals Used in Plastics and Elastomers
1986; 403 pages Sw. fr. 83.—

Volume 40 Some Naturally Occurring and Synthetic Food Components, Furocoumarins and Ultraviolet Radiation
1986; 444 pages Sw. fr. 83.—

Volume 41 Some Halogenated Hydrocarbons and Pesticide Exposures
1986; 434 pages Sw. fr. 83.—

Volume 42 Silica and Some Silicates
1987; 289 pages Sw. fr. 72.

Volume 43 Man-Made Mineral Fibres and Radon
1988; 300 pages Sw. fr. 72.—

Volume 44 Alcohol Drinking
1988; 416 pages Sw. fr. 83.

Volume 45 Occupational Exposures in Petroleum Refining; Crude Oil and Major Petroleum Fuels
1989; 322 pages Sw. fr. 72.—

Volume 46 Diesel and Gasoline Engine Exhausts and Some Nitroarenes
1989; 458 pages Sw. fr. 83.—

Volume 47 Some Organic Solvents, Resin Monomers and Related Compounds, Pigments and Occupational Exposures in Paint Manufacture and Painting
1989; 536 pages Sw. fr. 94.—

Volume 48 Some Flame Retardants and Textile Chemicals, and Exposures in the Textile Manufacturing Industry
1990; 345 pages Sw. fr. 72.—

Volume 49 Chromium, Nickel and Welding
1990; 677 pages Sw. fr. 105.-

Volume 50 Pharmaceutical Drugs
1990; 415 pages Sw. fr. 93.-

Volume 51 Coffee, Tea, Mate, Methylxanthines and Methylglyoxal
1991; 513 pages Sw. fr. 88.-

Volume 52 Chlorinated Drinking-water; Chlorination By-products; Some Other Halogenated Compounds; Cobalt and Cobalt Compounds
1991; 544 pages Sw. fr. 88.-

Volume 53 Occupational Exposures in Insecticide Application and some Pesticides
1991; 612 pages Sw. fr. 105.-

Volume 54 Occupational Exposures to Mists and Vapours from Strong Inorganic Acids; and Other Industrial Chemicals
1992; 336 pages Sw. fr. 72.-

Volume 55 Solar and Ultraviolet Radiation
1992; 316 pages Sw. fr. 65.-

Volume 56 Some Naturally Occurring Substances: Food Items and Constituents, Heterocyclic Aromatic Amines and Mycotoxins
1993; 600 pages Sw. fr. 95.-

Volume 57 Occupational Exposures of Hairdressers and Barbers and Personal Use of Hair Colourants; Some Hair Dyes, Cosmetic Colourants, Industrial Dyestuffs and Aromatic Amines
1993; 428 pages Sw. fr. 75.-

Volume 58 Beryllium, Cadmium, Mercury and Exposures in the Glass Manufacturing Industry
1993; 426 pages Sw. fr. 75.-

Supplement No. 1
Chemicals and Industrial Processes Associated with Cancer in Humans (IARC Monographs, Volumes 1 to 20)
1979; 71 pages (*out of print*)

Supplement No. 2
Long-term and Short-term Screening Assays for Carcinogens: A Critical Appraisal
1980; 426 pages Sw. fr. 40.-

Supplement No. 3
Cross Index of Synonyms and Trade Names in Volumes 1 to 26
1982; 199 pages (*out of print*)

Supplement No. 4
Chemicals, Industrial Processes and Industries Associated with Cancer in Humans (IARC Monographs, Volumes 1 to 29)
1982; 292 pages (*out of print*)

Supplement No. 5
Cross Index of Synonyms and Trade Names in Volumes 1 to 36
1985; 259 pages (*out of print*)

Supplement No. 6
Genetic and Related Effects: An Updating of Selected IARC Monographs from Volumes 1 to 42
1987; 729 pages Sw. fr. 80.-

Supplement No. 7
Overall Evaluations of Carcinogenicity: An Updating of IARC Monographs Volumes 1-42
1987; 440 pages Sw. fr. 65.-

Supplement No. 8
Cross Index of Synonyms and Trade Names in Volumes 1 to 46
1990; 346 pages Sw. fr. 60.-

IARC TECHNICAL REPORTS*

No. 1 Cancer in Costa Rica
Edited by R. Sierra,
R. Barrantes, G. Muñoz Leiva, D.M.
Parkin, C.A. Bieber and
N. Muñoz Calero
1988; 124 pages Sw. fr. 30.-

**No. 2 SEARCH: A Computer
Package to Assist the Statistical
Analysis of Case-control Studies**
Edited by G.J. Macfarlane,
P. Boyle and P. Maisonneuve
1991; 80 pages (*out of print*)

**No. 3 Cancer Registration in the
European Economic Community**
Edited by M.P. Coleman and
E. Démaret
1988; 188 pages Sw. fr. 30.-

**No. 4 Diet, Hormones and Cancer:
Methodological Issues for
Prospective Studies**
Edited by E. Riboli and
R. Saracci
1988; 156 pages Sw. fr. 30.-

No. 5 Cancer in the Philippines
Edited by A.V. Laudico,
D. Esteban and D.M. Parkin
1989; 186 pages Sw. fr. 30.-

**No. 6 La genèse du Centre
International de Recherche sur le
Cancer**
Par R. Sohier et A.G.B. Sutherland
1990; 104 pages Sw. fr. 30.-

**No. 7 Epidémiologie du cancer dans
les pays de langue latine**
1990; 310 pages Sw. fr. 30.-

**No. 8 Comparative Study of Anti-
smoking Legislation in Countries of
the European Economic Community**
Edited by A. Sasco, P. Dalla Vorgia
and P. Van der Elst
1992; 82 pages Sw. fr. 30.-

**No. 9 Epidemiologie du cancer dans
les pays de langue latine**
1991 346 pages Sw. fr. 30.-

**No. 11 Nitroso Compounds:
Biological Mechanisms, Exposures
and Cancer Etiology**
Edited by I.K. O'Neill & H. Bartsch
1992; 149 pages Sw. fr. 30.-

**No. 12 Epidémiologie du cancer dans
les pays de langue latine**
1992; 375 pages Sw. fr. 30.-

**No. 13 Health, Solar UV Radiation
and Environmental Change**
By A. Kricker, B.K. Armstrong, M.E.
Jones and R.C. Burton
1993; 216 pages Sw.fr. 30.—

**No. 14 Epidémiologie du cancer dans
les pays de langue latine**
1993; 385 pages Sw. fr. 30.-

**No. 15 Cancer in the African
Population of Bulawayo, Zimbabwe,
1963–1977: Incidence, Time Trends
and Risk Factors**
By M.E.G. Skinner, D.M. Parkin, A.P.
Vizcaino and A. Ndhlovu
1993; 123 pages Sw. fr. 30.-

**No. 16 Cancer in Thailand,
1988–1991**
By V. Vatanasapt, N. Martin, H.
Sriplung, K. Vindavijak, S. Sontipong,
S. Sriamporn, D.M. Parkin and J.
Ferlay
1993; 164 pages Sw. fr. 30.-

DIRECTORY OF AGENTS BEING TESTED FOR CARCINOGENICITY (Until Vol. 13 Information Bulletin on the Survey of Chemicals Being Tested for Carcinogenicity)*

No. 8 Edited by M.-J. Ghess,
H. Bartsch and L. Tomatis
1979; 604 pages Sw. fr. 40.-

No. 9 Edited by M.-J. Ghess,
J.D. Wilbourn, H. Bartsch and
L. Tomatis
1981; 294 pages Sw. fr. 41.-

No. 10 Edited by M.-J. Ghess,
J.D. Wilbourn and H. Bartsch
1982; 362 pages Sw. fr. 42.-

No. 11 Edited by M.-J. Ghess,
J.D. Wilbourn, H. Vainio and
H. Bartsch
1984; 362 pages Sw. fr. 50.-

No. 12 Edited by M.-J. Ghess,
J.D. Wilbourn, A. Tossavainen and H.
Vainio
1986; 385 pages Sw. fr. 50.-

No. 13 Edited by M.-J. Ghess,
J.D. Wilbourn and A. Aitio 1988; 404
pages Sw. fr. 43.-

No. 14 Edited by M.-J. Ghess,
J.D. Wilbourn and H. Vainio
1990; 370 pages Sw. fr. 45.-

No. 15 Edited by M.-J. Ghess, J.D.
Wilbourn and H. Vainio
1992; 318 pages Sw. fr. 45.-

NON-SERIAL PUBLICATIONS

Alcool et Cancer†
By A. Tuyns (in French only)
1978; 42 pages Fr. fr. 35.-

**Cancer Morbidity and Causes of
Death Among Danish Brewery
Workers†**
By O.M. Jensen
1980; 143 pages Fr. fr. 75.-

**Directory of Computer Systems Used
in Cancer Registries†**
By H.R. Menck and D.M. Parkin
1986; 236 pages Fr. fr. 50.-

**Facts and Figures of Cancer in the
European Community***
Edited by J. Estève, A. Kricker, J.
Ferlay and D.M. Parkin
1993; 52 pages Sw. fr. 10.-
